# HEAD AND NECK CANCER: SCIENTIFIC PERSPECTIVES IN MANAGEMENT AND STRATEGIES FOR CURE

# HEAD AND NECK CANCER: SCIENTIFIC PERSPECTIVES IN MANAGEMENT AND STRATEGIES FOR CURE

Edited by

## John R. Jacobs, MD
Associate Professor
Department of Otolaryngology
Wayne State University School of Medicine
Detroit, Michigan

## John D. Crissman, MD
Vice Chairman of Anatomic Pathology Laboratories
Division of Anatomic Pathology
Department of Pathology
Henry Ford Hospital
Detroit, Michigan

## Frederick A. Valeriote, PhD
Associate Director
Division of Medical Oncology
Wayne State University School of Medicine
Detroit, Michigan

## Muhyi Al-Sarraf, MD
Professor
Division of Oncology
Department of Internal Medicine
Wayne State University School of Medicine
Detroit, Michigan

**Elsevier**

New York • Amsterdam • London

Elsevier Science Publishing Co., Inc.
52 Vanderbilt Avenue, New York, New York 10017

Sole distributors outside the United States and Canada:

Elsevier Science Publishers B.V.
P.O. Box 211, 1000 AE Amsterdam, the Netherlands

Library of Congress Cataloging in Publication Data

Head and neck cancer.

Includes index.
1. Head — Cancer.   2. Neck — Cancer.   I. Jacobs, John R.
[DNLM: 1. Head and Neck Neoplasms — therapy.
WE 707 H43172]
RC280.H4M3863   1987          616.99′491          87-6873
ISBN 0-444-01213-3

Current printing (last digit):
10 9 8 7 6 5 4 3 2 1

Manufactured in the United States of America

# Contents

# Preface

The management of carcinoma of the head and neck long has been regarded as one of the more difficult problems in oncology. In addition to disappointing cure rates, the disease can be associated with significant functional and cosmetic problems that are often aggravated by the recommended treatment. Carcinoma of the head and neck most commonly is seen in a patient population that has multiple coexisting medical problems often related to long-standing abuse of alcohol and tobacco products. Not the least of these problems is the distressing tendency to develop a second carcinoma of the upper aerodigestive tract once the first one is successfully treated.

Perhaps as a result of these difficulties, the combined modality approach to the treatment of head and neck carcinoma is widely practiced. The modalities employed are not only therapeutic, but also focused on the prevention and ultimate rehabilitation of the patient. The contributions to this book represent current thinking regarding the scientific foundations upon which many of the current, and perhaps future, practice techniques are based.

# Contributors

Muhyi Al-Sarraf, MD
Professor
Division of Oncology
Department of Internal Medicine
Wayne State University School of Medicine
Detroit, Michigan

Madeline Bauer, PhD
Statistician
Statistical Office
Radiation Therapy Oncology Group
Philadelphia, Pennsylvania

Oliver H. Beahrs, MD
Emeritus Professor of Surgery
Mayo Medical School;
Emeritus Consultant
Section of Gastroenterologic and General Surgery
Mayo Clinic and Mayo Foundation
Rochester, Minnesota

Joseph R. Bertino, MD
American Cancer Society Professor
Department of Medicine
Memorial Hospital–Sloan Kettering Institute
New York, New York

Stephen K. Carter, MD
Senior Vice President, Anti-Cancer Research
Pharmaceutical Research and Development Division
Bristol-Myers Company
New York, New York

## Yu-Ming Chang, MD
Visiting Research Scientist
Department of Pharmacology
Yale University School of Medicine
New Haven, Connecticut

## Marc S. C. Cheah
Medical Staff Fellow
Laboratory of Cellular and Molecular Biology
National Cancer Institute
National Institutes of Health
Bethesda, Maryland

## Dennis Cooper, MD
Assistant Professor of Medicine
Department of Internal Medicine
Yale University School of Medicine
New Haven, Connecticut

## Thomas H. Corbett, PhD
Associate Professor
Division of Medical Oncology
Department of Internal Medicine
Wayne State University School of Medicine
Detroit, Michigan

## Lawrence R. Crane, MD, FACP
Associate Professor
Department of Internal Medicine
Wayne State University School of Medicine;
Chief of Infectious Disease
Harper-Grace Hospitals
Detroit, Michigan

## John D. Crissman, MD
Vice Chairman of Anatomic Pathology Laboratories
Division of Anatomic Pathology
Department of Pathology
Henry Ford Hospital
Detroit, Michigan

## Lawrence W. DeSanto, MD
Professor
Department of Otolaryngology
Mayo Medical School;
Consultant
Department of Otorhinolaryngology
Mayo Clinic and Mayo Foundation
Rochester, Minnesota

Isaiah W. Dimery, MD
Assistant Professor
Section of Head and Neck Medical Oncology
Department of Medical Oncology
The University of Texas System Cancer Center
M.D. Anderson Hospital and Tumor Institute
Houston, Texas

James A. Duncavage, MD, FACS
Associate Professor
Department of Otolaryngology
Vanderbilt University School of Medicine
Nashville, Tennessee

Bahman Emami, MD
Associate Professor
Division of Radiation Oncology
Mallinckrodt Institute of Radiology
Washington University School of Medicine
St. Louis, Missouri

John F. Ensley, MD
Assistant Professor
Division of Oncology
Department of Internal Medicine
Wayne State University School of Medicine
Detroit, Michigan

Karen K. Fu, MD
Professor
Department of Radiation Oncology
University of California, San Francisco, School of Medicine
San Francisco, California

Mary Ann Hederman, BS
Division of Radiation Oncology
Mallinckrodt Institute of Radiology
Washington University School of Medicine
St. Louis, Missouri

Frank R. Hendrickson, MD
Radiation Oncologist
Neutron Therapy Facility
Midwest Institute for Neutron Therapy at Fermilab
Batavia, Illinois

Waun Ki Hong, MD
Professor of Medicine
Chief, Head and Neck and Thoracic Oncology
Department of Medical Oncology
Section of Head and Neck Medical Oncology and Thoracic Oncology
University of Texas System Cancer Center
M. D. Anderson Hospital and Tumor Institute at Houston
Houston, Texas

Ned B. Hornback, MD
Chairman, Radiation Oncology
Department of Radiation Oncology
Indiana University Medical Center
Indianapolis, Indiana

Hisanaga Igarashi, PhD
Assistant Professor
Department of Bacteriology
Nagasaki University School of Medicine
Nagasaki, Japan

John R. Jacobs, MD
Associate Professor
Department of Otolaryngology
Wayne State University School of Medicine
Detroit, Michigan

Toshiaki Kawakami, MD, PhD
Visiting Fellow
Laboratory of Cellular and Molecular Biology
National Cancer Institute
National Institutes of Health
Bethesda, Maryland

Julie A. Kish, MD
Assistant Professor
Division of Oncology
Department of Internal Medicine
Wayne State University School of Medicine
Detroit, Michigan

Alfred J. Lawson, PhD
Administrative Director
Department of Radiation Oncology
Jackson-Madison County General Hospital
Jackson, Tennessee

Fernando Leal, PhD
Associate Professor
Department of Microbiology
Universidad de Salamanca
Salamanca, Spain

Wilbur R. Leopold III, PhD
Research Associate
Tumor Biology Section
Pharmaceutical Research Division
Warner Lambert/Parke Davis
Ann Arbor, Michigan

Zosia Maciorowski
Research Associate
Division of Oncology
Department of Medicine
Wayne State University School of Medicine
Detroit, Michigan

JoAnne Mansell, RN, PA
Clinical Research Coordinator
Neutron Therapy
Fermi National Accelerator Laboratory
Batavia, Illinois

Robert H. Ossoff, DMD, MD
Guy M. Maness Professor and Chairman
Department of Otolaryngology
Vanderbilt University Medical College
Nashville, Tennessee

Claire Y. Pennington, MS
Research Technician
Laboratory of Cellular and Molecular Biology
National Cancer Institute
National Institutes of Health
Bethesda, Maryland

Carlos A. Perez, MD
Professor of Radiology
Director
Radiation Oncology Center
Division of Radiation Oncology
Mallinckrodt Institute of Radiology
Washington University School of Medicine
St. Louis, Missouri

## Keith C. Robbins, PhD
Chief
Molecular Genetics Section
Laboratory of Cellular and Molecular Biology
National Cancer Institute
National Institutes of Health
Bethesda, Maryland

## Billy J. Roberts, BS
Senior Associate Scientist
Tumor Biology Section
Pharmaceutical Research Division
Warner Lambert/Parke Davis
Ann Arbor, Michigan

## Martin C. Robson, MD
Professor
Department of Surgery
Wayne State University School of Medicine;
Chief
Division of Plastic and Reconstructive Surgery
Wayne State University Health Center
Detroit, Michigan

## Stephen A. Sapareto, PhD
Associate Professor
Division of Hematology/Oncology
Department of Internal Medicine
Wayne State University School of Medicine
Detroit, Michigan

## K. R. Saroja, MD
Radiation Oncologist
Neutron Therapy Facility
Midwest Institute for Neutron Therapy at Fermilab
Batavia, Illinois

## Gisele Sarosy, MD
Senior Investigator
Investigational Drug Branch
National Cancer Institute
Bethesda, Maryland

## Ronald S. Scott, MD, PhD
Assistant Professor
Department of Radiation Oncology
University of Washington School of Medicine
Seattle, Washington

## Laurie Smaldone, MD
Assistant Clinical Professor
Yale University School of Medicine
New Haven;
Director
Clinical Cancer Research
Bristol-Myers Company
Wallingford, Connecticut

## Efstathios Tapazoglou, MD
Assistant Professor
Division of Oncology
Department of Internal Medicine
Wayne State University School of Medicine
Detroit, Michigan

## Frederick A. Valeriote, PhD
Associate Director
Division of Medical Oncology
Wayne State University School of Medicine
Detroit, Michigan

## Steven E. Vogl, MD
Associate Clinical Professor of Medicine
Albert Einstein College of Medicine
Bronx;
President
Cancer Treatment Research Foundation of New York
Scarsdale, New York

## Debbie VonGerichten, BS
Division of Radiation Oncology
Mallinckrodt Institute of Radiology
Washington University School of Medicine
St. Louis, Missouri

## Arthur W. Weaver, MD
Professor
Department of Surgery
Wayne State University School of Medicine
Chief, Head and Neck Service
Allen Park Veterans' Administration Medical Center
Detroit, Michigan

## Richard J. Zarbo, MD, DMD
Assistant Professor
Department of Pathology
Wayne State University School of Medicine
Director of Immunocytochemistry
Harper Hospital
Detroit, Michigan

# CHAPTER 1

# Treatment of Head and Neck Cancer: The Research and Patient Care Interaction

*Stephen K. Carter, MD*

## INTRODUCTION

Symposia such as this one on head and neck cancer are designed to achieve a mixture of objectives. The most important of these objectives involves professional education. This education is geared to two audiences, which can overlap, and are usually not fully delineated. The first audience is the clinical researcher in head and neck cancer. These individuals are coming to hear the latest research results with the goal of using that information in either the planning of their own new research or the modulation of their current research. The second audience is the practicing physician who has to develop appropriate treatment recommendations for patients outside of a clinical research milieu. While an individual physician attending the symposium may combine aspects of both audiences, there is an important separation between them that is often not recognized. It is the purpose of this introductory paper to focus on the differences between the research-oriented and patient care-oriented perspectives of the data base to be presented, and to outline some of the critical issues in this group of tumors.

The treatment of head and neck cancer can have one of two goals. The first is cure, and if that is not deemed possible, then palliation becomes the next hope. The therapeutic end points for both goals can be viewed in research-oriented and patient care-oriented terms (Table 1.1).

**TABLE 1.1** Therapeutic End-Points in the Treatment of Head and Neck Cancer

| Cure | | Palliation | |
|---|---|---|---|
| Research Oriented | Patient Care Oriented | Research Oriented | Patient Care Oriented |
| 1. Local control | 1. Survival | 1. Tumor shrinkage | 1. Survival |
| 2. Relapse-free survival | 2. Quality of life | 2. Progression-free interval | 2. Quality of life |

## THE THERAPEUTIC INDEX

All cancer therapy carries with it risks to the patient. Cancer is a devastating disease which, if left untreated, will kill rapidly in the great majority of cases. Cure for an individual requires total eradication of all malignant cells. Three approaches are now considered to be able to accomplish this eradication, in selected tumor types, with selected stages of spread. These approaches are surgical extirpation, radiation therapy and chemotherapy.[1-3] Each of these therapies damages normal tissues. The surgeon must remove normal tissue and, at times, entire organs. Irradiation damages normal tissues, and it is this damage which limits the amount of x-ray that can be delivered to a particular area of tumor. Chemotherapy also damages normal tissues and, again, the limitation of dose to the neoplastic cells is the tolerance of the particular normal tissues which are most sensitive to the action of the drug(s) used. All cancer therapy, therefore, must be evaluated utilizing a risk-benefit analysis which translates into the therapeutic index. The benefit involves the lengthening of survival the patient achieves and the quality of life involved in that gain. The risk involves the possibility of acute or chronic treatment-related mortality or morbidity. The acute aspect may include surgical mortality or a drug-related death due to toxicity. It may also include the morbidity of a major surgical procedure or severe vomiting caused by a cytotoxic drug. The chronic aspect may involve functional failure of a critical organ damaged by irradiation or drugs or the induction of second malignancy by the carcinogenic potential of the modalities.

Clinical research develops a probability analysis for the therapeutic index of a given regimen by detailed observation of its efficacy and side effects in the selected populations utilized for the clinical trials. For any individual patient, the therapeutic index may turn out to be superior or inferior to the mean (or median) figure which is derived from the trial analysis. The practicing oncologist must integrate the probability concerns of clinical trials with his own clinical experience and intuition when the decision is made for an individual patient's therapeutic prescription.

A major problem in the clinical research literature is that the therapeutic index is often not specifically analyzed or discussed. It must be derived from a careful reading of the efficacy results balanced against the side effects reported. Both the efficacy and the toxicity tend to be reported in research terms, and rarely, if ever, is the therapeutic index detailed from the perspective of what a practicing physician ought to do for the next patient who might be a candidate for the treatment approach in question.

The therapeutic index, while often mathematically calculated in mice and rats with tumors, is rarely delineated in patients. There is no accepted definition of the therapeutic index in clinical research, and, as already mentioned, it is rarely discussed directly in the papers which report on clinical trials.

## PATIENT CARE DECISION-MAKING

The ultimate goal of clinical research in head and neck cancer is to enable a physician to develop an optimal therapeutic prescription for an individual patient. Patient care-oriented therapeutic decision-making involves three broad sets of factors (Table 1.2). The first set of factors involves the tumor itself, and includes aspects such as histologic type, differentiation, and the extent of tumor spread. The extent of tumor spread is usually classified by a clinical staging system which details the primary tumor size (T), the lymph node involvement (N), and whether widespread metastases are found (M).

The second set of factors is physician-related. The practicing physician develops a probability analysis for the therapeutic index (Table 1.3) of various treatment options. This probability analysis utilizes the physician's understanding of the research data base modulated by past clinical experi-

**TABLE 1.2** Factors in Patient Care-Oriented Therapeutic Decision-Making

| Tumor | Physician | Patient |
|---|---|---|
| 1. Extent of tumor spread | 1. Probability analysis for therapeutic index based on: | 1. Co-morbidity |
| 2. Histology | a) understanding of research data base | 2. Psycho-social status |
| | b) past clinical experience | 3. Socioeconomic status |
| | 2. Training and other biases | 4. Understanding of therapeutic index options |

**TABLE 1.3** Cost-Benefit Analysis of a Therapeutic Approach to Head and Neck Cancer

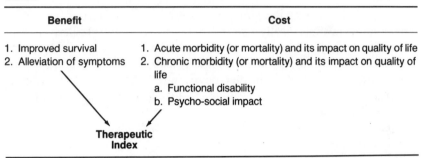

| Benefit | Cost |
|---------|------|
| 1. Improved survival | 1. Acute morbidity (or mortality) and its impact on quality of life |
| 2. Alleviation of symptoms | 2. Chronic morbidity (or mortality) and its impact on quality of life |
| |    a. Functional disability |
| |    b. Psycho-social impact |

Therapeutic
Index

ence and his or her training bias. As mentioned previously, one of the difficulties faced by the physician in making this probability analysis is that the literature is dominated by reports which utilize research-oriented criteria and often ignore discussions of the patient care-oriented therapeutic index.

The third set of factors is patient-related. It includes the unique set of psycho-social and socioeconomic situations that an individual patient brings into the decision-making equation. In addition, there are the physical aspects of co-morbidity and cultural and psychological aspects of the patient's ability to understand the therapeutic options presented.

## MODALITY VS. DISEASE-ORIENTED RESEARCH

The research thrusts in head and neck cancer involve the integration and timing of a range of modality-oriented and disease-oriented strategies.[4] Every one of the manifold diseases called Cancer are impacted upon by an ever increasing and diversified group of modality-oriented thrusts. These are geared to evaluate whether a new drug, surgical technique, radiation delivery system, or biologic approach has a role to play in cancer treatment, in general, and within a disease such as head and neck cancer, in particular. A selected list of generalized modality research opportunities is given in Table 1.4.

The disease-oriented strategy considers the unique tumor and treatment factors for head and neck cancer and poses a series of questions which can be answered by appropriately designed clinical trials. Some of these questions are outlined in Table 1.5 with respect to both practical and research-oriented formulations.

The attempted integration of modality- and disease-oriented strategies in head and neck cancer leads to a series of critical interactive questions

**TABLE 1.4** Selected List of Generalized Modality-Oriented Research Opportunities

I. Surgery

    1. More radical procedure
    2. Less radical procedure
    3. Cytoreductive procedure
    4. Resection of metastases

II. Radiation

    1. High LET delivery
       A. Neutrons
       B. Pi-mesons
       C. Heavy ions
    2. Radiation sensitizers
    3. Radiation protectors
    4. New fractionation schedules
    5. Hemi-body and total body irradiation
    6. Brachytherapy
    7. Intra-operative radiation

III. Chemotherapy

    1. New chemotypes
    2. Analogs
    3. New schedules of administration
    4. New routes of administration
       A. Intra-arterial
       B. Intraperitoneal
    5. New delivery systems
    6. Activity modulators
    7. Toxicity modulators

IV. Biological Therapy

    1. Interferons
       A. Alpha
       B. Beta
       C. Gamma
    2. Interleukins
       A. IL-1
       B. IL-2
       C. IL-3
    3. Other lymphokines and cytokines
    4. Immune modulators
    5. Lymphokine-cytokine stimulators
    6. Monoclonal antibodies
       A. Alone
       B. Radiolabelled
       C. Linked to toxins
       D. Linked to cytotoxics

*(continued)*

**TABLE 1.4** Selected List of Generalized Modality-Oriented Research Opportunities *(continued)*

IV. Biological Therapy *(continued)*
  7. Redifferentiating agents
  8. Anti-metastatic agents

V. New Modalities

  1. Hyperthermia
    A. Superficial
    B. Deep-seated
    C. Localized
    D. Whole Body
    E. Combined with irradiation
  2. Photodynamic therapy

**TABLE 1.5** Broad Care Critical Questions in Head and Neck Cancer

| Practical Formulation | Research Formulation |
|---|---|
| Can the disease be easily and routinely diagnosed at any earlier point in time allowing for curative therapy with diminished functional disability? | Does a biologic or immunological marker exist which will allow for screening and/or early diagnosis at a stage amenable for cure with minimal morbidity? |
| Can an individualized patient treatment prescription be developed which optimizes long-term survival and diminished functional disability? | Does a biologic or immunologic marker exist or does a diagnostic test exist which can more accurately clinically stage patients? |
| For early stage disease, which option for therapy offers the best therapeutic index, i.e., long-term disease-free survival with minimal functional disability? | Which local control modality, surgery or radiotherapy or the combination, offers the best local control rate and RFS rate and the least treatment-related morbidity and mortality? |
| For advanced stage disease, can the addition of systemic therapy either before, after, or concomitant with surgery and/or radiotherapy improve the long-term survival to the degree that the increased acute and chronic toxicities still result in a positive therapeutic index? | 1. Will neo-adjuvant therapy improve the local control, RFS, and overall survival rates with acceptable treatment-related morbidity and mortality?<br>2. Will adjuvant therapy improve the RFS and OS rates with acceptable treatment-related morbidity and mortality?<br>3. Will radiation-sensitizer treatment improve the local control rate, RFS, and OS with acceptable treatment-related morbidity and mortality? |

(Table 1.6). These interactive questions have as their bottom line the priority decisions which have to be made for the clinical research resources existing within a given stage of disease. An example of the complexity of options is shown in Table 1.7; it lists some possible phase 2 and phase 3 clinical questions which could be posed for the subset of patients who present with advanced disease and no prior systemic therapy. The phase 2 studies are predominantly modality-oriented, while the phase 3 questions tend to be a mixture of the drug-oriented and disease-oriented type.

In attempting to make the priority decisions between modality- and disease-oriented research thrusts, important questions to consider are what can be currently accomplished and what the research opportunities are perceived to be. When the current treatment results are poor and in plateau, it does not make much sense to emphasize disease-oriented questions which focus on modulations of the existing therapeutic tools. An example would be palliation of advanced disease with chemotherapy. Protocols which test various combinations of the currently active list of drugs (cisplatin, bleomycin and methotrexate) would appear to have only a minimal chance of improving the therapeutic index. The best hope for progress would be to utilize the lowest risk patients in this category to test new drugs or biologicals or combined therapeutic approaches in a phase 2 or pilot fashion.

The area which is currently receiving a very high priority for disease-oriented studies is stage III – IV disease. Patients in this stage of disease achieve a low rate of local control after surgery and/or x-ray used alone. It is hoped that combined modality strategies which add systemic therapy into the mix will offer a meaningful opportunity to improve the results. At this time, three strategies are being tested (Table 1.8). Each of these strategies has its own theoretical basis, and involves a variety of potential sequences for the three critical modalities (Chemotherapy [C], Surgery [S] and Radiation[R]). In addition, there are specific research-oriented therapeutic end-points for each

**TABLE 1.6** Critical Interactive Questions for the Modality and the Disease-Oriented Strategies in Head and Neck Cancer

1. What types of patients are appropriate for phase 1 studies?
2. Where is the most appropriate place to perform phase 2 studies within the sequential flow of therapy for a given site and stage?
3. What should be the priority for phase 2 studies within a given site and stage?
4. What should be the priority between phase 2 studies and phase 3 studies within a given site and stage?
5. What should be the priority between modality-oriented and pure disease-oriented phase 3 studies?

**TABLE 1.7** Some Possible Studies for Advanced Disease Patients with No Prior Systemic Therapy

| Phase 2 | Phase 3 (limited to two arms) |
| --- | --- |
| 1. New chemotype finishing phase 1 | 1. Platinol + 5-FU<br>vs.<br>Carboplatin + 5-FU |
| 2. New analog finishing phase 1<br>Folate antagonist<br>Anthracycline<br>Alkylating agent<br>Bleomycins<br>Platinum derivative<br>Mitomycin | 2. Platinol + 5-FU<br>vs.<br>Platinol + 5-FU + Bleomycin |
| 3. New combination regimen<br>Platinol + 5-FU + other agent(s)<br>Carboplatin + Bleomycin | 3. High dose Platinol ± 5-FU<br>vs.<br>Low or standard dose Platinol ± 5-FU |
| 4. Combination of chemotherapy<br>plus biological<br>Platinol + 5-FU + Interferon<br>or            or<br>MTX         Interleukin-2 | 4. Platinol + 5-FU<br>vs.<br>Platinol + MTX + Bleomycin |
| | 5. Platinol + 5-FU vs. MTX |
| | 6. Platinol vs. Carboplatin |
| | 7. Platinol + 5-FU vs. Platinol |
| | 8. Platinol + 5-FU vs. 5-FU |

which partially overlap. This multiplicity of strategies leads to a mélange of potential options for both care and research decision-making (Table 1.9).

At this time, there are no clear answers to many of the questions posed. Hopefully, the on-going clinical trials will resolve some of the combined modality issues in a manner which will be helpful for the practicing physician. The physicians listening to the research results reported at this symposium will have to remember that there is a selection bias in clinical research, and that the methodology for translating research findings to everyday care is still rudimentary.

## THE SELECTION BIAS IN CLINICAL RESEARCH

There are differences between clinical research and routine patient care which can be important in the translation of clinical research findings to everyday patient care. Clinical research takes place in selected patients whose epidemiological and prognostic factors are rigidly defined by the protocol document. Exclusions are commonly made for patients with certain prior treatments, poor performance status, co-morbidity, disease extent, and for inability to participate in the protocol. When these exclusions are made, combined with the selection of patients who eventually give informed consent, the percentage of patients within an institution who are actually entered into a protocol may be only a small fraction of those patients who are generally seen with the same disease and stage. A critical, unanswered question is how representative are these patients for the population who will be treated in a non-research setting? The practitioner of oncology does not select patients for a regimen with protocol guidelines in hand. Patients who would be deemed "ineligible" or "non-assessable" if approached for the

**TABLE 1.8** Combined Modality Strategies Under Test in Head and Neck Cancer

| Strategy | Theoretical Basis | Potential Sequences | Research-Oriented Therapeutic End-Point |
|---|---|---|---|
| Neo-Adjuvant Chemotherapy | 1. Drug treatment will shrink primary thus making local control easier to obtain<br>2. Potential eradication of micrometastatic disease in regional and/or distant sites<br>3. Early attack on micrometastatic disease before mutation to resistance (Goldie-Coldman hypothesis) | 1. C→S<br>2. C→S→R<br>3. C→R<br>4. C→R→S | 1. Local control<br>2. Relapse-free survival |
| Adjuvant Chemotherapy | 1. Drug treatment after local control will eradicate micrometastatic disease which would otherwise lead to a relapse<br>2. Micrometastatic disease will be kinetically more responsive to drugs (cell kill hypothesis) | 1. S→C<br>2. R→C<br>3. R→S-→C<br>4. S→R→C | 1. Relapse-free survival |
| Radiation Sensitization | 1. Drugs can enhance cell kill of radiation by damaging cells or inhibiting repair of damaged cells<br>2. Drugs can kill cells which will not be killed by irradiation | 1. R + C<br>2. C→R<br>3. C→R + C | 1. Local control<br>2. Relapse-free survival |

**TABLE 1.9** Potential Options for a Patient with Stage III-IV Head and Neck Cancer

---

**Clinical Staging**

---

I. Neoadjuvant or Induction Therapy

   1. Regimen*
   2. Number of courses

II. Local Control

   1. Surgery
   2. X-ray ± Sensitizer
   3. Sequential combination ± radiation sensitizer
     A) S→X
     b) X→S

III. Adjuvant Therapy

   1. Regimen*
   2. Number of courses

---

*Regimen options: 1. single agent chemotherapy; 2. combination chemotherapy; 3. biological; 4. combined chemotherapy and biological.

protocol study (whose literature report is guiding the therapeutic decision in question) may well be administered a regimen. In clinical trials, the therapy administered is tightly quality-controlled. The protocol clearly defines the dosage regimen, and the adjustments for toxicity, when chemotherapy is being used. With radiation therapy, the port and technique is carefully defined and the port films may be reviewed for their correctness. In routine care, this same level of quality control does not exist, and dosages may be modified or treatment ports changed at the discretion of the practicing physician. These changes might well make the patient "non-assessable" if they were in a clinical trial.

    Clinical trials are carefully analyzed for the literature reports which are made. These publications usually occur at some interim point in the trial when the results are felt to be mature enough to be disseminated. An obvious bias is that the more positive the trial, the earlier the publication will occur. It is distinctly uncommon to see publications of trials which are fully mature, with every patient off study and fully assessable for survival. While the early publication of interim positive results may be justifiable from a research (and investigator ego) perspective, the value in terms of population-based patient care is less obvious, and a case can be made for it being detrimental in some cases. The reporting of clinical trials often involves a process of lowering the denominator as patients are excluded for being non-assessable due to factors such as early death, early severe toxicity resulting in an inadequate therapy duration, and being lost to follow-up. These exclusions, which may again have some validity from a research point of view, may have less validity from the patient care perspective. The interpretation of the literature is further complicated by the lack of any widely accepted standard definition for response, toxicity, and the statistical methodology to be used for analyzing the survival curves. This interpretive problem is magnified even further for the practicing physician by the total failure of most papers to even discuss a patient care-oriented therapeutic index.

## POPULATION-BASED PATTERNS OF CARE

How can the scientific community determine the results of cancer treatment? How well are we actually doing and how can cancer theory be analyzed? Several approaches exist. One approach is to evaluate the results of clinical trials, as reported in the journals, and to assume that the mean of the cumulative results (for a given regimen or for a given disease and stage) will be representative of what is actually happening in the entire country or within a given state, county or city. This approach has never been validated, and I suspect would give us an overly optimistic view of what is actually happening.

A second approach would be to analyze the results from population-based tumor registries. Such data bases suffer from a significant lack of detail concerning the therapy given and the adequacy of its delivery, but are reflective of the real world to the extent that these registries are complete. Another problem with tumor registry data is that it cannot reflect today, but only what has happened years earlier. There is a significant lag phase between a new treatment impacting upon survival and that impact showing up in tumor registry data.

A third approach would be to perform population-based patterns of care studies which would develop a level of detail somewhere in between the massive number of items in a protocol flow sheet and the paucity of items in a tumor registry form. These patterns of care studies could evaluate the appropriateness of the staging and the therapeutic prescription, the adequacy of therapy delivery and follow-up, and the therapeutic index (or at least the survival) in relation to the other factors. Only then would we know how well the literature reflects patient care reality, and, if it doesn't, why and what needs to be done about it.

# REFERENCES

1. Carter SK, Glatsten E, Livingston RB: Principles of cancer treatment. New York: McGraw-Hill, 1982.
2. DeVita VT, Hellman SH and Rosenberg SA: Cancer: principles and practice of oncology, 2nd Ed. Philadelphia: Lippincott, 1985.
3. Calabresi P, Schein PS, Rosenberg SA: Medical oncology: basic principles and clinical management of cancer. New York: Macmillan, 1985.
4. Carter SK: The Role of Clinical Trials, in Veronesi U, Bonadonna G (eds): Clinical trials in cancer medicine. New York: Academic Press, 1985. pp 1–21.

# CHAPTER 2

# Current Progress in Head and Neck Cancer: The Wayne State University Experience

*Muhyi Al-Sarraf, MD, Julie A. Kish, MD,*
*John F. Ensley, MD, and*
*Efstathios Tapazoglou, MD*

## INTRODUCTION

Cancers of the head and neck are estimated to be the most prevalent cancers in the world. Cancer of the oral cavity is the most common site among the head and neck tumors. The most common histopathological type is squamous cell carcinoma. In the United States, head and neck cancer accounts for only 5% of all malignancies. Because of the location of these tumors and current progress in their treatment (including the combined modality approach and the team concept), there has been a greater scientific and medical interest in head and neck cancers than incidence data might suggest. Overall, head and neck cancer is becoming a model to be applied to other solid tumors.

The majority of the patients (70%–80%) present with locally advanced (stage III and IV) disease. Because of the high incidence of advanced disease at presentation, the management of these patients (i.e., providing the best cure rate and the improvement of survival and quality of life) has become a great challenge.

The results of traditional treatments for patients with locally advanced squamous cell cancer of the head and neck are poor and not acceptable today.[1-10] For those patients with operable and resectable stage III or IV, the most commonly employed therapies are the following: (1) surgery alone, (2) pre-operative radiation followed by surgery, (3) surgery followed by radiotherapy, and (4) radiotherapy alone with salvage surgery for persistent disease. Most investigators agree that the results of radiotherapy alone in the same group of patients are inferior to the results obtained with surgery with or without radiation therapy.[3,4] In patients with recurrent head and neck cancer after definitive treatment, the chances of salvage is less than 10% and most of these patients are then treated with systemic chemotherapy for palliation.

Considering all of the above, when the organized Head and Neck Cancer Program started at Wayne State University ten years ago, our major goals were to change the natural history of head and neck cancers and to improve the quality of life of head and neck cancer patients. To achieve such important objectives and goals, our program grew and expanded to cover a wide scope of activities. The most important concepts governing these efforts were

1. total patient care;
2. total cancer-related activities;
3. multidisciplinary team approach; and
4. the benefits of first-planned effective treatment(s).

Our overall activities included the following:

1. Clinical research;
2. Basic research;
3. Rehabilitation research and related programs;
4. Educational efforts; and
5. Administrative activities.

In this chapter, we will cover only the programs and the concepts applicable to clinical research at Wayne State University. Many areas of our basic research are covered in other chapters by the members of the head and neck cancer programs.

The scope of clinical research activities is shown in Table 2.1. Our therapeutic trials and treatment and the concepts concerning recurrent and metastatic cancer are covered in Chapter 15 (Kish et al.), our studies involving prognostic factors are covered in Chapter 3 (Ensley et al.), and our continuing efforts to improve the present staging systems will be covered in the Chapter 5 (Jacobs and Al-Sarraf).

**TABLE 2.1** Clinical Research

I. Therapeutic Trials

    A. Recurrent and Metastatic Cancer
    B. Previously Untreated Cancer
       1. Resectable and Operable Disease
       2. Unresectable and/or Inoperable Cancer
    C. Nasopharyngeal Cancer

II. Prognostic Factors

    A. Clinical
    B. Morphologic
    C. Biologic
    D. Tumor Markers

III. Improve Staging Systems

# RECURRENT AND METASTATIC CANCER

It is very important to define the disease status and the patients comprising this disease category (Table 2.2). The majority of the patients fall in the group with loco-regional recurrence due to failure of our "standard" treatment. It is also important to emphasize three critical concepts in this group of patients.

## The Need for Assessment of the Amount of Disease

During our last 10 years of experience, and as has been confirmed by many other investigators in this area, the need to re-stage and reassess the amount of disease in patients with recurrent and/or systemic cancer is becoming clear. The amount of disease can be categorized as: minimal, intermediate, or bulky.

**TABLE 2.2** Treatment of Recurrent and/or Systemic Disease

| Types and Definition |
| --- |

I. Local-Regional (Due to Failure of Definitive Treatment)

    1. Recurrent
    2. Grossly Persistent

II. Systemic

    1. In Patients Receiving Systemic Adjuvant Therapy
    2. In Patients Not Receiving Systemic Adjuvant Therapy
    3. As First Presentation

Past experience with the treatment of patients with leukemia, lymphoma, and multiple myeloma has shown that the response to therapy and survival are related to the extent of the disease. Recently, the same findings were reported in clinical trials for patients with testicular cancer. Response to chemotherapy in patients with recurrent head and neck cancer is better, the chance of complete response (CR) is higher, and the possibilities of stopping chemotherapy and long palliation are existing and hopeful. Furthermore, the investigation of new agents may be halted, and it is quite possible that we may miss active drug(s) in patients with head and neck cancers by always studying patients with bulky disease and poor performance status in such trials.

In our randomized Phase II trials, it is also possible that we may not have observed differences between therapeutic regimens used if we lumped all patients together regardless of their disease extent.

The need for better tumor mass assessment and detection of earlier recurrent disease necessitates a better and closer follow-up. This will require the early performance of triple endoscopy and possible biopsy of any suspicious lesion(s).

The assessment of recurrent tumor masses requires that the following be reported: number and site of lesions; number of organ(s) involved; and size of all measurable lesions. Additional techniques in certain patients may be required for optimum assessment of tumor mass. These include CAT scan, NMR, tumor marker(s), etc.

## Prognostic Factors

These factors play an important role in determining the response to systemic chemotherapy and/or overall survival of patients with recurrent cancer. We have identified and reported some of these prognostic factors,[15] and continue to identify other factors based on our experience in clinical trials with these patients.[16-19] These findings have been accepted and confirmed by many investigators.[20] Therefore, it is important to update and report the present status of prognostic factors. Tables 2.3 and 2.4 show the good and poor prognostic factors that we feel are important in assessing the response to chemotherapy and survival in these patients.

## Definition of Effective Therapy

To continue to improve our therapeutic modalities and optimize chemotherapy, it is important to define what we mean by "effective" meaningful therapy. This definition is to include the following: type of response to chemotherapy i.e., CR (complete response) vs <CR duration of response for

**TABLE 2.3** Recurrent and/or Systemic Head and Neck Cancer

| Good Prognosis |
| --- |
| Good performance status |
| Minimal disease |
| Local recurrence only |
| No bony erosion |
| Good response to induction (adjuvant) chemotherapy |
| Good response to previous radiotherapy |
| Long DFI |
| First line chemotherapy |
| Good organ(s) function |
| CR to chemotherapy |

the CR patients; and duration of survival of the CR patients vs <CR patients. It is clear to us, based on solid evidence, that the only meaningful response of any malignant disease treated with chemotherapy is the achievement of CR, and especially a CR that could be confirmed histologically by restaging and biopsy. This is also, without exception, the case in head and neck cancer patients with recurrent and/or distant metastasis.

The achievement of partial response (PR) is important in assessing the biological effectiveness of anti-cancer chemotherapeutic agent(s). But, as in patients with malignant diseases such as leukemia, lymphoma or testicular cancers, PR response does not influence survival. In control clinical trials, if we believe that the amount of tumor mass present is the most important

**TABLE 2.4** Recurrent and/or Systemic Disease Head and Neck Cancer

| Poor Prognosis |
| --- |
| Poor performance status |
| Bulky disease |
| Systemic/visceral disease |
| Bone metastasis and/or hypercalcemia (and local bone invasion) |
| Lymphangitic spread (skin) |
| Failure of radiotherapy (persistent disease) |
| Failure of induction (adjuvant) chemotherapy |
| Patients receiving first line chemotherapy for recurrent and/or systemic cancer |
| Organ(s) impairment |
| Less than CR to chemotherapy |

factor in determining patient survival, then some, if not the majority of PR patients, may have more tumor mass than non-responding patients. This of course depends on the amount of tumor mass present before the start of systemic chemotherapy. Agent(s) producing PR will continue to be investigated alone or in combination with other agent(s), to improve our therapeutic effectiveness by achieving a high CR rate.

This means we have to stop comparing the survival of all responders (CR + PR) between trials, and we should only compare CR rate and the survival of these patients in our randomized trials or in pilot studies from different institutions. The majority of patients (70%–80%) with recurrent head and neck cancer treated with chemotherapy had less than CR to such treatment. Therefore, the median survival of these patients is poor and not expected to be different between the different groups in pilot trials. We do feel strongly that randomized Phase III trials (the end points of which compare survival) are a waste of effort and are not warranted due to the need of large numbers of patients in order to answer such an objective. We strongly recommend comparison of response rate and especially CR and toxicities in Phase II randomized trials which require fewer patients and much less time to reach our objectives. Phase III studies in recurrent disease are worthwhile and more meaningful to do at times when we have a better and more effective CR rate to systemic chemotherapy. Table 2.5 summarizes our clinical trials over the last 10 years (1976–1986) in patients with recurrent cancer.

## PREVIOUSLY UNTREATED HEAD AND NECK CANCER

As we mentioned earlier, patients with locally advanced, previously untreated head and neck cancer have a poor outcome with our presently available definitive treatments. This is especially true in those patients with inoperable and/or unresectable disease. Since we believe that the best therapy for these patients is the first planned and effective treatment, and because of low salvage rates in recurrent cases, our efforts have been concentrated upon this group of patients. Since an important part of our goals and objectives is the quality of life of these patients, we feel that the most meaningful factor involving quality of life is the successful treatment of their cancer (cure).

The main objective, then, is to improve the cure rate of patients with head and neck cancer. To achieve this important goal, we need the following: (1) Early detection of these cancers; and (2) To continue to optimize the effectiveness of our therapeutic modalities (surgery, radiotherapy, chemotherapy, and other modalities).

In patients with locally advanced (stage III and IV) head and neck

**TABLE 2.5** Prospective Chemotherapy Trials in Patients with Recurrent Cancer

| | Reference |
|---|---|
| 1. First Line Therapy | |
|   a. Cisplatin, Oncovin, and bleomycin (COB) | 16 |
|   b. methotrexate / COB | 17,21 |
|   c. 5-FU infusion and cisplatin | 18 |
|   d. methotrexate / 13-cis-retinoic acid | |
|   e. 5-FU bolus and cisplatin / 5-FU infusion and cisplatin | 19,22,23 |
|   f. CBDCA / CHIP | 24 |
| 2. Second Line Therapy | |
|   Ftorafur | 25 |
|   m-AMSA | 26 |
|   Aclacinomycin | 27 |
|   AZQ | 28 |
|   5-FU infusion | 29 |

cancer, "adequate" surgical resection of all gross disease and involved regional lymph nodes with negative margins is an important part of therapy. Such surgery should be performed by an individual possessing the expertise to perform "adequate" reconstruction. To compromise the surgical resection for cosmetic or functional benefit is ultimately of no real advantage to the majority of such patients. This topic is covered by other chapters.

Attempts to improve radiotherapy are continuing both locally and nationally. Some of these important efforts and their results are discussed in the following chapters in this book.

Therefore, we will discuss our efforts to optimize chemotherapy results and theoretically improve our present definitive therapy. To achieve such a goal we need the following:

**1.** To continue to identify the most effective and safest agent(s) and combination(s);

**2.** To identify prognostic factors; and

**3.** To continue to conduct and improve our combined modality trials.

## Induction Chemotherapeutic Trials

Since late 1976 and the early part of 1977, with the introduction of cisplatin as an active agent for squamous cell cancer of the head and neck, high overall response rates were observed when cisplatin combinations were used in previously untreated patients. This led to our continued efforts to identify the most effective and safe combination chemotherapy to be used as part of a multimodality treatment (Table 2.6).

Our three most publicized trials are the two courses of COB,[30,31] two courses of cisplatin and 96 hour 5-FU infusion,[32,33] and three courses of cisplatin and 120 hour 5-FU infusion.[34] Table 2.7 shows the overall response rate to each of these pilots. It became clear, following these three trials, that hope existed, and that more effective chemotherapy (represented by higher CR rates) could be achieved.

It is important to mention that patients treated with two courses of cisplatin and 96 hour 5-FU infusion all had advanced stage IV disease,[32,33] and $^{13}/_{26}$ (50%) had multiple primary cancers of the head and neck, esophagus, or lung. Stage III disease was present in $^{16}/_{77}$ COB patients and $^{17}/_{88}$ patients receiving three-course cisplatin and 120 hour 5-FU infusion.[30,31,34] The incidence of second primary cancers in these two trials was $^{10}/_{77}$ and $^{15}/_{88}$, respectively.[30,31,34]

We previously reported that many factors influence the response rate (CR) to induction chemotherapy as part of multimodality therapy.[37] It is important to mention that, in assessing the CR rate after each course of chemotherapy, the increased duration and amount of 5-FU infusion (1000 mg/$M^2$)/24 hour (from 96 hour to 120 hour) and the increased number of

**TABLE 2.6** Prospective Induction Chemotherapy Trials in Patients with Previously Untreated Cancer

| Type of Combination | No. of Courses | References |
|---|---|---|
| 1. Cisplatin, Oncovin, bleomycin (COB) | 2 | 30,31 |
| 2. COB-methotrexate | 2 | — |
| 3. Cisplatin, 5-FU, 92 hr. infusion | 2 | 32,33 |
| 4. Cisplatin, 5-FU, 120 hr. infusion | 3 | 34 |
| 5. Cisplatin, 5-FU 120 hr. infusion | 6 | — |
| 6. Cisplatin 40 mg/$M^2$ D1-5, and 5-FU 120 hr. infusion | 3 | 35 |
| 7. Sequential cisplatin, 5-FU 120 hr. infusion and methotrexate and 5-FU* | 5 | 36 |

*Cisplatin, 5-FU course 1,3, and 5, and high dose methotrexate, 5-FU bolus, leucovorin weekly for 3 weeks course 2 and 4.

**TABLE 2.7** Response to Induction Chemotherapy in Previously Untreated Cancer Patients

| | COB (2 courses) | Cisplatin-5-FU (2 courses) | Cisplatin-5-FU (3 courses) | |
|---|---|---|---|---|
| | | | | p Value |
| CR 22 (28.6%) | | 5 (19.3%) | 48 (54.5%) | 0.04 |
| PR 39 (50.6%) | | 18 (69.2%) | 35 (39.8%) | |
| NR 16 (20.8%) | | 3 (11.5%) | 5 (5.7%) | |
| CR + PR/Total | 61/77 (79.2%) | 23/26 (88.5%) | 83/88 (94.3%) | N.S. |

courses (from two to three) had elevated the clinical complete response rate.[38] For patients with clinical complete response who underwent surgical resection after induction chemotherapy, the histological CR's were $\frac{1}{10}$, $\frac{2}{2}$ and $\frac{10}{20}$, respectively, with each chemotherapy treatment (Table 2.8).[39] The type of induction chemotherapy influenced the overall survival of these patients regardless of the subsequent definitive therapy.[40,45]

Also, patients achieving clinical CR to the initial chemotherapy had significantly longer survival than those patients with lesser CRs, regardless of the subsequent definitive therapy.[37,49,40,46] More importantly, those CR patients who were found to have no microscopic disease after surgical resection, had statistically superior survival when compared to those clinical CR's who had residual disease at surgery.[39]

The above has led to the theory that response to induction chemotherapy has only prognostic value and may not have a real impact on the survival of these patients. And this has led to the notion that patients who have CR to chemotherapy will do better, regardless of the chemotherapy, if only definitive surgical therapy and/or radiotherapy are used.

In spite of our strong belief that only properly conducted stratified and

**TABLE 2.8** Incidence of Histological CR in Complete Responders to Induction Chemotherapy Who Underwent Surgical Resection

| | COB (2 courses) | Cisplatin-5-FU (2 courses) | Cisplatin-5-FU (3 courses) | Sequential Cisplatin-5-FU (3) and MTX-5-FU (2) |
|---|---|---|---|---|
| No. Operation | 10 | 2 | 20 | 7 |
| No. no viable cancer | 1 | 2 | 10 | 5 |
| | 10% | 100% | 50% | 71% |

randomized trials will prove or disprove the impact of chemotherapy as part of multimodality treatment (provided we have used our best chemotherapy and addressed the question of timing combined modality therapy—see below), the following evidence may support the beneficial effect of chemotherapy:

1. There was better survival in the cisplatin-5-FU trials, as compared to COB, because of a better regimen used as manifested by better clinical and/or histological CR.[41,43]

2. The only real impact of induction chemotherapy was on histological CR following such treatment, in spite of adequate surgical resection followed by postoperative chemotherapy for those patients with clinical CRs who went directly to surgery.[39]

3. Survival of patients treated with COB was significantly better ($p \leq 0.05$) for well- and moderately differentiated cancers.[30] This difference disappeared with more effective induction chemotherapy with cisplatin and 5-FU.

4. Clinical CR patients had survival rates that differed according to tumor differentiation. Patients with poor morphology had poorer survival rates when compared to patients with moderately and well-differentiated tumors. The overall clinical CR rates were the same among the three morphological groups.

5. Patients with stage III disease had better overall clinical CR rates than those with stage IV disease, when the results of all the three pilot studies were combined. In patients with stage III disease, the clinical CR to three courses of cisplatin and 5-FU infusion was 76% ( 13/17 ) versus 49% for stage IV disease. In evaluating the survival of patients according to chemotherapeutic response, no survival advantages were found in patients with stage III, clinical CR, as compared to patients with PR or no response to chemotherapy. Patients with stage IV and clinical CR have statistically longer survival than those with PR or NR to such chemotherapy.

6. When the survivals of patients on an RTOG non-randomized protocol receiving three courses of cisplatin and 5-FU infusion either before or after surgical resection were compared, the survival was better for the "sandwich" chemotherapy group, despite the observations that these patients had higher stage IV disease (especially N disease), and most of them had a poorer performance status.[47]

These points, along with many other findings derived from our clinical trials (including trials with recurrent cancer patients), and data from other investigators, lead us to believe that chemotherapy-induced CR is not only prognostic but many have impact on the natural history of these patients.

This fact will perhaps be proven by national randomized trials which we have supported and participated in with all our efforts and capacity. Of course, it will be contingent upon our use of the best chemotherapy possible to achieve the highest clinical and histological CR. Furthermore, in resectable and operable patients, these studies will explore the problem of the best timing of chemotherapy as part of definitive therapy.

As shown in Table 2.6, attempts to improve the COB combination were conducted by adding methotrexate without changing the doses of the COB agents. A small number of patients were treated with highly toxic drug levels (myelosuppression, mucositis), without producing a better response.

We attempted to give cisplatin and 5-FU 120 hour infusion for six courses in those patients who refused further therapy (surgery and/or radiation). Again, a small number of patients were treated, and a higher incidence of side effects (myelosuppression, alopecia, and, especially, peripheral neuropathy) was observed; therefore, in spite of possible better PRs and possible higher clinical CRs, we stopped pursuing this pilot.

With the report of higher CR rates in testicular cancer patients treated with high dose cisplatin in combination with other agents, we initiated our pilot of cisplatin 40 mg/$M^2$ I.V. D1-5 with mannitol and hypertonic saline with 5-FU 120 hour infusion for three courses.[35] The incidence and degree of myelosuppression was prohibitive, and the dose of cisplatin had to be reduced to 30 mg/$M^2$, and then to 25 mg/$M^2$ D1-5, without overall improvement in the CR rate.

Due to the reports of high response rates obtained with high dose methotrexate followed 1 hour later with a 5-FU bolus and 24 hours later with leucovorin rescue, as well as the possible synergism of this combination and the lack of cross-resistance with cisplatin and 5-FU, our present trial was activated to incorporate three courses of cisplatin and 5-FU and two courses of MTX and 5-FU (Table 2.6).[36] The clinical complete response rate obtained with this combination was 68% ($^{17}/_{25}$). Also, we were able to achieve high histological CR of those clinical CR patients who underwent surgical resection after induction chemotherapy (Table 2.8).

## Chemotherapy after Surgery

In patients with previously untreated, locally advanced, resectable and operable head and neck cancer, the timing and sequence of effective chemotherapy as part of multimodality treatment needs to be investigated. Besides the obvious importance of the sequence of chemotherapeutic agents, the following problems exist with induction chemotherapy when given as the initial treatment in combined modality therapy:

1. Patients' refusal of surgical resection or other further therapy, especially by those achieving the best response to chemotherapy (CR).
2. The surgery planned after initial chemotherapy, especially after achieving good response to treatment (CR), may not be the same surgery previously performed by a surgeon on identical untreated tumors of same site and T and N stage.
3. Local-regional failure, in spite of adequate surgery and postoperative radiotherapy, may occur. In patients with resectable cancer, one would not expect the results of surgery after three courses of chemotherapy and achievement of up to 50% clinical CR to be any different from those of adequate surgery without preoperative treatment. In both instances, the gross disease is removed and the surgeons obtain a negative margin.
4. Present evidence indicates a higher clinical response rate with smaller tumor masses (stage III vs stage IV), therefore, the effectiveness of chemotherapy on minimal residual disease after surgery (microscopic) is expected to be more beneficial than the effect of induction chemotherapy on gross bulky disease.
5. In induction chemotherapy trials of resectable patients having surgery and radiotherapy vs the standard treatment of surgery and radiation therapy alone, in the experimental group, about 30% will refuse the "best" therapy i.e., surgery overall, and about 50% of the clinical CR will do so. Also, the stratification will be done based on the clinical staging, with a certain percent of under-staging as compared to postoperative, pathological staging.

Because of these factors, and in order to determine the actual T & N stage before chemotherapy, we initiated a pilot study for patients with locally advanced but resectable cancer; three courses of cisplatin and 120 hour 5-FU infusion were given after surgery and before radiotherapy.[47] Following a demonstration of the feasibility of this type of multimodality treatment, two pilots were simultaneously begun by the RTOG in 1981. One study of resectable patients utilized induction chemotherapy followed by surgery and postoperative radiotherapy. The second pilot utilized the same chemotherapy applied after surgery and before radiotherapy. The side effects of chemotherapy were the same regardless of the sequence of chemotherapy in relation to the definitive treatments. Patient survival favored chemotherapy in the middle (sandwich), in spite of higher stage IV and poorer performance status in this group.[46]

## Combined Cisplatin and Radiotherapy

Since the late 1960's, efforts to simultaneously administer single or combination chemotherapeutic agents with radiotherapy were tested.[14, 37] In randomized trials, the use of Hydrea, methotrexate, 5-FU, or bleomycin with radiotherapy led to increased oral cavity side effects, problems in continuation of treatments, and problems with compliance, without improved survival.[37] The possible combination of cisplatin with radiotherapy seemed very attractive. A small pilot was conducted at Wayne State University combining cisplatin (100 mg/M$^2$ I.V. – Day 1, every three weeks for three courses) with radiotherapy (up to 70 Gy) in patients with unresectable and/or inoperable head and neck cancer. With the feasibility of this combined modality treatment being established, the same trial was activated in the RTOG in late 1981.[49,50] This combination has a clinical CR of about 70% on the cooperative group level, with reversible and acceptable side effects.

## Cooperative Groups and Head and Neck Cancer Inter-Group Activities

In spite of continuing efforts to improve the effectiveness and safety of our chemotherapy, determining the timing of chemotherapy as part of multimodality treatments and testing the combination of cisplatin and radiotherapy, we were very active participants in nationally randomized trials. As shown in Table 2.9, the extent of our past and present cooperative group and inter-group activities is obvious. Many of these trials were activated by the members of our Head and Neck Cancer Program.

## COMBINED MODALITY THERAPY: CONCEPTS AND THE ROLE OF CHEMOTHERAPY

Our definition of combined modality therapy is the incorporation of effective chemotherapy as part of the definitive treatment of surgery and/or radiotherapy in patients with locally advanced head and neck cancer. The obvious reasons for the combined modality trials is the unacceptable, poor results (failure) obtained with definitive treatments in this group of patients.

It is very important to understand and to discuss the concepts and the role of chemotherapy as part of combined modality therapy. Tables 2.10 – 2.15 summarize the concepts and questions that need to be answered in the future about the role of chemotherapy as part of the multimodality treatments.

**TABLE 2.9** Cooperative and Inter-Group Activities

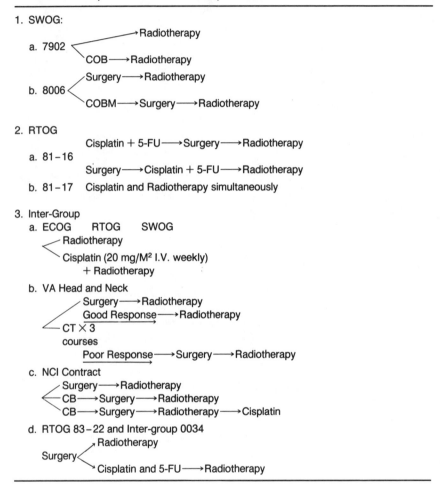

1. SWOG:
   a. 7902 → Radiotherapy / COB → Radiotherapy
   b. 8006 → Surgery → Radiotherapy / COBM → Surgery → Radiotherapy

2. RTOG
   a. 81-16 — Cisplatin + 5-FU → Surgery → Radiotherapy / Surgery → Cisplatin + 5-FU → Radiotherapy
   b. 81-17 Cisplatin and Radiotherapy simultaneously

3. Inter-Group
   a. ECOG RTOG SWOG
      Radiotherapy / Cisplatin (20 mg/M² I.V. weekly) + Radiotherapy
   b. VA Head and Neck
      Surgery → Radiotherapy
      CT × 3 courses — Good Response → Radiotherapy
      Poor Response → Surgery → Radiotherapy
   c. NCI Contract
      Surgery → Radiotherapy
      CB → Surgery → Radiotherapy
      CB → Surgery → Radiotherapy → Cisplatin
   d. RTOG 83-22 and Inter-group 0034
      Surgery — Radiotherapy / Cisplatin and 5-FU → Radiotherapy

---

**TABLE 2.10** Multimodality Therapy: The Best Chemotherapy Combination

Questions That Need to be Answered About The Role of Chemotherapy
  I. The best chemotherapy combination
 II. When to be included in multimodality treatment
III. Timing and sequence of chemotherapy as part of multimodality treatment
IV. Efficacy of chemotherapy in multimodality treatment
 V. Delay or less extensive definitive treatment

**TABLE 2.11** Multimodality Therapy: The Best Chemotherapy Combination

A. Effectiveness

    1. Incidence of clinical complete response
    2. Incidence of histological complete response after resection or "adequate" biopsy

B. Safety

    1. Incidence of transient and acute side effects
       Nausea and/or vomiting
       Myelosuppression
       Renal impairment
       Hair loss
       Other G-I toxicities
    2. Incidence of subacute side effects
       Peripheral neuropathy
    3. Incidence of chronic side effects
       Deafness
       Renal impairment
       "Pulmonary failure"
       (Second Primary Malignancy)

C. Administration

    1. Number of courses overall and to induce CR
    2. Number of courses after clinical CR achieved
    3. Total dose of more "toxic" agent(s)
    4. Frequency and duration of the chemotherapy

D. Tolerance
    1. Patients acceptance
    2. Incidence of patient exclusion
    3. Delay of definitive therapy—surgery and/or radiation
    4. Acceptance by the multimodality team

E. Cost

    1. Inpatient vs outpatient administration
    2. Central I.V. line
    3. Lab tests needed
    4. Supportive care needed
    5. Days lost from work
    6. Days of treatment

## The Best Chemotherapy Combinations

Prior to investigating the value of chemotherapy as part of multimodality treatment, it is crucial to identify and employ the most active chemotherapy regimen possible. At the time of surgical resection, the surgeon removes all

**TABLE 2.12** Multimodality Therapy: When to be Included in Multimodality Therapy

A. Incidence of clinical CR rate

B. Incidence of histological CR rate

C. Incidence of side effects that may delay or prevent other treatment

the gross tumor with a healthy margin, then obtains multiple frozen biopsies; if all biopsies are negative, he will reconstruct the surgical deficit. This is considered adequate resection.

The radiotherapist delivers the highest tolerable dose, using a port to cover all known disease sites and drainage lymph nodes. This is considered adequate radiotherapy.

As medical oncologists, we have to be allowed to utilize the best and the most adequate chemotherapy, especially when there is a question of the value of this modality of treatment as an adjunct to other definitive therapies. Table 2.11 defines the best and most adequate chemotherapy for use in randomized trials. One of the most important factors in selecting chemotherapy is the incidence of clinical and histological CR achieved by such agents. About 10–20% of patients with advanced cancer will not respond ( < PR) to combination cisplatin chemotherapy. It is hoped that future regimens will convert all possible responders to clinical CR and most of the clinical CR to histological CR. It is important to stress the time when clinical CR was achieved in relation to the number of courses of chemotherapy given. This is critical in determining the incidence of histological CR and possible influence on overall survival. A clinical CR occurring after one course of chemotherapy, when additional courses of the same chemotherapy are planned, is a more favorable prognostic factor than clinical CR occurring at the end of the last planned course of chemotherapy. When evaluating the best chemotherapy to be used as part of multimodality treatment, it is important to determine the number of courses needed to achieve clinical CR and the additional courses to be given after a clinical CR, and to obtain the highest possible histological CR.

**TABLE 2.13** Timing and Sequence of Chemotherapy

A. Induction, pre-definitive treatment

B. Post-Surgery

C. Post-Radiotherapy

D. Combined with radiation (simultaneous)

E. Combination of the above

**TABLE 2.14** Multimodality Therapy: Efficacy of Chemotherapy

A. Effect on Disease-Free Survival

B. Effect on Overall Survival

C. Effect on Quality of Life

D. Incidence of Chronic or Delayed Side Effects

E. Change of Pattern of Recurrence

## When To Include Chemotherapy in Multimodality Treatment

At what stage of drug development and at what level of antitumor activity should we introduce these agents into multimodality treatment and begin testing their value?

We believe in the necessity of obtaining maximum clinical complete response rates. Additional courses of chemotherapy given before definitive therapy will enable us to obtain the highest rate of true histological complete response. This should be done without jeopardizing or delaying definitive treatments like surgery or radiotherapy. Poor results (in particular, low overall survival rates), the high incidence of local-regional failure, and the possibility of systemic metastases after our present "definitive" treatments, raise a moral and ethical issue in withholding combination chemotherapy from multimodality therapy.

As was mentioned earlier, we are in the tenth year of clinical trials, and we do not feel the optimum effective chemotherapeutic regimen has been produced even when added to other definitive treatments in patients with locally advanced head and neck cancer. The number of additional years needed to develop such a regimen is unknown and is dependent on many factors including resources, new agent(s), safer agent(s), investigators, and institutional commitment. In addition, all pilot studies from single institutions must be tested and accepted by other institutions and by national cooperative multi-institutional groups.

**TABLE 2.15** Multimodality Therapy: Delay or Less Extensive Definitive Treatment

A. Less surgical resection

B. Selective radical surgical resection

C. "Salvage" surgery only

D. Less "radical" radiation therapy

E. Delay ("salvage") radiotherapy

F. Combinations of the above

In 1978, with activation of the NCI Head and Neck cancer contract, one course of cisplatin and bleomycin was used as initial therapy in the experimental arms followed by surgery and postoperative radiotherapy. This chemotherapy produced an approximate 50% overall response and only a 5% clinical complete response.[50]

In 1979, the Southwest Oncology Group (SWOG) performed a randomized trial in patients with inoperable locally advanced head and neck cancer. Two courses of cisplatin, Oncovin and bleomycin followed by radiotherapy were compared to radiotherapy alone. The overall response rate with this combination was approximately 80% and the clinical CR was 20–30%.

In 1983, the Radiation Therapy Oncology Group (RTOG) performed a randomized trial in resectable cancer patients to test the efficacy of three courses of cisplatin and 5-FU infusion as part of combined modality therapy. This protocol of the Head and Neck Cancer Intergroup (Protocol #0034) is now used nationwide. It has produced a 90% overall response and up to a 50% clinical CR, with 50% of these achieving a histological CR.

The problem that we have to study in the future is the value of chemotherapy. The following questions must be answered: If no real advantage can be presently obtained, is this due to the fact that chemotherapy may not have a place in combined modality settings, or that we have not found the most active and effective chemotherapy? The latter possibility means we still have a long road ahead of us in order to continue to improve on the effectiveness and safety of our chemotherapy.

## Delay or Less Extensive Definitive Treatment

The goals of testing chemotherapy as part of multimodality treatment in locally advanced head and neck cancer patients are better overall survival and/or quality of life. When the time comes that the best chemotherapy may be used in the best sequence with other definitive multimodality therapies of proven value, then the next possible investigation should consider the delay or utilization of less extensive definitive treatment, especially surgery. The main purpose of this would be to lessen the cosmetic and/or functional morbidity caused by such radical procedures without jeopardizing the survival of these patients.

Since all of this may take years, many trials to minimize surgical resection at the institutional and national level are already under way and are being carried out by the Veterans Administration Laryngeal Cancer Group (Table 2.9).[51-53]

## SUMMARY AND FUTURE CHALLENGES

It is clear that we must increase our cure rate for patients with locally advanced head and neck cancer. This can only be accomplished by optimizing and improving all modes of therapy available to us.

Adequate surgery is a very important treatment in patients with resectable and operable cancer. Radiotherapy is also important for treatment of these patients and many attempts are underway to improve its effectiveness. These include: radiosensitizers, radioprotectors, hyperfractionation, hyperthermia, neutron therapy, etc.

The need to improve the effectiveness of present chemotherapy and safety is part of our future challenge. Another important issue is investigating the timing and the value of such effective chemotherapy as part of the multimodality treatment.

It is also important to continue to identify prognostic factors that may effect the complete response (CR) to chemotherapy and the overall survival of these patients. There is also a need to improve our present staging systems, especially for stage III, IV, T4 and N3 cancers. Equally significant are our efforts to improve the quality of life of these patients by better, more effective, and safer therapy combined with active rehabilitation and nutritional programs.

The most important challenge, however, is the need of real prevention efforts (primary, secondary, and tertiary) at all levels and throughout the United States and the world, to decrease the incidence of head and neck cancers by decreasing the consumption of the most commonly used carcinogen: tobacco.

## REFERENCES

1. Cachin Y, Eschwage F: Combination of radiotherapy and surgery in the treatment of head and neck cancer. Cancer Treat Rev 1975;2:177–191.
2. Fletcher GH, Jesse RH: The place of irradiation in the management of the primary lesion in head and neck cancer. Cancer 1977;39:862–867.
3. Hintz B, Charyulu K, Chandler JR, et al: Randomized study of control of the primary tumor and survival using pre-operative radiation, radiation alone or surgery alone in head and neck carcinomas. J Surg Oncol 1979;12:75–85.
4. Schuller DE, McGuirt WF, Krause CJ, et al: Symposium: Adjuvant cancer therapy of head and neck tumors. Increased survival with surgery alone vs. combined therapy. Laryngoscope 1979;89:582–594.
5. Vandenbrouck C, Sancho H, LeFur R, et al: Results of a randomized clinical trial of pre-operative irradiation vs. post-operative in treatment of tumors of the hypopharynx. Cancer 1977;39:1445–1449.
6. Snow JB, Gelber RD, Kramer S, et al: Randomized pre-operative and post-operative

radiation therapy for patients with carcinoma of the head and neck. Preliminary report. Laryngoscope 1980;90:930–945.

7. Kramer S, Gelber RD, Snow JB, et al: Pre-operative vs. post-operative radiation therapy for patients with carcinoma of the head and neck. Progress report. Head and Neck Surg 1985;3:255.

8. Vikram B, Strong EW, Shah JP, et al: Failure at the primary site following multimodality treatment in advanced head and neck cancer. Head and Neck Surg 1984;6:720–723.

9. Vikram B, Strong EW, Shah JP, et al: Failure in the neck following multimodality treatment for advanced head and neck cancer. Head and Neck Surg 1984;6:724–729.

10. Vikram B, Strong EW, Shah JP, et al: Failure at distant sites following multimodality treatment for advanced head and neck cancer. Head and Neck Surg 1984;6:730–733.

11. Probert JC, Thompson RW, Bagshaw MA: Patterns of spread of distant metastases in head and neck cancer. Cancer 1974;33:127–133.

12. O'Brien P, Carlson R, Steubner F, et al: Distant metastases in epidermoid cell carcinoma of the head and neck. Cancer 1971;27:304–307.

13. Papal JR: Distant metastases from head and neck cancer. Cancer 1984;53:342–345.

14. Fazekos JT, Sommer C, Kramer S: Tumor regression and other prognosticators in advanced head and neck cancers. Int J Rad Oncol Biol Phys 1983;9:957–959.

15. Amer MH, Al-Sarraf M, Vaitkevicius VK: Factors that effect response to chemotherapy and survival of patients with advanced head and neck cancer. Cancer 1979;43:2202–2206.

16. Amer MH, Izbicki RM, Vaitkevicius VK, et al: Combination chemotherapy with cis-diaminedichloroplatinum, Oncovin, and bleomycin (COB) in advanced head and neck cancer—Phase II. Cancer 1980;45:217–223.

17. Drelichman A, Cummings G, Al-Sarraf M: A randomized trial of the combination of cis-platinum, Oncovin and bleomycin (COB) versus Methotrexate in patients with advanced squamous cell carcinoma of the head and neck. Cancer 1983;52:399–403.

18. Kish JA, Weaver A, Jacobs J, et al: Cis-platinum and 5-fluorouracil infusion in patients with recurrent and disseminated epidermoid cancer of the head and neck. Cancer 1984;53:1819–1824.

19. Kish JA, Ensley JF, Jacobs J, et al: A randomized trial of cis-platinum (CACP) plus 5-fluorouracil (5-FU) infusion and CACP plus 5-FU bolus for recurrent and advanced squamous cell carcinomas of the head and neck. Cancer 1985;56:2740–2744.

20. Jacobs C, Meyers F, Henderickson C, et al: A randomized phase II study of cisplatin with or without methotrexate for recurrent squamous cell carcinoma of the head and neck. A Northern California Oncology Group Study. Cancer 1983;52:1563–1569.

21. Al-Sarraf M: The cost and clinical value of combination of cis-platinum, Oncovin and bleomycin (COB) vs. methotrexate in patients with advanced head and neck epidermoid cancer (Abstr). Proc Amer Soc Clin Oncol 1980;21:198.

22. Kish J, Decker D, Bergsman K, et al: Preliminary reports of treatment of recurrent squamous carcinoma of the head and neck with cis-platinum (CACP) + 5-FU infusion vs. CACP + 5-FU bolus (Abstr). Proc Amer Soc Clin Oncol 1983;2:163.

23. Kish J, Ensley J, Weaver A, et al: Superior response rate with 96 hour 5-Fluorouracil (5-FU) infusion vs. 5-FU bolus combined with cis-platinum (CACP) in a randomized trial for recurrent and advanced squamous head and neck cancer (Abstr). Proc Amer Soc Clin Oncol 1984;3:179.

24. Kish J, Ensley J, Al-Sarraf M, et al: Activity of CHIP and CBDCA (platinum analogs) in recurrent epidermoid cancer of the head and neck (HNC)-randomized phase II trial of WSU and SWOG. Proc Amer Soc Clin Oncol 1985;4:130.

25. Campbell M, Al-Sarraf M: Phase II ftorafur therapy in previously treated squamous cell cancers of the head and neck. Cancer Treat Rep 1980; 64:713–715.

26. Ratanatharathorn V, Drelichman A, Sexon-Porte M, et al: Phase II evaluation of 4'-(9-

acridinylamino)-methanesulfon-m-anisidine (AMSA) in patients with advanced head and neck cancers. Am J Clin Oncol (CCT) 1982;5:29–32.

27. Kish JA, Al-Sarraf M: Aclacinomycin: Phase II evaluation in advanced squamous carcinoma of the head and neck. Am J Clin Oncol (CCT) 1984;7:535–537.

28. Kish JA, Ensley JF, Al-Sarraf M: Phase II evaluation of AZQ in recurrent head and neck cancer. Cancer Treat Rep (in press).

29. Tapazoglou E, Kish J, Ensley J, et al: The activity of a single agent 5-fluorouracil (5-FU) infusion in advanced and recurrent head and neck cancer. Cancer 1986;57:1105–1109.

30. Al-Sarraf M, Binns P, Vaishampayan G, et al: The adjuvant use of cis-platinum, Oncovin and bleomycin (COB) prior to surgery and/or radiotherapy in untreated epidermoid cancer of the head and neck, in Jones SE, Salmon SE (eds): Adjuvant Therapy of Cancer II. New York: Grune & Stratton, Inc., 1979. pp 421–428.

31. Al-Sarraf M, Drelichman A, Jacobs J, et al: Adjuvant chemotherapy with cis-platinum, Oncovin, and bleomycin followed by surgery and/or radiotherapy in patients with advanced previously untreated head and neck cancer. Final Report, in Jones SE, Salmon SE (eds): Adjuvant Therapy of Cancer III. New York: Grune & Stratton Inc., 1981. pp. 145–152.

32. Al-Sarraf M, Drelichman A, Peppard S, et al: Adjuvant cis-platinum and 5-fluorouracil 96 hour infusion in previously untreated epidermoid cancers of the head and neck. Proc Amer Assn Clin Res 1981;22:428.

33. Kish J, Drelichman A, Jacobs J, et al: Clinical trials of cis-platinum and 5-FU infusion as initial treatment for advanced squamous carcinoma of the head and neck. Cancer Treat Rep 1982;66:471–474.

34. Al-Sarraf M, Kish J, Ensley J, et al: Induction cis-platinum and 5-fluorouracil infusion before surgery and/or radiotherapy in patients with locally advanced head and neck cancer. Progress Report. Proc Amer Assn Cancer Res 1984;25:196.

35. Kish J, Ensley J, Jacobs J, et al: Investigation of optimal initial chemotherapy in patients with advanced head and neck cancer (HNC) utilizing "high dose" cis-platinum (CACP)-phase I–II. Proc Amer Assn Cancer Res 1984;25:173.

36. Ensley J, Kish J, Jacobs J, et al: The use of a five course, alternating combination chemotherapy induction regimen in advanced squamous cell cancer of the head and neck (SCC of H&N). Proc Amer Soc Clin Oncol 1985;4:143.

37. Al-Sarraf M: Chemotherapy strategies in squamous cell carcinoma of the head and neck. CRC Critical Rev in Oncol/Hematol 1984;1:323–355.

38. Al-Kourainy K, Crissman J, Ensley J, et al: Achievement of superior survival of histologically negative vs. histologically positive clinically complete responders to cis-platinum (CACP) combinations in patients with locally advanced head and neck cancer. Proc Amer Assn Cancer Res 1985;26:164.

39. Schwert R, Jacobs JR, Crissman J, et al: Improved survival in patients with advanced head and neck cancer achieving complete clinical response to induction chemotherapy. Proc Amer Soc Clin Oncol 1983;2:159.

40. Weaver A, Fleming S, Ensley J, et al: Superior complete clinical response and survival rates with initial bolus cis-platinum and 120 hour 5-FU infusion before definitive therapy in patients with locally advanced head and neck cancer. Am J Surg 1984;148:525–529.

41. Rooney M, Stanley R, Weaver A, et al: Superior results in complete response rate and overall survival in patients with advanced head and neck cancer treated with three courses of 120 hour 5-FU infusion and cis-platinum. Proc Amer Soc Clin Oncol 1983;2:159.

42. Rooney M, Kish J, Jacobs J, et al: Improved complete response rate and survival in advanced head and neck cancer after 3 course induction therapy with 120 hour 5-FU infusion and cis-platinum. Cancer 1985;55:1123–1128.

43. Amrein P, Weitzman S: 24-Hour infusion cisplatin (ACP) and 5 day infusion 5-fluoura-

cil (5-FU) in squamous cell carcinoma of the head and neck (SCC H&N). Proc Amer Soc Clin Oncol 1985;4:133.

44. Kies MS, Lester EP, Gordon LI, et al: Cisplatin and infusion 5-FU fluorouracil (5-FU) in stage III and IV squamous cancer of the head and neck. Proc Amer Soc Clin Oncol 1985;4:139.

45. Kies MS, Gordon GI, Hauck WW, et al: Analysis of complete responders after initial treatment with chemotherapy in head and neck cancer. Otolaryngol Head and Neck Surg 1985;93:199–205.

46. Al-Sarraf M, Pajak T, Laramore G: Timing of chemotherapy as part of definitive treatment for patients with advanced head and neck cancer. An RTOG Study. Proc Amer Soc Clin Oncol 1985;4:141.

47. Al-Sarraf M, Kinzie J, Jacobs J, et al: New way of giving chemotherapy as part of multi-disciplinary treatment for patients with head and neck cancers. Preliminary Report. Proc Amer Assn Cancer Res 1982;23:134.

48. Al-Sarraf M, Jacobs J, Kinzie J, et al: Combined modality therapy utilizing single high intermittent dose of cis-platinum and radiation in patients with advanced head and neck cancer. Proc Amer Soc Clin Oncol 1983;2:159.

49. Al-Sarraf M, Marcial V, Mowry P, et al: Superior local control with combination of high dose cis-platinum and radiotherapy. An RTOG Study. Proc Amer Assn Cancer Res 1985;26:169.

50. Baker SR, Makuch RW, Wolf G: Pre-operative cisplatin and bleomycin therapy in head and neck squamous carcinoma. Prognostic factors for tumor response. Arch Otolar 1981;107:683–689.

51. Ensley J, Kish JA, Jacobs JR, et al: Superior survival in complete responders achieved with chemotherapy alone compared to those requiring chemotherapy and radiotherapy in patients with advanced squamous cell cancer of the head and neck. Proc Amer Soc Clin Oncol 1984;3:181.

52. Ensley JF, Jacobs JR, Weaver A, et al: The correlation between response to cis-platinum combination chemotherapy and subsequent radiotherapy in previously untreated patients with advanced squamous cell cancers of the head and neck. Cancer 1984;54:811–814.

53. Jacobs C, Goffinet D, Fee W, et al: Chemotherapy as a substitute for surgery in the treatment of advanced operable head and neck cancer. An NCOG Pilot. Proc Amer Soc Clin Oncol 1985;4:137.

# CHAPTER 3

# The Significance of Pretreatment Identification of Prognostically Important Subgroups of Squamous Cell Cancers of the Head and Neck

*John F. Ensley, MD, Julie A. Kish, MD,*
*Efstathios Tapazoglou, MD,*
*Zosia Maciorowski, and Muhyi Al-Sarraf, MD*

## INTRODUCTION

The treatment status of advanced squamous cell cancer of the head and neck (SCC of the H&N) has evolved to the point where it is realistic to consider cure as the goal of current and future therapeutic strategies. Progress towards this goal has occurred in steps that are analogous to therapy regimens for other cancers which are now curable in the advanced state with combination chemotherapy either alone or as part of a multimodality treatment program. The process of developing successful combination chemotherapy regimens in advanced SCC of the H&N will be defined by achieving the following objectives: production of high clinical response rates; production of high clinical complete response rates; and the translation of clinical complete response to histologically negative resected specimens. Certain of these objectives have been achieved with regimens currently in use. Overall clinical response rates of 75–98% have been and are being achieved with both platinum and non-platinum based combination chemotherapy.[1,2] Clinical complete response rates ranging from 40–60% have been reported particularly with platinum based combinations.[3,4] Preliminary reports of complete clinical response rates of 80% or better have been described in certain pilot studies of induction regimens including simultaneous platinum-radiotherapy or five courses of alternating combination chemotherapy.[5,6] In current induction trials in SCC of the H&N, histologically negative tumor resections are being reported in 30–50% of those complete responders following induction chemotherapy.

The importance of response to induction regimens in advanced SCC of the H&N has been stressed in numerous trials.[7] Clear advantages have been reported for responders versus non-responders, complete responders versus partial responders, and most significantly, the group of complete responders with histologically negative versus positive surgical resections in which cures may have been achieved.[8] Additionally, initial response to platinum based induction regimens has been shown to predict for subsequent response to radiation and survival of those patients requiring radiation for complete response following chemotherapy.[9,10] The response patterns of patients with advanced SCC of the H&N treated with induction chemotherapy fall into four major categories:

1. complete clinical response with negative histological resections;
2. complete clinical response with positive histological resections;
3. initial response (PR or MR) followed by a plateau of response and residual resistant tumor; and
4. complete or nearly complete resistance from the onset of therapy which may include frank progression during therapy.

Given the variety of response patterns demonstrated in chemotherapy trials in advanced SCC of the H&N and the prognostic implications of such patterns in terms of successful treatment and survival, it becomes vitally important to identify these response groups pre-therapeutically. Indeed, current induction trials in advanced SCC of the H&N are reporting as high as 20% long term survivors, particularly among those patients in which induction chemotherapy has eliminated tumors at the microscopic level.[8] The task of interested oncologists from all specialties will be to increase this percentage to a range consistent with other chemotherapeutically curable tumors (50–60%). To accomplish this, it will be necessary to pre-therapeutically identify these response and prognostic subgroups. Such identification would then permit the following to occur:

1. stratification of clinical trials based upon known criteria for resistance.
2. the ability to study tumor biology, including the mechanisms of resistance or response, in these subgroups.
3. the design of more intensive treatment regimens for resistant subgroups.

4. the prevention of overly aggressive regimens for the treatment of subgroups that easily achieve a histological CR.
5. the ability to rationally design multimodality treatment plans, to determine their proper sequence, and to decide whether a particular treatment modality is necessary.
6. the possible development of a model to study the chemo-curability of other solid tumors.
7. the more accurate determination of natural history and prognosis in this disease.

The ability to pre-therapeutically identify tumors having a high potential for aggressiveness, persistance or recurrence would have applications for patient subgroups other than those with advanced tumors. Conceptually, patients can be divided into four groups on the basis of presentation, natural history and treatment.

1. Early tumors, equally curable with surgery or radiation, without functional or cosmetic sequelae.
2. More advanced tumors that are curable with surgery and/or radiation but have undesirable functional and cosmetic sequelae.
3. More advanced tumors that are considered curable with surgery and/or radiation at presentation, but routinely reoccur.
4. Tumors presenting in the advanced state that are considered incurable (using conventional methods of treatment) at the time of presentation.

In each of these four groups, a definite and increasing percentage of patients will fail conventional therapy. The reasons for such failure are not always due to obvious causes such as positive margins at the time of surgery. The ability to pre-therapeutically identify response groups, and the successful design of curative regimens in the advanced state, would have definite applicability in groups 3 and 2, but also for a small percentage (15%) in group 1 as well.

## TRADITIONAL APPROACHES TO PRE-THERAPEUTIC IDENTIFICATION OF PROGNOSTIC SUBGROUPS IN SCC OF H&N

In clinical trials, it has been customary to attempt to correlate clinical features of patients with SCC of the H&N with treatment and survival outcome.[11] Indeed, features such as performance status, stage, site, and morphology have, in some instances, been the basis of stratification of such trials. Clinical parameters so employed may be divided into three categories: patient-related, tumor-related, and treatment-related. Tables 3.1, 3.2, and 3.3 list those parameters that have most frequently been either examined or studied in these clinical trials.

Of all the patient-related factors listed in Table 3.1, the one that is most consistently associated with prognostic outcome, including both response and survival, is performance status.[11,12] In trials of patients with both untreated and recurrent tumors, performance status has been a significant factor in determining not only the ability to treat, but the outcome of treatment as well. Additionally, the inability to alter the life styles of patients with head and neck cancers, particularly those who continue to smoke and drink, is responsible for the occurrence of second cancers in up to 30% of these patients.[13]

Table 3.3 examines various aspects of diagnosis, treatment, and support, that when done improperly, may negatively impact on treatment outcome and survival. The issues listed in the table seem self-evident, but it is interesting to note the frequency with which they are violated as evidenced by patients seen in major head and neck cancer referral centers such as ours. The last issue listed in the table may not be as self-evident as it appears. To date, there is no chemotherapeutically curable tumor that has achieved that status without the oncologists' willingness and ability to intensively support these patients both medically and nutritionally. Given the patient population in which this tumor occurs, where advanced age, poor nutritional status, and serious concomitant medical problems are the rule, it becomes imperative that this support be provided. Additionally, intensive and prolonged induction regimens are either being contemplated or are currently in use for the treatment of advanced SCC of the H&N. Our institution has recently gained experience with a five course alternating combination chemotherapy regimen which is given over a 4 to 5 month period in such patients.[6] During this trial, we have demonstrated that increased complete response rates and improved quality of these responses are possible in patients that complete

**TABLE 3.1** Factors Related to Patient

---

Age
Sex
Race
Performance status
   Other medical conditions
   Nutrition
Social habits
   Tobacco
   Alcohol
Compliance

---

**TABLE 3.2** Factors Related to Tumor

Stage
   Primary size (T)
   Lyrnph node status (N)
   Distant metastasis (M)
   Multiple primaries
Untreated vs. previously treated
Site of tumor
Tumor-related products
   Hypercalcemia
   Alkaline phosphatase
Tumor morphology

such therapy. We have also learned that, in certain patients with this disease, concurrent medical problems, or inability to comply, may preclude them from such intensive chemotherapy trials. Indeed, this issue may become the critical factor that ultimately determines whether this tumor is chemo-curable as more intensive and prolonged regimens are tested.

Table 3.2 reviews the commonly studied tumor parameters that have been variously correlated with treatment outcome and survival. Table 3.4 summarizes the experience with using these parameters to predict response in five large chemotherapy induction trials.[1,2,4,11-13] At best, one may conclude that certain tumor parameters, such as degree of lymph node involvement, may statistically correlate with treatment outcome and survival in a

**TABLE 3.3** Factors Related to Diagnosis and Treatment

1. Diagnostic
   Proper diagnosis with histological confirmation
   Upper aerodigestive panendoscopy
   Surgically violated neck
2. Surgery:
   Considerations and determination of resectability for cure
   Adequately planned surgical resection
3. Radiotherapy:
   Adequate radiation ports
   Adequate dosage and fractionization
4. Chemotherapy:
   Type of single agents employed
   Single vs. combination chemotherapy
   Optimum sequence in multimodality treatment plans
   Number of courses of chemotherapy
5. Adequate nutritional/medical support

**TABLE 3.4** Effect of Prognostic Indicator on Response to Adjuvant Combination Chemotherapy

| Study | No. Pts. | Type Chemotherapy | Response% | PS | Stage | T | N | Site | Morphology |
|---|---|---|---|---|---|---|---|---|---|
| W.S.U. (1) | 164 un-resectable | (77) COB-2 courses<br>CACP 100 mg/M² dl<br>VCR 2 mg/dl<br>BLEO 15 μ/M² dl-7 | CR-29<br>PR-51 | — | NO | NO | *YES*<br>RR & CR<br>dec<br>$N_3$ vs<br>$N_1$ & $N_2$ | NO | NO |
| | | (23) 5-FU/CACP-2 courses<br>5-FU 1000 mg/M² × 96 hrs.<br>CACP 100 mg/M² dl | CR-19<br>PR-69 | | | | | | |
| | | (61) 5-FU/CACP-3 courses<br>5-FU 1000 mg/M² × 120 hrs.<br>CACP 100 mg/M² dl | CR-54<br>PR-39 | | | | | | |
| N.C.I. Contract (11) | 282 resectable | 1 course<br>CACP 100 mg/M² dl<br>BLEO 15 μ/M² d3-7 | *Primary*<br>CR-8<br>PR-40<br>*Nodes*<br>CR-15<br>PR-37 | NO | NO | *YES*<br>RR & CR<br>dec<br>$T_3$ & $T_4$<br>vs<br>$T_1$ & $T_2$ | *YES*<br>RR dec<br>$N_3$ vs<br>$N_1 N_2$<br>RR dec<br>$N_3 N_2 N_1$ | NO | NO |
| Hill et al. (8) | 200 un-resectable | 2 courses | | | | | | | |

| Study | Regimen (n) | Response | | | | | | |
|---|---|---|---|---|---|---|---|---|
| | VCR 2 mg<br>MTX 100 mg/M² hrs. 12,15,18<br>BLEO 60 μ(I) hr 12–18<br>5-FU 500 mg hr.18 | CR + PR = 66 | — | YES<br>II 71%<br>III 70%<br>IV 56% | — | — | YES<br>RR inc<br>Oral cavity<br>RR dec<br>Hypopharynx | NO |
| Hong et al. (4)<br>104 advanced | (23) BLEO 15 μ/M² × 7d | CR-4<br>PR-30 | NO | NO | — | NO | NO | |
| | (17) CACP 100 mg/M² dl<br>BLEO 15 μ/M² × 6d | CR-6<br>PR-65 | | | | | | |
| | (69) CACP 120 mg/M² dl & 22<br>BLEO 15 μ/M² × 7d | CR-20<br>PR-54 | | | | | | |
| S.W.O.G. (13)<br>172 un-<br>resectable | 3 courses<br>CACP 50 mg/M² dl<br>MTX 40 mg/M² dl | CR-29<br>PR-46 | NO<br>for (sig)<br>survival | NO<br>(PR Stg III<br>inc vs<br>Stg IV NSD) | NO | NO | NO | |
| | (79 on adj.<br>chemo arm) | BLEO 15 μ/M² d1 & 8<br>VCR 2 mg dl | | | | | | |

W.S.U. = Wayne State University, Detroit, Michigan; SWOG = Southwest Oncology Group, Houston, Texas March 6–8, 1986 Annual Meeting; NCI = National Cancer Institute Head and Neck Contract; CACP - cisplatin; BLEO - bleomycin; 5-FU - 5-fluorouracil; MTX - methotrexate; VCR - vincristine.

large group of patients. For an individual patient, these factors, either singly or in combination, are not sufficiently predictive. Tumor morphology and grade have proven useful in the prediction of response and survival in several human malignancies. Data exist that support the notion that morphological features of early SCC of the H&N may be of value in this regard.[14,15] Our center has studied this question in patients with advanced SCC of the H&N over the last decade. Tumor morphology in this group has been examined with respect to both conventional grades (WD, MWD, PD) and specific histological parameters. The conclusions reported from these investigations indicate that, in the advanced state, neither conventional grade nor specific histological features of these tumors are successful in predicting chemotherapeutic response or survival. Table 3.5 summarizes our institution's analysis of conventional morphological grades of SCC of the H&N and their correlation with overall and complete response rates in patients undergoing induction chemotherapy. It is evident from this data that these tumor grades do not predict overall or complete response rates. Figure 3.1 examines survival differences for these patients based on the morphological grades of their tumors; it clearly demonstrates that morphological grade of tumor does not predict survival in patients with advanced SCC of the H&N treated with induction chemotherapy.

Correlations of clinical parameters, i.e., stage, size of the primary (T), and degree of lymph node involvement (N), with chemotherapeutic response and survival are summarized in Tables 3.6–3.9 and Figures 3.2–3.5. Table 3.6, which examines response by stage, reveals a small, 13%, difference in complete response rate and no difference in overall response rates. No survival differences are noted between patients with stage III or IV disease. Survival differences are clearly evident, though, when one subdivides even a single stage into T, N, and M groupings, such as in Figure 3.2, where stage IV patients are so analyzed. When stage IV patients are similarly subdivided by TNM and correlated with response (as in Table 3.7), a 28% difference (46% vs 18%) in CR rates is evident between $T_4N_0$ and $T_4N_3$, respectively, although no differences in overall response rates are seen.

Figure 3.3 compares survival differences in this patient group with the

**TABLE 3.5** Morphology and Response to Chemotherapy

|             | Well          | Moderate       | Poor          |
|-------------|---------------|----------------|---------------|
| CR          | 8 (47.1%)     | 39 (34.8%)     | 28 (45.2%)    |
| PR          | 8 (47.1%)     | 59 (52.7%)     | 25 (40.3%)    |
| NR          | 1 (5.9%)      | 14 (12.5%)     | 9 (14.5%)     |
| CR + PR/Total | 16/17 (94.1%) | 98/112 (87.5%) | 53/62 (85.5%) |

## Survival For 191 Patients By Differentiation

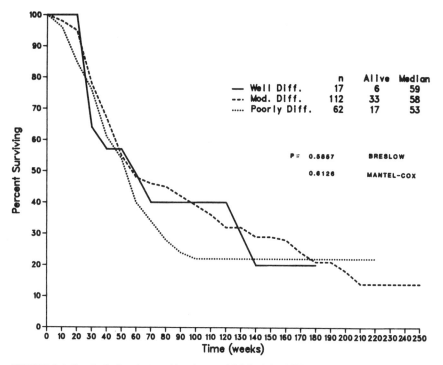

**FIGURE 3.1** Survival of patients with advanced SCC of the H&N by morphological groups.

**TABLE 3.6** Stage and Response to Chemotherapy

|              | II        | III          | IV             |
|--------------|-----------|--------------|----------------|
| CR           | 2 (67%)   | 15 (50%)     | 58 (37%)       |
| PR           | 0 (0%)    | 11 (37%)     | 81 (51%)       |
| NR           | 1 (33%)   | 4 (13%)      | 19 (12%)       |
| CR + PR/Total| 2/3 (67%) | 26/30 (87%)  | 139/158 (88%)  |

**TABLE 3.7** TNM Stage IV Groups and Response

|  | $T_4N_0$ | $T_4N_1$ | $T_4N_2$ | $T_4N_3$ |
|---|---|---|---|---|
| CR | 17 (46%) | 3 (43%) | 8 (50%) | 6 (25%) |
| PR | 15 (40%) | 4 (57%) | 7 (44%) | 16 (67%) |
| NR | 5 (14%) | 0 (0%) | 1 (6%) | 2 (8%) |
| CR + PR/Total | 32/37 (94%) | 7/7 (100%) | 15/16 (94%) | 22/24 (92%) |

degree of response to induction chemotherapy. Statistically significant survival differences are seen only in those patients who achieve a complete clinical response to such therapy. Tables 3.8, and 3.9 and Figures 3.4 and 3.5 summarize response and survival correlations with patients grouped by size of primary tumor (T) and degree of lymph node involvement (N). No survival differences are noted in this series when patients are grouped by the size of their primary. On the other hand, significant decreases in CR rates and survival are noted in patients with advanced nodal disease. Of the clinical and morphological parameters analyzed, only advanced nodal states has a clear negative impact on CR rates and survival. It is also quite clear that failure to report stage by TNM categories will result in the loss of prognostically important data.

In summary, then, it may be possible to identify certain clinical features or tumor parameters that may be statistically correlated with treatment response and survival in large patient populations. However, they do not have the ability to predict such outcome for an individual patient. In particular, they cannot pre-therapeutically predict the crucial issue of tumor response or resistance. While it may be possible, using these parameters, to describe a patient with a very high or low potential for response or survival, such analysis does not serve the vast majority of these patients.

**TABLE 3.8** Size of Primary and Response

|  | $T_0$ | $T_1$ | $T_2$ | $T_3$ | $T_4$ |
|---|---|---|---|---|---|
| CR | 0 (0%) | 2 (40%) | 8 (67%) | 31 (36%) | 34 (40%) |
| PR | 3 (75%) | 3 (60%) | 2 (17%) | 41 (48%) | 42 (50%) |
| NR | 1 (25%) | 0 (0%) | 2 (17%) | 14 (16%) | 8 (10%) |
| CR + PR/Total | 3/4 (75%) | 5/5 (100%) | 10/12 (83%) | 72/86 (84%) | 76/84 (91%) |

**TABLE 3.9** Degree of Lymph Node Involvement and Response

|  | $N_0$ | $N_1$ | $N_2$ | $N_3$ |
|---|---|---|---|---|
| CR | 26 (49%) | 11 (45%) | 22 (46%) | 16 (24%) |
| PR | 19 (36%) | 11 (45%) | 20 (42%) | 41 (62%) |
| NR | 8 (15%) | 2 (8%) | 6 (13%) | 9 (14%) |
| CR + PR/Total | 45/53 (85%) | 22/24 (92%) | 42/48 (88%) | 57/66 (86%) |

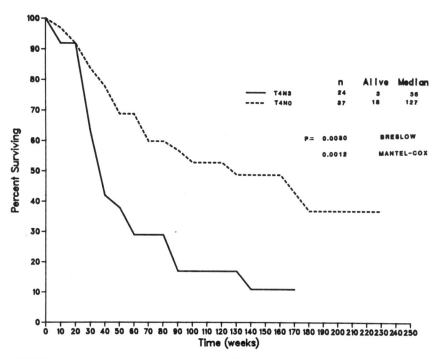

**FIGURE 3.2** Survival of patients with advanced SCC of the H&N Stage IV by TNM groups.

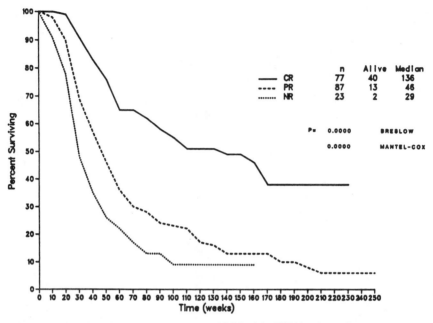

FIGURE 3.3 Survival of patients with advanced SCC of the H&N by chemotherapy response.


## CURRENT AND FUTURE APPROACHES TO PRE-THERAPEUTIC IDENTIFICATION OF PROGNOSTIC SUBGROUPS IN SCC OF THE H&N

In light of the preceding discussion, it becomes imperative to investigate and develop newer techniques for the pre-therapeutic identification of prognostic subgroups in advanced SCC of the H&N. One approach to the problem has been the development of pre-therapeutic, in vitro drug sensitivity testing of human tumors, as initially described by Hamburg and Solomon.[18] Such techniques have the following inherent conceptual drawbacks:

1. inability to culture specimens in a large percentage of human tumors.
2. inability to produce viable, unaltered, single cell suspensions from many solid human tumors.
3. anticipated differences in the biology of isolated cancer cell responses versus the native solid tumor.

4. differences in drug metabolism and activation in vitro compared to in vivo.
5. the inhibition of growth in culture versus the prediction of gross tumor response.
6. in vitro drug time/concentration correlations with drugs administered clinically.
7. definitions and confirmation of cancer growth and response.

In one retrospective analysis and one prospective trial,[19,20] the human tumor stem cell assay was predictive of human tumor response 60% of the time, and was predictive of resistance 90% of the time. Variations of this technique have evolved that attempt to circumvent many of the drawbacks listed above. Van Hoff has developed a capillary tube method for the growth of human tumors, and reports a significant increase in the number of tumors that can be cultured.[21] Corbett et al. have developed a modification of the

## Survival For Complete Responders By T

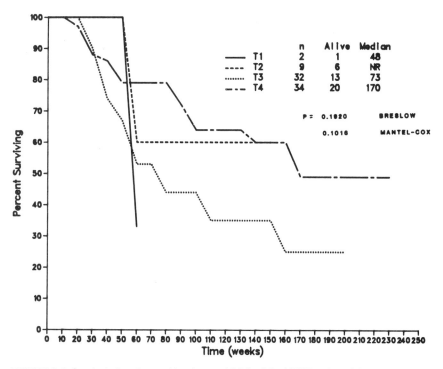

FIGURE 3.4 Survival of patients with advanced SCC of the H&N by size of the primary (T).

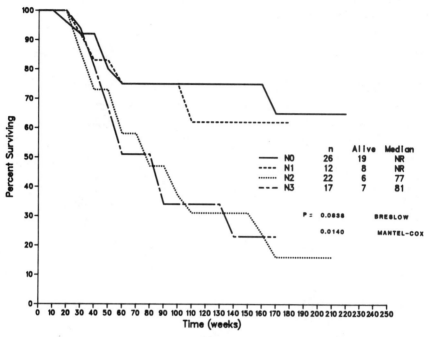

**FIGURE 3.5** Survival of patients with advanced SCC of the H&N by degree of lymph node involvement (N).

Kiby-Bauer technique (for human tumor drug testing) that quickly and inexpensively identifies new cancer drug activity in a panel of standard, resistant human tumors.[22] Xenographs of human tumors have been implanted in nude mice (either subcutaneously or by sub-renal capsule) to develop murine models of human solid tumors for the determination of human tumor response.[23] Neither technique has been tested in sufficiently large numbers in prospective trials to establish its value as a predictor of human tumor chemotherapeutic response.

Two new techniques, alkaline elution and magnetic resonance imaging (MRI),[24-26] are being studied for their potential use as pre-therapeutic indicators of tumor response. Alkaline elution is a technique whereby the effect of chemotherapeutic drugs or radiation on tumor cells is measured by the degree of DNA strand breakage induced either in vitro or in vivo; correlations between this data and clinical tumor response can then be made. One would anticipate that the inability to produce DNA breakage would correlate with clinical tumor resistance. MRI is a technique in which the spin resonance orientation of various nuclei from elements such as hydrogen or phosphorus may be measured in the native, unperturbed state following exposure to a magnetic field. This technique has applications for tumor spectroscopy and imaging. Preliminary studies in laboratory models indicate that differences in MRI parameters can be identified in responsive and resistant tumor lines prior to therapy. Should this hold true for human neoplasms, a non-invasive, non-toxic technique may be employed for the detection of tumor response in cancer patients early in the course of their treatment.

The detection and measurement of tumor parameters by flow cytometry has evolved over the last three to four decades.[27,28] The principle of this technique involves the interruption of a beam of light by a passing cell. Light scatter parameters so produced can be used to determine cell size and density. In addition, the incident light may be used to activate naturally occurring or added cellular fluorochromes. In theory, any feature of a cell that can be caused to fluoresce may be detected and measured. This includes ultrastructural components, DNA/RNA parameters, cytochemical reactions, or cell surface markers. In addition, under certain conditions, this technique has the potential to perform these measurements on living cells. Depending on the complexity of these interrogations, from 3–10,000 cells may be examined per second. These data are converted by photomultiplier tubes into electrical signals and are instantaneously recorded and collated by sophisticated computers. On the basis of predetermined cellular features of interest, cells may be sorted out and retrieved for further studies or analysis.

At present, the application of this technique to human tumors has its greatest utility in hematological malignancies.[29] Solid tumor flow cytometry (FCM) is hindered by the problem of producing high yield, unaltered, viable single cell preparations. Table 3.10 reviews the currently available information concerning the correlation, in human tumors, of FCM cellular nucleic acid determinations with various prognostic measurements. Following extensive investigations to determine optimum techniques for the production of single cell suspensions,[30,31] nearly 230 patient specimens of human SCC of the H&N in our center have been examined for cellular DNA characteristics by FCM. Tables 3.11, 3.12, and 3.13 list the patient characteristics, tumor preparation data, and DNA cellular characteristics of the first 232 specimens.

Table 3.12 indicates that the average combined mechanical-enzymatic cellular yield per gram is $71.2 \times 10^6$ for all specimens with an average dye exclusion viability of greater than 90% for enzymatically dissociated cells. DNA histograms so produced have a mean coefficient variation of 4.1. In addition, 65% of these dissociated specimens were successfully cultured in in vitro systems.

**TABLE 3.10** Prognostically Significant FCM-Determined Parameter in Human Malignancies

| Tumor | Prognostic Factor Association | DNA H | Index L | RNA H | Index L | SPF H | SPF L |
|---|---|:-:|:-:|:-:|:-:|:-:|:-:|
| Leukemia | | | | | | | |
| All | | | | | | | |
| Childhood | Inc. remission rate | * | | | | | |
| | Inc. remission duration | * | | | | | |
| Adult | Inc. remission rate | * | | | | * | |
| | Inc. survival | * | | | | * | |
| | Inc. remission duration | | | | | | * |
| AML | Inc. remission rate | | * | * | | | |
| | Inc. remission duration | | | * | | | |
| | Inc. survival | | * | * | | | |
| Myeloma | Inc. tumor | * | | | | | |
| | Inc. renal failure | * | | | | | |
| | Dec. survival | * | | | * | | |
| | Dec. dfi | * | | | | | |
| | Chemotherapy resistance | * | | | | | |
| | Inc. remission rate | | | * | | | |
| | Inc. remission duration | | | | | | * |
| Lymphoma | Higher grade | * | | | | * | |
| | Dec. survival | * | | * | | * | |
| Sezary synd. | Dec. d.f. survival | * | | | | * | |
| Lung | Dec. survival | * | | | | * | |
| Breast | Dec. ER/PR | * | | | | | |
| | Poor. diff. tumors | * | | | | | |
| | Dec. survival | * | | | | * | |
| Bladder | High grade | * | | | | * | |
| | Degree invasiveness | * | | | | | |
| | Dec. survival | * | | | | * | |
| Prostate | Higher stage | * | | | | | |
| | Inc. metastatsis | * | | | | | |
| | Higher grade | * | | | | | |
| | Inc. hormone response | | * | | | | |
| | Dec. survival | * | | | | * | |
| Renal | Increased postoperative recurrance rates and dissemination | * | | | | | |
| Ovarian | Dec. survival | * | | | | * | |
| Colon | Dec. survival | * | | | | | |
| | High grade | * | | | | | |
| Melanoma | Dec. survival | | | * | | | |
| Brain | Inc. relapse rate | * | | | | | |
| Heterogeneous | | | | | | | |
| Solid | Higher stage | * | | * | | | |
| Tumors | Shorter survival | * | | * | | | |

**TABLE 3.11** Patient Characteristics

| Number Patients = 194 | Number Specimens = 232 |
|---|---|
| New = 119 | Multiple = 38 |
| Recurrent = 75 | |

| Age | Sex | Race |
|---|---|---|
| Median = 59 | M = 82% | W = 66% |
| Range = 35–85 | F = 18% | B = 34% |

| Stage | T | N | Morphology |
|---|---|---|---|
| I = 6% | 0 = 3% | 0 = 48% | WD = 15% |
| II = 5% | 1 = 10% | 1 = 18% | MWD = 53% |
| III = 35% | 2 = 16% | 2 = 22% | PD = 32% |
| IV = 54% | 3 = 42% | 3 = 12% | |
| | 4 = 29% | | |

Table 3.13 describes the cellular DNA characteristics of these tumor specimens. Basically, two cytological parameters based on cellular DNA content were determined. The degree of aneuploidy, as defined by the DNA index and the degree of cellular proliferation (% S phase fraction), may be determined from a single DNA histogram, as is shown in Figure 3.6. Cells in various parts of the cell cycle may be defined by their cellular DNA content; i.e., $G_0/G_1$ cells have diploid DNA contents (DI = 1.0), those in $G_2/M$ have tetraploid DNA contents (DI = 2.0), and those in S phase have DNA con-

**TABLE 3.12** Comparative Specimen Preparation Data

| Dissociation Technique | All Specimens | Primary | Lymph Nodes | Recurrent |
|---|---|---|---|---|
| **Mechanical** | | | | |
| Ave. Total Yield ($\times 10^6$/gm) | 31.3 | 18.7 | 88.1 | 31.3 |
| Ave. Viable Yield ($\times 10^6$/gm) | 15.9 | 9.4 | 46.1 | 14.2 |
| Ave. Viability (%) | 50.8 | 50.2 | 52.3 | 45.2 |
| Ave. C.V. | 4.27 | 4.4 | 3.74 | 4.3 |
| **Enzymatic** | | | | |
| Ave. Total Yield ($\times 10^6$/gm) | 39.3 | 37.2 | 51.6 | 40.0 |
| Ave. Viable Yield ($\times 10^6$/gm) | 35.9 | 33.6 | 46.5 | 35.2 |
| Ave. Viability (%) | 91.4 | 90.3 | 89.7 | 87.7 |
| Ave. C.V. | 4.10 | 4.11 | 4.01 | 4.06 |
| **Combined** | | | | |
| Ave. Total Yield ($\times 10^6$/gm) | 71.2 | 46.9 | 139.7 | 71.3 |
| Ave. Viable Yield ($\times 10^6$/gm) | 51.8 | 43.0 | 92.6 | 49.4 |

**TABLE 3.13** DNA Content Squamous Cell Cancer of Head and Neck

Number specimens = 230
% Diploid (DI of 1.10) = 22.5
% Aneuploid (DI of 1.10) = 77.5

% DI of 1.10 − 1.50 = 30.3
% DI of 1.50 − 2.00 = 38.0
% DI of 2.0          = 9.0

% SPF Distribution:

| | | |
|---|---|---|
| 10% | | 13.4% |
| 10% but | 20% | 35.4% |
| 20% but | 30% | 48.3% |
| 30% but | 40% | 7.1% |
| 40% | | 0.01% |

tents (and DNA indices) between these two extremes. Cellular subpopulations that demonstrate aneuploidy are identified by a second DNA histogram (Fig. 3.7) with a $G_0/G_1$ DI different from the diploid standard. The SPF is that fraction of cells located within the S phase portion of the histogram as compared to the total number of cells. The DI and SPF of such an aneuploidal cell subpopulation are then compared to human diploid standards.

Approximately three-fourths of SCC of the H&N specimens demonstrated aneuploidy, while one-fourth were cytologically confirmed diploid malignancies. Nearly 50% of these specimens had SPF between 20 and 30%.

**FIGURE 3.6** DNA histogram of monoclonal-diploid cell line with cell cycle fractions as labeled

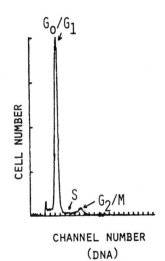

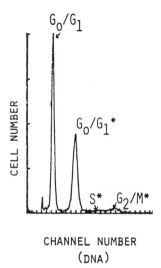

CHANNEL NUMBER
(DNA)

**FIGURE 3.7** DNA histogram of biclonal-diploid aneuploid cell lines with * indicating cell cycle fractions of the aneuploid cell line

This was significantly higher than one might expect from a tumor such as SCC of the H&N, since it is usually presumed to be slow – growing. Attempts to correlate degree of aneuploidy and SPF with clinical features such as stage, T, N, or morphology, have not yet been productive. Data from a larger group of patients than this, and, in particular, more data from early stages, will be necessary for this analysis to be performed. Statistically, conclusions concerning disease-free interval or survival are at present premature due to an inadequate period of follow-up. Intriguing, but preliminary, data from two sources may be evolving concerning tumor response or resistance.

Following induction chemotherapy, microscopically positive or gross residual specimens tend to be predominately diploid. Tumors initially resistant to induction chemotherapy likewise are predominately diploid. A comparison of recurrent tumors following radiation or surgery with untreated tumors indicates that the percentage of tumors that are diploid is 50% versus 25% in the non-recurrent groups. These diploid tumor lines tend to have a relatively low SPF. Much larger numbers of patients will need to be studied to confirm these preliminary observations. It would be naive to believe that cellular DNA parameters alone will be sufficient to characterize clinical prognostic subgroups in SCC of the H&N.

Several other known markers of keratinocytes are undergoing preliminary studies in our laboratory, such as those detailed for DNA determinations for future use in prognostic studies. It is hoped that one or probably a combination of such features will be capable of defining tumor subgroups in such an assay as to allow correlation with important prognostic subgroups.

Theoretically, FCM has a limitless potential for examining such cellular parameters. Much needs to be learned concerning the production of unaltered, representative single cell suspensions and the identification of those cellular parameters that are potentially discriminatory, before FCM reaches this potential.

## SUMMARY

The treatment of advanced SCC of the H&N has reached the stage where chemotherapy may be potentially curative in a significant percentage of patients. The ability to pre-therapeutically identify various response and survival groups and to determine the tumor's natural history would be of use in reaching this goal. The successful development of chemotherapeutic regimens that are curative in the advanced state would have a significant impact on the treatment of many non-advanced patients. Previous attempts to employ clinical or morphological features for the pre-therapeutic identification of prognostically important subgroups have not been successful. Currently we are exploring the use of newer techniques such as MRI and FCM for this purpose, with the hope that the identification of tumor or cellular parameters may be applied.

## REFERENCES

1. Al-Sarraf M: Chemotherapeutic strategies in squamous cell carcinomas of the head and neck. CRC critical review in Oncology/Hematology 1984;1:323–355.
2. Hill BT, Price LA, Busey E, et al: Positive impact of initial 24 hour combination chemotherapy without cisplatinum on 6 year survival figures in advanced squamous cell carcinomas of the head and neck, in: Jones SE, Solomon SE (eds): Adjuvant Therapy of Cancer, 4th ed. Orlando: Grune & Stratton, 1984. pp 97–106.
3. Weaver A, Fleming S, Ensley J, et al: Superior complete clinical response and survival rates with initial bolus cisplatinum and 120 hour infusion before definitive therapy in patients with locally advanced head and neck cancer. Am J Surg 1984;148:525–529.
4. Hong WK, Poplin J, Shapshays Hoffer S, et al: Adjuvant chemotherapy as initial treatment of advanced head and neck cancer: survival data at three years, in: Jones SE, Solomon SE (eds): Adjuvant Therapy of Cancer, 4th ed. Orlando: Grune & Stratton, 1984. pp 127–133.
5. Al-Sarraf M, Kinzie J, Marcial V, et al: Combination of cisplatinum and radiotherapy in patients with advanced head and neck cancers. An RTOG report (Abstr). Proc Amer Soc Clin Oncol 1984; 3:180.
6. Ensley J, Kish J, Jacobs J, et al: The use of an S course alternating combination chemotherapy induction regimen in advanced squamous cell cancer of the head and neck (Abstr). Proc Amer Soc Clin Oncol 1985;4:143.
7. Schwert R, Jacobs J, Crissman J, et al: Improved survival in patients with advanced head

and neck cancer achieving a complete response to induction chemotherapy. Proc Amer Soc Clin Oncol 1983;2:195.

8. Al-Kourainy K, Crissman J, Ensley J, et al: Achievement of superior survival in histologically negative versus histologically positive clinical complete responses to cisplatinum (CACP) combinations in patients with locally advanced head and neck cancer (Abstr). Proc Amer Assn Cancer Res 1985;C:648.

9. Ensley J, Jacobs J, Weaver A, et al: Correlation between response to cisplatinum combination chemotherapy and subsequent radiotherapy in previously untreated patients with advanced squamous cell cancers of the head and neck. Cancer 1984;54:811–814.

10. Ensley J, Kish J, Jacobs J, et al: Incremental improvements in median survival in patients with advanced squamous cell cancer of the head and neck, in: Jones SE, Solomon SE (eds): Adjuvant Therapy of Cancer, 4th ed. Orlando: Grune & Stratton, 1984. pp 117–125.

11. Wolf GT, Makoch R, Baker S: Predictive factors for tumor response to preoperative chemotherapy in patients with head and neck squamous carcinomas. Cancer 1984;55:2869–2877.

12. Amer MH, Al-Sarraf M, Vaitkevicius VK. Factors that affect response to chemotherapy and survival of patients with advanced head and neck cancer. Cancer 1979;43:2202.

13. Schuller DE, Wilson HE, Smith RE, et al: Preoperative reductive chemotherapy for locally advanced carcinomas of the oral cavity, oropharynx and hypopharynx. Cancer 1983;51:15–19.

14. Crissman JD, Liu WY, Gluckman JL, et al: Prognostic value of histopathologic parameters in squamous cell carcinoma of the oropharynx. Cancer 1984;54:2995–3001.

15. Jakobsson PA: Histological grading of malignancy and prognosis in glottic carcinoma of the larynx. Workshop No. 14, in: Albert PW, Bryer DP (eds): Centennial Conference on Laryngeal Cancer, New York: Appleton-Century Crofts, 1976. pp. 847–852.

16. Ensley J, Crissman J, Kish J, et al: The impact of conventional morphological analysis in response rates and survival in patients with advanced head and neck cancers treated initially with cisplatinum containing combination chemotherapy. Cancer 1986;57:711–717.

17. Ensley J, Crissman J, Weaver A: The impact of tumor morphology in the response rate and overall survival of patients with head and neck cancer treated with cisplatinum combination chemotherapy (Abstr). Proc Amer Soc Clin Oncol 1983;2:C658.

18. Hamburger AW, Solomon SE: Primary bioassay of human tumor stem cells. Science 1977;197:461–463.

19. Johnson P, Kassof AH: The role of the human tumor stem cell assay in medical oncology. Arch Int Med 1983;143:111–119.

20. Von Hoff DD, Clark GM, Stagdill BJ, et al. Prospective clinical trials of a human tumor cloning system. Cancer Res 1983;43:1926–1931.

21. Von Hoff D, Buchok J, Knight W: Use of in-vitro dose response curves to select anti-neoplastics for high dose or regional perfusion regimens (Abstr). Proc Amer Assn Cancer Res 1985;1439.

22. Corbett TH, Wozniak A, Gerpheide S, et al: A selective two-tumor soft agar assay for drug discovery, in: White R (ed): In-Vitro and In-Vivo Models for Detection of New Antitumor Drugs. 14th International Congress of Chemotherapy. (in press).

23. Overjera AA, Houchens DP: Human tumor xenographs in athymic nude mice as a preclinical screen for anticancer agents. Sem Oncol 1981;8:836–893.

24. Kohn K: DNA as a target in cancer chemotherapy measurement of macromolecular DNA damage produced in mammalian cells by anticancer agents and carcinogens, in: Methods of Cancer Research, Vol. 16, Academic News, Inc., 1979. pp 29–345.

25. Buddiuger TF, Lautesbor PC: Nuclear magnetic resonance technology for medical studies. Science 1984;226:228–297.
26. Bounanno FS, Pykett IC, Brady TJ, et al: Clinical applications of nuclear magnetic resonance. Disease of the Mouth. Chicago: Year Book Medical Publishers. 1983. pp 1–81.
27. Laerum OD, Farsund T: Clinical applications of flow cytometry. A review. Cytometry 1981;2:1.
28. Lovett EJ, Schnitzer B, Keren DF, et al: Application of flow cytometry to diagnostic pathology. Lab Invest 1984;50:115–140.
29. Barlogie B, Raber MN, Schuman J, et al: Flow cytometry in clinical cancer research. Cancer Res 1983;43:3977–3982.
30. Ensley JF, Maciorowski Z, Crissman J, et al: Clinical correlation and technical problems encountered in flow cytometric examination of clinical specimens of advanced squamous cell carcinoma of the head and neck (Abstr). Proc Internatl Conf Head Neck Cancer 1984;C:94.
31. Ensley J, Maciorowski Z, Crissman J, et al: Inferior cell yields and alterations in histograms produced by technical differences in tissue preparations employing a standard reference murine tumor (Abstr). Proc Amer Assn Cancer Res 1984;25:33.

# CHAPTER 4

# Squamous Cell Carcinoma: Progression and Invasion

*John D. Crissman, MD and*
*Richard J. Zarbo, MD, DMD*

Precursor intraepithelial alterations preceding the development of invasive squamous cell carcinoma (SCC) have been described but not well defined. Physical examination of squamous mucosa of the upper aerodigestive tract (UADT) often reveals mucosal alterations, especially in individuals with high risk factors. These factors are well characterized and consist of heavy and prolonged alcohol exposure combined with tobacco abuse, usually in the form of habitual cigarette use. The cocarcinogens found in alcohol and tobacco exposure are not completely defined, but their relationship to the subsequent development of SCC in the UADT mucosa is recognized.[1]

Squamous mucosa responds to injury by cell proliferation, usually resulting in epithelial thickening or hyperplasia. In most regions of the UADT, especially anatomic areas associated with the trauma of mastication, swallowing, voice production, etc., the hyperplastic epithelium often develops extensive surface keratinization. This is a common reaction to any form of injury and is usually caused by mechanical trauma, but may also develop secondary to carcinogenic influences. The development of surface keratin is common in all forms of reaction to injury in the UADT mucosa and differs from other mucosal surfaces such as found in the uterine cervix where surface keratinization is uncommon.[2]

The most common form of mucosal alteration or reaction to injury in the UADT mucosa takes the form of leukoplakia. This is a description term meaning white patch. It represents a form of hyperplasia with thick epithelium and prominent surface keratin formation. For the most part, leukoplakia is the result of non-carcinogenic influences and is secondary to various types of mechanical traumas. The histologic expression most commonly encountered in leukoplakia is orderly maturation of a hyperplastic epithelium with prominent surface keratinization (Table 4.1).[3] However, leukoplakia does not always represent benign hyperplasia. Approximately 8 – 10% of leukoplakic mucosal changes have epithelial changes of dysplasia, especially in leukoplakic changes found in the thin mucosa of the retromolar palatine tonsil, floor of the mouth, and ventral tongue.[4] Leukoplakic mucosal changes occurring in these locations should always be viewed with suspicion (Table 4.2).

Erythroplasia or red mucosal changes represent thin mucosa which is commonly associated with dysplasia, carcinoma in situ (CIS) and/or invasive carcinoma.[5,6] The red or erythroplastic mucosal alterations are most common in palatine tonsil, floor of mouth, and ventral tongue. However, erythroplastic changes in any UADT mucosal site must be strongly suspected to contain dysplasia, CIS or invasive carcinoma. The speckled or mixed leukoplakic-erythroplastic mucosal changes are probably the most common change, depending on the examiner, and must be viewed as variants of erythroplasia.[5] Invariably, the red areas in the speckled mucosa are associated with dysplastic/CIS changes and have a high frequency of association/transformation to invasive carcinoma. In the past, speckled lesions were not recognized as a serious mucosal change and were commonly grouped with leukoplakia. This may be the primary reason leukoplakic mucosal changes were considered to represent a major source of mucosal alterations preceding invasive carcinoma in the past.

**TABLE 4.1** Intraepithelial Neoplasia Associated with Mucosal Appearance

|  | Dysplasia | Carcinoma |
|---|---|---|
| **Leukoplakia** | | |
| Waldron and Shafer (1975)[3] | 153/3256 (5%) | 104/3256 (3%) |
| Mashberg (1978)[6] | 3/43 (7%) | 3/43 (7%) |
| Silverman et al. (1984)[4] | 2/107 (2%) | 7/107 (7%) |
| **Speckled Leukoplakia and Erythroplasia** | | |
| Mashberg (1978)[6] | 6/58 (10%) | 33/58 (57%) |
| Silverman et al. (1984)[4] | 20/128 (16%) | 30/128 (23%) |
| **Erythroplasia** | | |
| Shafer and Waldron (1975)[5] | 26/65 (40%)† | 33/65 (51%) |
| Mashberg (1978)[6] | 1/44 (2%) | 28/44 (64%)†† |

†65 biopsies in 58 specimens from a series of 64,354 biopsy specimens.
††Includes both CIS and invasive cancer.

TABLE 4.2 Distribution of Intraepithelial Neoplasia of Oral Cavity: Number of Patients (% of total)

| | Tonsil Retromolar Trigone | Floor of Mouth | Oral Tongue | Palate | Buccal | Alveolar Ridge | Lip |
|---|---|---|---|---|---|---|---|
| **Histopathology** | | | | | | | |
| Oral Dysplasia | | | | | | | |
| Mincer et al (1978)[8] | 3 (4.5) | 11 (16.4) | 8 (11.9) | 4 (6.0) | 9 (13.4) | 18 (26.9) | 14 (21) |
| Oral Dysplasia/CIS | | | | | | | |
| Waldron and Shafer (1975)[3] | 10 (3.3) | 45 (15) | 22 (7.3) | 34 (11.3) | 54 (17.9) | 51 (16.9) | 75 (25) |
| Oral CIS | | | | | | | |
| Shafer (1975)[7] | 6 (7.3) | 19 (23.2) | 18 (22) | 5 (6.1) | 9 (11) | 9 (11) | 16 (19.5) |
| **Mucosal Appearance** | | | | | | | |
| Erythroplasia | | | | | | | |
| Shafer and Waldron (1975)[5] | 12 (18.8) | 18 (28.1) | 8 (12.5) | 8 (12.5) | 5 (7.8) | 13 (20.3) | — |
| Leukoplakia | | | | | | | |
| Waldron and Shafer (1975)[3] | 197 (5.9) | 289 (8.6) | 277 (6.8) | 361 (10.7) | 736 (21.9) | 1204 (35.9) | 346 (10.3) |

## HISTOLOGIC MANIFESTATION OF INTRAEPITHELIAL NEOPLASIA

The differentiation of neoplastic and non-neoplastic or "reactive" hyperplasias of the squamous mucosa remains one of the most difficult tasks encountered in head and neck pathology. The most common reaction of squamous mucosa of the UADT to any form of injury is cell proliferation or epithelial hyperplasia. The development of surface keratin is common in all histologic patterns in reaction to injury. When the mucosa has a normal pattern of maturation with little cytologic atypia, a confident diagnosis of benign hyperplasia can be rendered, and this pattern of injury commonly appears as a white patch or leukoplakic change on physical examination. Conversely, when the mucosa is thin or irregular with altered or irregular maturation and prominent cytologic atypia, a diagnosis of severe dysplasia or CIS is in order. Thin mucosa invariably has a red or erythroplastic appearance on physical examination. The major problem for the surgical pathologist is the intermediate mucosal changes of moderate dysplasia in which the alterations are not easily interpreted and the differentiation of neoplastic from reactive hyperplasia is nearly impossible.[9]

Reactive hyperplasia of the squamous mucosa is characterized by epithelial thickening, often with surface keratin production. The basal layer is usually intact and readily identified. Normal maturation of the cells with an orderly matrix of cell distribution is the rule. Cytologic atypia, as defined by nuclear variation in size, staining intensity, and location within the cell, is not present. Mitotic figures are normally found adjacent to the basal layer and never in the upper portion of the epithelium. DNA analysis of epithelium of this type invariably reveals either a diploid or normal DNA content.[10]

Epithelium with changes of severe dysplasia/CIS are of two types. The "classic" type is characterized by the full thickness of the epithelium being replaced by a proliferation of small "basal-like" cells. This is the common histologic type found in severe dysplasia/CIS of the uterine cervix; similar histological counterparts have been found in all squamous mucosa. However, in our experience, this histologic expression of intraepithelial neoplasia is rare and seldom encountered in the UADT mucosa. The "classic" histological appearance of CIS is in association with adjacent invasive carcinomas and is seldom encountered as an isolated finding.

The most common histological form of intraepithelial neoplastic change in our experience is hyperplastic epithelium, usually with prominent keratinization. The keratin is almost always present on the surface, and abnormal expression of keratin production is commonly found in the depths of the epithelium. This is either in the form of single cell keratinization (dyskeratosis) or extracellular keratin pearls.

The abnormal distribution of keratin represents a marker for disordered epithelial maturation.[11] Usually, this distinct maturation abnormality is associated with cytologic alterations that in reality are primarily nuclear changes, since keratin production is the major cytoplasmic feature recognizable at the light microscopic level. The usual nuclear alterations of atypia include increased nuclear size and variable nuclear contour in association with increased nuclear staining; they are all suggestive of aneuploidy or an abnormal increase in DNA content.

In addition, one of the most important clues to disordered (dysplastic) growth patterns is the loss of the orderly nuclear mosaic pattern. Normally, the nuclei are centrally placed within the cell and are equidistant from each adjacent cell's nucleus. In dysplastic epithelium, the number of nuclei per unit area usually increases (decreased nuclear/cytoplasmic ratio), and the equidistant placement or orderly mosaic pattern of the nuclei is lost due to irregular random placement. The nuclei tend to become crowded and commonly overlap — a sign of a marked growth disorder. Usually, the nuclei are pleomorphic in size and shape and hyperchromatic in staining — signs of aneuploidy. However, this is not always the case, and maturation abnormalities can exist with deceptively bland or apparently normal nuclei.

The problem of how to differentiate between intermediate histological patterns of disordered epithelial maturation (i.e., reactive and reversible changes) and irreversible neoplastic transformation remains. DNA analysis is one technique whereby abnormal or aneuploid DNA histograms may represent true intraepithelial neoplastic transformation. The majority of epithelia with aneuploid histograms are classified as severe dysplasia/CIS, and a minority fit into an intermediate or moderate dysplasia group.[10,12,13] These latter patterns can be confused with reactive, reversible epithelial changes, although this appears to be an uncommon problem.

In summary, the benign reversible hyperplasias are relatively easy to identify and are characterized by normal maturation and cytologic features. The marked dysplasias/CIS are also quite distinctive in their appearance and are usually not a diagnostic problem. However, it can be difficult to interpret occasional biopsies from foci with regenerative epithelia adjacent to ulcers or biopsies from post-radiation patients. The intermediate dysplasia group remains a diagnostic problem, and for the most part, the reversible reactive epithelial changes cannot be reproducibly distinguished from the persisting or progressive intraepithelial neoplastic alterations.

## EARLY INVASION WITH CARCINOMA IN SITU

Carcinoma in situ of squamous mucosa of the UADT invariably persists (non-reversible) and commonly progresses to invasive SCC.[14] The diagnosis of invasion is based on the light microscopic observation of penetration of the epithelial basement membrane by neoplastic cells.[15] Confident diagnosis of the earliest observed stages in tumor invasion is often difficult. The biopsy or cord stripping must be done with care by an experienced surgeon, and the proper orientation, embedding, cutting and examination of tissue sections must be performed by an experienced surgical pathologist. In selected instances, various forms of hyperplasia, including extension down submucosal or minor salivary gland ducts, pseudoepitheliomatous hyperplasias, and other bizarre epithelial reactions to injury (e.g., radiation), result in unusual growth patterns that are further confused by scant biopsy and the tangential plane of section.

Proper biopsies with appropriate orientation at embedding and comprehensive clinical histories will circumvent many of the pitfalls involved in the proper diagnosis of early invasive SCC. We continue to use the term early or microinvasive carcinoma and define it as invasive SCC confined to the adjacent submucosa and surrounded by non-neoplastic host stroma in the biopsy.[9,10] Adequate biopsies will, by our definitions, allow a confident diagnosis of early or microinvasion. In biopsies that are small or fragmented, often the only possible interpretation is of invasive cancer and small early carcinomas cannot be diagnosed with any accuracy. We feel that with strict application of our definition of microinvasive carcinoma, cure is imminent from the biopsy or excision. However, there is also the implication that the overlying epithelium has developed advanced intraepithelial neoplastic change (CIS) and additional invasive carcinoma will most likely develop in the immediate area or other portions of the affected (condemned) mucosa. For the most part, we feel that these early carcinomas are indicators of the presence or future development of additional malignant neoplasms. It is this latter characteristic that is the most significant feature of microinvasive neoplasms and that is, for the most part, an incidental finding in adequately sampled and prepared biopsy material.

The distribution of basement membrane in intraepithelial neoplasia including CIS and early or microinvasive carcinoma is quite variable.[15] We have recently completed a study of a variety of intraepithelial changes and invasive carcinomas using antibodies to laminin or type IV collagen, the primary constituents of basement membrane.[16] Unfortunately, our antibodies do not readily recognize formalin-fixed tissue due to the extensive cross-linking associated with aldehyde fixatives. We found that ethanol-fixed tissue was an excellent fixative with good preservation of laminin and type IV collagen antigens. We were able to identify all basement membrane structures in normal tissues, and this allowed a confident observation as to the presence (or absence) of basement membrane and its distribution in the intraepithelial and invading neoplastic tissues.

Basement membrane is readily identifiable in all mild and moderate dysplasias. Only in severe dysplasia/CIS are there discernible changes. In some of the advanced intraepithelial neoplastic changes, the basement membrane becomes attenuated and patchy in distribution.[15,16] This finding would suggest that penetration of basement membrane is not an important step in the development of invasive SCC, as it appears that the basement membrane is not present in intraepithelial changes preceding invasive carcinoma. Likewise, the identification and distribution of invasive SCC is also quite variable. In general, aggregates of invasive neoplasm that are cohesive with some identifiable organization, including large cords of neoplasm with well-defined tumor host stroma interface, usually produce basement membrane. In contrast, neoplastic cells that invade as single cells or small irregular cords seldom contain identifiable basement membrane separating the small aggregates of tumor from adjacent host stroma. In this instance, it could be hypothesized that basement membrane is a good marker of tumor differentiation, i.e., well-defined large cords of invading cells surrounded by basement membrane are better differentiated than single cells or small irregular cords of invading cells that seldom contain evidence of basement membrane at the light microscopic level.

The pattern in which invasive SCC infiltrates host stroma appears to be an important prognostic indicator. One of the major goals of an infiltrating neoplasm is to gain access to blood and lymphatic vessels, usually at the capillary or post-capillary venule.[17] It would be difficult to imagine that a cohesive tumor infiltrating in large organized aggregates or cords would be capable of vascular invasion. This does appear to be the case, as vascular permeation is most common in tumors invading as single cells or as small irregular cords of tumor.[18,19] One of the obstacles in the infiltration of blood vessels is penetration of vascular basement membrane.[17] Large cords of SCC with well-developed basement membrane separating tumor from host stroma would be less likely to manufacture the enzymes needed to penetrate the vascular basement membrane. Single cells or small cords of infiltrating tumor cells produce and/or maintain little or no basement membrane and are more likely to be capable of producing and excreting enzymes allowing vascular invasion.

## SUMMARY

The histological identification of events involved in the development and progression of squamous cell carcinoma of the UADT are slowly being defined. The definition of intraepithelial neoplastic change (dysplasia) has provided some insight into the natural history of SCC in this region. More specifically, the correlation of histologic alterations of dysplasia with the mucosal changes of leukoplakia and erythroplasia has been a major advanced in the identification of both "at risk" patient groups and the identification of individuals with multiple SCC arising from "condemned" UADT mucosa.

The identification of early or microcarcinoma has been made possible by adequate biopsy technique in conjunction with proper handling of the specimen. The development of early microinvasive carcinomas from overlying CIS has helped to better define the latter. While the treatment of intraepithelial neoplasia is controversial, it is readily treated by excision whenever focal in distribution. The application of radiotherapy to mucosal neoplasia is quite controversial, although intraepithelial neoplasia of a severe type (e.g., CIS) appears to be more radiosensitive than lesser degrees of dysplasia.[20] Once early or microinvasive SCC has developed, it is painfully clear that the overlying epithelium has reached the level of CIS regardless of histologic interpretation.

The progression to invasive cancer appears to occur in a stepwise, but unpredictable, time sequence. The presence and distribution of basement membrane was hypothesized as a potential indicator of early or microinvasion. However, subsequent study reveals that the distribution of basement membrane in both intraepithelial and invasive carcinoma is more an indicator of tumor differentiation than of tumor progression. The pattern of basement membrane distribution confirms the observation that the pattern of tumor invasion is an important indicator of tumor grade or differentiation. Squamous cell carcinomas invading with cohesive organized broad tumor fronts are better differentiated than neoplasms infiltrating as single cells or as small irregular cords. The latter appear to be more capable of penetration of both blood and lymphatic vascular structures.

## REFERENCES

1. Cann CI, Fried MP, Rothman KJ: Epidemiology of squamous cell cancer of the head and neck. Otolaryngol Clin North Am 1985;18:1–22.
2. Crissman JD: Laryngeal keratosis and subsequent carcinoma. Head Neck Surg 1979;1:386–391.
3. Waldron CA, Shafer WG: Leukoplakia revisited. A clinicopathologic study of 3256 oral leukoplakias. Cancer 1975;36:1386–1392.
4. Silverman S, Gorsky M, Lozada F: Oral leukoplakia and malignant transformation. Cancer 1984;53:563–568.
5. Shafer WG, Waldron CA: Erythroplakia of the oral cavity. Cancer 1975;36:1021–1028.
6. Mashberg A: Erythroplasia: The earliest sign of asymptomatic oral cancer. J Am Dent Assoc 1978;96:615–620.

7. Shafer WG: Oral carcinoma in-situ. Oral Surg 1975;39:227–238.
8. Mincer H, Coleman SA, Hopkins KP: Observations on the clinical characteristics of oral lesions showing histologic epithelial dysplasia. Oral Surg 1972;33:389–392.
9. Crissman JD: Histopathologic diagnosis of early cancer. Head Neck Cancer 1985;1:134–140.
10. Crissman JD, Fu YS: Intraepithelial neoplasia (CIS) of the larynx. A clinicopathologic study of six cases with DNA analysis. Arch Otolaryngol 1986;112:522–528.
11. Crissman JD: Laryngeal keratosis preceding laryngeal carcinoma. Arch Otolaryngol 1982;108:445–448.
12. Bocking A, Auffermann W, Vogel H, et al: Diagnosis and grading of malignancy in squamous epithelial lesions of the larynx with DNA cytophotometry. Cancer 1985;56:1600–1604.
13. Doseva D, Christov K, Kristeva K: DNA content in reactive hyperplasia, precancerosis, and carcinomas of the oral cavity. A cytophotometric study. Acta Histochem 1984;75:113–119.
14. Hellquist H, Lundgren J, Olofsson J: Hyperplasia, keratosis, dysplasia and carcinoma in-situ of the vocal cords—a follow-up study. Clin Otolaryngol 1982;7:11–27.
15. Bosman FT, Havenith M, Cleutjens JPM: Basement membranes in cancer. Ultrastruct Pathol 1985;8:291–304.
16. Sakr WA, Zarbo RJ, Jacobs JR, Crissman JD: Distribution of basement membrane in squamous cell carcinoma of the head and neck. Am J Surg Pathol. (in press).
17. Liotta LA, Rao CN, Barsky SH: Tumor invasion and the extracellular matrix. Lab Invest 1983;49:636–649.
18. Crissman JD, Liu WY, Gluckman JL, Cummings G: Prognostic value of histopathologic parameters in squamous cell carcinoma of the oropharynx. Cancer 1984;54:2995–3001.
19. Yamamoto E, Kohama G, Sunakawa H, Iwai M, Hiratsuka H: Mode of invasion, bleomycin sensitivity and clinical course in squamous cell carcinoma of the oral cavity. Cancer 1983;51:2175–2180.
20. Elman AJ, Goodman M, Wang CC, et al: In-situ carcinoma of the vocal cords. Cancer 1979;43:2422–2428.

# CHAPTER 5

# Problems in Staging: Prospects for Future Improvement

*John R. Jacobs, MD and Muhyi Al-Sarraf, MD*

It is generally agreed that the current staging system, while usable, is in need of improvement. The TNM system is based upon the concept that the larger the primary tumor and the increasing extent of lymph node involvement, the worse the ultimate prognosis. Under the current system, the staging information utilized is the clinical examination. The closer the clinical examination reflects the actual tumor extension, the higher the accuracy of the staging system relative to prognosis. Clearly, given the shortcomings of the clinical examination, it is unlikely that the known tumor heterogeneity can be encompassed under such a schema.

## BACKGROUND

The goals of an ideal staging system are multiple. It should provide prognostic information. This is important not only in treatment planning, but also in facilitating the design of clinical trials. Clearly, an essential element of any prospective randomized trial is the ability to select groups of patients with equivalent prognoses. The staging system should also act as a vocabulary between clinicians. This facilitates the interchange of information and reporting of results between colleagues. Finally, the ideal staging system should be easy to utilize and update.

The current TNM staging system has been in active use with refinements for better than 30 years.[1] During that time period, it has become apparent that there are multiple shortcomings to this system relative to an ideal one. Many of the problems appear to be inherent in the utilization of clinical examination as the basis of the staging system. They revolve around

**66**

problems of interobserver reliability variation, determination of fixation, the inability to classify accurately very large tumors, either in the primary site or neck, i.e., T3 and N3, and problems in accurately defining tumor extension in anatomical areas that resist clinical examination, such as paranasal sinuses. For example, the current staging system does not allow for differentiation between superficial and invasive carcinoma. Kaplan et al.,[2] reported on prognostic factors relative to survival in patients with Stage II glottic carcinoma. These patients were treated with surgery and/or radiotherapy. They found statistically different five year actual survival in patients with normal cord mobility versus hypomobility. Similar findings were reported by Platz et al.,[3] in analysis of patients with carcinoma of the oral cavity. What, therefore, are new techniques or alternative parameters that can be utilized to augment the clinical examiner in development of an improved staging system?

## ALTERNATIVE PARAMETERS
### Radiographic

There have been consistent improvements in the imaging sciences since the first radiograph was developed. Over the recent past few years, the potential of computer tomography (CT) has been explored. The level of resolution has improved dramatically with each new generation of CT scanner. The CT scanner has been found to be useful in the determination of cartilage invasion, invasion of paralaryngeal soft tissues, and intracranial extension. Currently on the horizon is the nuclear magnetic resonance (NMR) machine. The capability and clinical role of NMR have yet to be delineated. As with CT, it is expected that NMR will be of value in selected cases only. The current shortcomings of radiographic parameters is that it is only of value if the problem is visualized. There are a multitude of clinical and current technical problems that prevent visualization of the problem in each individual case. The incorporation of radiographic imaging, therefore, must at best be considered a supplement to the clinical examination.

### Pathologic Parameters

Rapidis et al.,[4] have developed a staging system for oral cavity carcinoma that incorporated pathologic characteristics along with the traditional categories. According to Wittes,[5] the resulting system has not shown to be superior to the current TNM system. Further work in the area has lead to interest in the development of new parameters that might improve upon the efforts of Rapidis et al.. Table 5.1 lists some of the items of interest. It is possible that,

**TABLE 5.1** Additional Pathologic Parameters

Vascular Invasion
Perineural Invasion
DNA Analysis
Extracapsular Tumor Spread
Basement Membrane Integrity

as these parameters are developed, an improvement in staging capability will result.

## Immune Parameters

Over the past 10 years, tremendous improvement has been made in our understanding of how the immune system works. As a result of these efforts, the production of monoclonal antibodies is now possible. This technique has clinical potential in three areas: in vitro tissue analysis, serological analysis, and in vivo radioimaging. Whether or not the promise of this technique will be fulfilled has yet to be determined. If successful, however, this might be able to significantly alter the current staging system parameters' selection.

## CONCLUSIONS

The TNM System has to be regarded as very successful despite its limitations. It does meet many of the goals of the ideal staging system. Unfortunately, the inability to account of the known tumor heterogeneity puts absolute limits on the system as currently formulated. A multivariate analysis of the TNM System by Jacobs et al.[6] suggests that any improvement of the system would have to come from the addition of new variables rather than reclassification of current ones. Hopefully, efforts in that direction will be successful in the near future. The prognostic signs are encouraging.

## REFERENCES

1. Sisson G, Pelzer H: Staging system by site: problems in refinement. Otolaryngol Clin N Am 1985;18:3:397–402.

2. Kaplan MJ, Johns ME, McLean WC, et al: Stage II glottic carcinoma: prognostic factors and management. Laryngoscope 1983;93:725–728.
3. Platz H, Fries F, Hudec J, et al: Carcinomas of the oral cavity: analysis of various pretherapeutic classifications. Head Neck Surg 1982;5:93–107.
4. Rapidis A, Langdon J, Patel M et al: STNMP: a new system for the clinico-pathological classification and identification of intraoral carcinomata. Cancer 1977;39:204.
5. Wittes R: Current problems in clinical staging, in Wittes, R: Head and Neck Cancer. New York: John Wiley and Sons, 1985. pp 37–51.
6. Jacobs J, Spitznagel E, Sessions D: Staging parameters for cancers of the head and neck: a multifactorial analysis. Laryngoscope 1985;95:1378–1381.

# CHAPTER 6

# Problems with the Multiple Primary: Role of Endoscopy

*Arthur W. Weaver, MD*

Squamous cell cancer of the head and neck is best understood as a local manifestation of a systemic disorder that affects all of the mucous membranes of the upper aerodigestive tract. The mucous membrane of the oral cavity, pharynx, larynx, esophagus, and bronchus is a communal spawning ground for multifocal squamous cell cancer. It is no longer reasonable to conceive of these cancers as a localized phenomenon of disordered cells. It is now painfully evident that all of the surface mucosal cells of the upper digestive tract are being modified by often identifiable carcinogens, and a malignant tumor may likely appear in any area of the mucosa exposed to these irritants.

Dentists, oral surgeons, head and neck surgeons, and thoracic surgeons are likely to have specific and limited geographical interests in malignancies of this region. Unfortunately, the principle carcinogens suffer no such jurisdictional boundaries, and many surgeons have been embarrassed to discover a second unanticipated tumor while focusing attention on an already evident cancer present in their area of special emphasis.

The transformation from benign, normal-appearing mucous membrane to malignant, rapidly invasive tumor occurs only after long term insult. The basic pathophysiologic processes that makes one susceptible to these carcinogens is not known. Several life style factors, however, have been demonstrated that play an important role in transformation of these cells.

Tobacco use seems to be primarily responsible in most of these tumors. Drs. Wynder and Graham first demonstrated the ability of cigarette smoke extract to produce squamous cell cancer in the skin of animals in areas where tobacco smoke extract is applied.[1] The ability of tobacco to produce squamous cell carcinoma has since been carefully demonstrated by many investigators.

Dr. Joseph S. Incze of the Veterans Administration Medical Center in Boston has published fascinating evidence of these induced cellular changes.[2] He has shown that biopsy specimens of grossly and histologically normal mucous membrane taken from patients with known head and neck cancer and from heavy smokers without cancer will demonstrate similar electron microscopic mucosal alterations. He has identified several tobacco-induced gradations of cellular change from normal to frankly malignant. Happily, he has also demonstrated that many of these changes are reversible in individuals who quit smoking. It seems appropriate, then, to view the mucosa of the heavy smoker and/or drinker as being in some stage of alteration on the road to malignancy.

While head and neck cancer accounts for approximately only 5% of all malignancies in the North American continent, it is far more significant from a worldwide epidemiological viewpoint.

In Bombay, India for instance, head and neck cancer accounts for more than 50% of all malignancies. The betel quid, prominently used throughout southern Asia, appears to be the primary etiological agent responsible for the preponderence of head and neck cancer in this region. It appears that the tobacco and lime used in the betel quid are responsible for this potent carcinogenicity.

In the western world, tobacco in all its forms has been implicated as a promoter of carcinoma in the head and neck area. Ingestion of alcoholic beverages appears to greatly potentiate the carcinogenic effect of the tobacco. The effect of alcohol appears to be multiplicative rather than additive. The heavy smoker will have at least a five times greater risk of developing one of these diseases than the general population. A person who drinks heavily as well as smokes heavily will carry a 22-fold risk of developing one of these tumors.

Dr. Condit Moore, in analyzing the sites of origin for cancer in the oral cavity, has pointed out that the floor of the mouth, retromolar trigone, the tonsillar fauces, and lateral tongue, are the sites for most frequent occurrence.[3]

We have observed that these sites, along with the larynx, pharynx, hypopharynx, and esophagus, appear to be the usual sites associated with malignant transformation in those of our patients who smoke cigarettes and drink significant amounts of alcohol. Those tumors associated with the use of smokeless tobacco, however, are nearly always located on the mucous membranes where the tobacco is held. The buccal mucosa, floor of the mouth, and alveolar ridges are the prominent sites of tumor formation in persons using chewing tobacco. The same areas are frequently affected by betel quid. It is not unusual to see squamous cell carcinoma developing on the inner surface of the lip among those who use this site to deposit their snuff.

Several years ago, we suggested that mouthwash might have a possible etiological role in the development of oral squamous cell cancer in the few persons who compulsively use these products. Various mouthwashes have an alcohol content varying from 15–28%. Several other substances, including cetylpyridinium chloride, thymol, eucalyptol, phenol, methylsalicylate and boric acid are frequent constituents. The irritating nature of mouthwash has been reported by Kowitz and others.[4] He has shown that an occurrence of epithelial peeling, mucosal ulceration, gingivitis, and petchia will be present in as many as 25% of normal individuals who use 20 milliliters of full-strength mouthwash for five second intervals twice daily throughout a two week period. These signs of acute inflammation completely disappeared when use of the mouthwash was discontinued.

There are a few individuals who neither smoke nor use alcoholic beverages who do develop squamous cell cancer. Such tumors usually occur in older women and are most frequently found in the oral cavity. We have found that most of these patients are compulsive mouthwash users who are afraid of offending others with their breath. We believe that long-term use of undiluted mouthwash may serve as a carcinogenic stimulus for some susceptible individuals. When we analyzed 200 consecutive patients with squamous cell cancer from our head and neck service, we found that 94% of them used beverage alcohol and tobacco regularly. There were 11 patients, however, without a history of beverage alcohol and tobacco use, who used mouthwash compulsively. When we included mouthwash as a possible etiological agent, we found only 1% of our patients for whom no known etiological factors were evident.[5]

## SCREENING TECHNIQUES FOR HEAD AND NECK CANCER

Careful and meticulous examination is necessary to identify premalignant changes or early malignancies of the upper aerodigestive tract, as these are usually asymptomatic. Early cancer and even carcinoma in situ are recognizable on gross examination; these changes, however, may be very subtle. The experienced examiner has a significant advantage in the gross diagnosis of these early changes. Physicians, as a group, do poorly when it comes to examination of the oral cavity. We might well learn from dental colleagues who emphasize a routine careful oral examination for cancer. This is particularly important in patients over 40 years of age who have a history of tobacco or alcohol use.

Appropriate examination of the oral cavity requires a relaxed patient, a good source of light, and appropriate equipment. Tongue blades, gauze, and laryngeal and nasopharyngeal mirrors are the other necessities for a routine examination of the head and neck area. The examination begins with a careful observation of the patient's face and neck for any possible asymmetry or identifyable lesions. Palpation of the neck may discover nodules within the thyroid or enlarged neck nodes. The oral cavity, pharynx, and hypopharynx should be examined systematically and thoroughly to include all the invisible mucous membranes. Palpation of any suspicious lesions within these areas may confirm visual conjectures. It is particularly important to palpate the posterior tongue, as this area is difficult to visualize. The laryngeal and nasopharyngeal mirrors should be used to examine the base of the tongue, larynx, hypopharynx, and nasopharynx.

Early carcinomas of the mucous membrane may present as white patches (leukoplakia), red patches (erythroplakia), and more frequently, as mixed red and white patches (erythro-leukoplakia). Carcinoma in situ frequently gives this variegated appearance. When the area is wiped with a gauze or a tongue blade, small petechial hemorrhages will occur from this minor trauma.

More advanced tumors will present as ulcerated lesions or nodular masses within the oral cavity. Larger tumors will frequently have considerably more disease submucosally than that which presents on the surface. In these situations, the lesion is often easier palpated than seen.

## AUXILIARY EXAMINATION TECHNIQUES

Various additions to the physical examination have been suggested as being of value for diagnosing early malignancies of the head and neck area. The magnification associated with the flexible bronchoscope or esophagoscope can be used with particular benefit for observing lesions around the larynx and hypopharynx. This is particularly beneficial in individuals who are difficult to observe indirectly or with rigid equipment.

Toluidine blue application to suspected areas of cancer will stain the area of the carcinoma and any adjacent carcinoma in situ. This dye will not stain normal mucosa, but will, however, color inflammatory benign lesions and leukoplakias. This technique is of more value for the physician who sees occasional cases of head and neck cancer than for more experienced examiners. The experienced examiner can identify the subtle changes seen with mucosal dysplasia and carcinoma in situ that would likely be missed by the less experienced professional. Exfoliative cytology has been used for diagnosis of cancer of the oral cavity and pharynx. Malignant cells are shed from carcinoma in situ and invasive cancer. There are, however, false positive and false negative results with this technique, and it is necessary to identify the suspect area in order to obtain good biopsies.

A high index of suspicion is the physician's best aid in the diagnosis of early head and neck cancer. The patient who uses a significant amount of alcohol and tobacco is a prime suspect, and any patient who has a current or previous diagnosis of squamous cell head and neck cancer of the upper aerodigestive tract remains suspect until he has had a complete lifestyle change for several years.

## TRIPLE ENDOSCOPY

We began in October, 1976 to do laryngoscopy, flexible esophagoscopy, and bronchoscopy on all patients admitted to our unit with suspected head and neck cancer. We adopted this examination technique after having been deceived several times by treating small, readily evident cancers only to discover we had missed other cancers of the bronchus, esophagus, or hypopharynx that obviously had been incipient or present at the time of our initial examination. We have now used this examination technique on more than 800 patients. In more than 10% of these patients, multiple synchronous carcinomas were identified. Many of these patients had more than two sites involved, some as many as five. In more than 5% of the cases, the second primary carcinoma was discovered in the esophagus or bronchus. Several patients each year have carcinoma identified as originating in the lung, esophagus, and head and neck area, all present at the same time.

Discovery of these additional lesions has in many cases completely changed our therapeutic approach to tumor management. In some cases, the lesion discovered at endoscopy carries a significantly greater prognostic implication for the patient than the lesion for which the endoscopy was performed. In other cases, small, early carcinomas have been found, particularly in the bronchus or esophagus, that could be treated with laser therapy or radiotherapy to preserve these organs. Indeed, we have diagnosed carcinoma in situ in several lesions found within the bronchus and the esophagus.

We generally perform our endoscopic examinations under local anesthesia with a premedication administered one hour prior to endoscopy. The recommended preoperative sedation for the well-developed, well-nourished male consists of 100 mg of pentobarbital sodium (Nembutol), 100 mg of meperidine (Demerol) and 0.6 mg of atropine. These doses are adjusted downward according to the age and general condition of the patients. Intravenous sedation has been a necessary supplement in only a few patients.

The internal branch of the superior laryngeal nerve is blocked bilaterally by 1% lidocaine with adrenalin, administered transcutaneously. The glossopharyngeal plexus is similarly anesthetized by injecting the glossopharyngeal plexus behind the posterior tonsillar pillar using an angulated tonsil needle. Tracheal anesthesia is obtained using 4 – 5 cc of 4% lidocaine topical anesthesia injected transtracheally. Jafek and Bauknight et al.[6] published a good description of the technique for giving superior laryngeal and glossopharyngeal blocks.

Laryngoscopy is performed using a Jako and/or Jackson anterior commisure scope. The bronchoscopy and esophagoscopy are accomplished using flexible fiberoptic equipment. This equipment gives a far superior view and produces much less discomfort to the patient than rigid endoscopes.

Metachronous carcinomas will occur in patients with previous head and neck cancer at the rate of approximately 7% a year for those individuals who do not change their lifestyle. There is unquestionably a marked reduction in metachronous carcinomas in those individuals who totally quit smoking and drinking. In fact, new cancers of this area are unlikely in individuals who have not been irradiated and have given up their tobacco and alcohol habits for a period of greater than 5 years. Most of the long term suvivors (greater than 10 years) in our clinic have given up both smoking and use of alcholic beverages.

The cost benefit ratio of doing a triple endoscopy on all head and neck cancer patients has been questioned. In the Veteran's Hospital setting where I do most of my work, the additional expense would be minimal. Most of these patients would necessarily come for laryngoscopy and biopsy of the lesion. The addition of esophagoscopy and bronchoscopy is a matter only of setting up the instruments and an additional 15 to 20 minutes of operating room time. There is an added educational benefit in that many of our residents can become proficient in flexible esophagoscopy and bronchoscopy while examining these patients. Most insurance companies deeply discount second and third procedures done in the same operating room setting, so the triple endoscopy may be accomplished at the same setting without the surgeon realizing excessive professional fee benefits. In order to truly determine an accurate cost benefit ratio from this examination, it would be necessary to demonstrate that the ultimate salvage rate varied from that for patients who did not have these procedures done. We do not have and are unlikely to obtain such figures.

We would hesitate now to go back to the era of unpleasant surprises that we had before we instituted this rather thorough examination. In over 800 examinations, we have had no perforations of the esophagus or pharynx.

There have been a few patients who had a tracheostomy done following endoscopy either because of compromised airway during the procedure or anticipated compromised airway. Most of the patients have felt that the examination was acceptable and have submitted to multiple examinations when that has been recommended.

## FOLLOW UP FOR HEAD AND NECK CANCER PATIENTS

The patient who has been treated for head and neck cancer is at significant risk for recurrent disease at the primary site or the neck. He must also be watched for a metachronous primary in the head and neck area, lung, or esophagus. As our treatment protocols have improved, we have seen more and more patients with second primary lesions and/or distant metastasis as the ultimate cause of death. Our routine follow-up of patients includes a thorough examination of the head and neck area with indirect laryngoscopy once each month for the first year, every 2 months during the second year, and every 3 months through the fifth year post-treatment. Every patient with a new or recurrent lesion is reendoscoped by triple endoscopy. So also are patients with new symptoms of dysphagia, chronic soreness, or hoarseness, where a tumor is not visualized by indirect examination.

Since we have instituted triple endoscopy for our patients, we are no longer often surprised by a carcinoma of the esophagus or new primaries of the oral cavity or laryngopharynx during the early follow-up period. Carcinoma of the bronchus, however, still is a cause of occasional and sometimes early failure, since the tracheobronchial tree is not entirely visualized even by flexible endoscopy. In fact, a carcinoma of the lung is the second most common reason for treatment failure in our patients. Careful and meticulous follow-up has, however, permitted long term survival for many of our patients who have experienced multiple primary disease.

We have a few surviving patients who have had head and neck cancer associated with cancer of the lung or esophagus, and several patients who have had long–term survival in spite of multiple head and neck primaries. We had one patient who may have set a world's record with 30 distinct and separate head and neck primary lesions diagnosed over an 11 year period. We have another patient who has had eight separate head and neck cancers over a 20-year period, including cancer of the larynx, pharynx, piriform sinus, plus several cancers of the mouth and tongue. He still has all of his teeth, and his larynx and tongue are basically intact. Most of these lesions were diagnosed at a very early stage and treated by cryotherapy. For head and neck cancer, eternal vigilance must be a life long commitment for both the treating professional and the patient.

# REFERENCES

1. Wynder EL, Graham EA, Kroniger AB: Experiments for production of carcinoma with cigarette tar. Cancer Res 1953;13:855–864.
2. Incze J, Vaughan CW, Lui P, et al: Malignant changes in normal appearing epithelium in patients with squamous cell carcinoma of the upper aerodigestive tract. Am J Surg 1982;144:401–405.
3. Moore C, Catlin D: Anatomic origins of oral cancer. Am J Surg 1967;114:510–513.
4. Kowitz GM, Lucatorto FM, Cherrick HM: Effects of mouthwashes on the oral soft tissues. J Oral Med 1976;31:47–50.
5. Weaver A, Fleming SM, Smith DB: Mouthwash and oral cancer: Carcinogen or coincidence? J Oral Surg 1979;37:250–253.
6. Jafek BW, Bauknight RS, Calcaterra TC: Percutaneous anesthesia for endoscopy. Arch Surg 1972;104:658–661.

# CHAPTER 7

# The Pathologist's Role in Diagnosis and Staging of Upper Aerodigestive Tract Carcinoma

*Richard J. Zarbo, MD, DMD and*
*John D. Crissman, MD*

## CONFIRMATION OF MALIGNANCY AND CELL TYPE

One of the major roles of the pathologist is the diagnosis of malignancy, and, specifically, the determination of cell type. The latter is of utmost importance since modern therapeutic strategies are often directed by cell type. Neoplasms derived from the squamous epithelium greatly outnumber malignancies derived from the hard and soft tissues in the head and neck region, and in most instances, the histologic diagnosis of carcinoma is not difficult. However, undifferentiated carcinoma of the large or small cell type in the head and neck region can be simulated histologically by a number of malignant neoplasms, usually large cell lymphoma and less commonly malignant melanoma, undifferentiated sarcoma, or esthesioneuroblastoma. A diagnosis of undifferentiated malignancy is insufficient for the clinician, since effective therapies can be directed against undifferentiated carcinoma (lymphoepithelioma) and toward large cell lymphoma. Undifferentiated large or small cell malignancies at the light microscopic level often require special diagnostic techniques to identify the precise cell of origin. Electron microscopy can be of great value in distinguishing carcinoma from small or large cell lymphoma and other undifferentiated malignancies by resolving the ultrastructure of specific cellular organelles and intercellular attachments indicative of an epithelial malignancy.[1,2] Poorly differentiated carcinomas can be further subclassified by ultrastructural features, e.g., poorly differentiated adenocarcinoma with glandular lumens, terminal junction complexes, and the presence of basement membrane, or squamous cell carcinoma with desmosome attachments and cytoplasmic tonofilament bundles representing aggregated keratin intermediate filaments. The small cell malignancies of the head and neck region — neuroendocrine carcinoma, esthesioneuroblastoma, Merkel cell carcinoma, rhabdomyosarcoma and Ewing's sarcoma — also display distinctive electron-optic features, as do the histologically similar appearing melanoma, angiosarcoma, and paraganglioma that are ennumerated in Table 7.1. Drawbacks of the use of electron microscopy include: the requirement that tissue be submitted fresh to Pathology for proper EM fixation at the time of the biopsy; the sampling artifact inherent to the examination of small pieces of tissue; and the time delay associated with this relatively time-consuming and expensive technique.

More recently, immunohistochemical techniques (commonly utilizing the immunoperoxidase method) are being used to discern cellular antigens in routinely processed, paraffin embedded, or fresh frozen tissues.[3] This recent advance in diagnostic surgical pathology can make use of routinely processed biopsy specimens, and because of the numerous diagnostic monoclonal antibodies available, is rapidly developing into the most popular method for identification of neoplasms. Many of the antigens indicative of epithelial, mesenchymal, or lymphoreticular differentiation can be demonstrated in fixed, paraffin embedded tissues. At present, many of the lymphoid cell surface differentiation antigens and cell surface immunoglobulins cannot be demonstrated in fixed tissues, as the antigens do not survive tissue fixation. For this reason, proper immunophenotyping of lymphoreticular proliferation still requires the use of snap frozen tissues. Therefore, pathologists familiar with these techniques who encounter an undifferentiated malignancy at the time of frozen section consultation will preserve a portion of the biopsy in the frozen state in order to exclude or confirm a diagnosis of lymphoma.

The most sensitive immunocytochemical means of diagnosing an epithelial malignancy is the detection, in fixed and paraffin embedded tissues, of one of the 19 known cytoplasmic intermediate filaments of the cytokeratin family.[4] The cytoskeletal keratin filaments detected in a primary malignancy of the head and neck are very specific for the diagnosis of carcinoma, and exclude from the diagnosis similar appearing lymphomas, melanomas, or sarcomas.[5] At this time, immunohistochemical distinction of poorly differentiated squamous cell carcinoma from adenocarcinoma is not possible. Detection of other cytoplasmic intermediate filament classes, such as the muscle filament desmin, have been used in subtyping sarcomas like rhabdo-

**TABLE 7.1** Undifferentiated Malignant Neoplasm of the Head and Neck

| | Antigens | | | | | | | | | | | | Electron Microscopy |
|---|---|---|---|---|---|---|---|---|---|---|---|---|---|
| | cytokeratin | vimentin | desmin | neurofilament | S-100 protein | premelanosome | chromogranin | Ulex europaeus Factor VIII | Leukocyte Common Ag | NSE | myoglobin | Immunoglobulin (Surface) | |
| Lymphoma | | +[1] | | | | | | | +/0[4] | | | +[3] | absence of specific features; variable organelles |
| Undifferentiated carcinoma (squamous and glandular) | + | | | +[2] | | | +[2] | | | +[2] | | | filopodia, desmosomes or primitive junction complexes, occasional tonofilaments or intracellular lumen |
| Merkel cell carcinoma | +[5] | | | +[6] | | | + | | | + | | | dense core granules just beneath plasmalemma, balls of paranuclear intermediate filaments |
| Melanoma | | + | | | + | + | | | | + | | | premelanosomes and melanosomes |

| | | | | | | | EM features |
|---|---|---|---|---|---|---|---|
| Esthesioneuroblastoma | | + | + | + | + | | dense core granules, neurites with microtubules, cell junctions neurofilaments |
| Rhabdomyosarcoma | + | | +[7] | | | +/o | parallel array of myofilaments, Z bands, glycogen, basal lamina cell processes, primitive junctions |
| Angiosarcoma | + | + | + | +/o | | | Weibel-Palade body, basal lamina pinocytosis, tight junctions, intermediate filaments |
| Ewing's sarcoma | + | | | | | | pools of glycogen, sparse organelles, rare primitive junctions |
| Paraganglioma | | + | +[8] | + | + | | dense core granules (eccentric norepinephrine) desmosomes, golgi; Sustentacular cells |

1. especially large cells; 2. some small cell anaplastic carcinomas; 3. frozen tissue required; 4. immunoblastic and lymphoblastic lymphomas often negative; 5. paranuclear blobs; 6. balls of intermediate filaments on EM; 7. sustentacular-Schwann cells; 8. sustentacular cells only.

myosarcoma. Use of antibodies directed against leukocyte common antigen and monoclonal antibodies directed against premelanosome granules are proving to be an effective, sensitive, and specific means of detecting lymphomas and amelanotic melanomas, respectively. Esthesioneuroblastomas also display characteristic immunologically detectable antigens that enable these tumors to be distinguished from other small cell malignant neoplasms of the region. By immunological probing of undifferentiated neoplasms for numerous antigens, immunoprofiles can be developed to exact a specific tissue and cell oriented diagnosis of many histologically similar appearing tumors (Table 7.1). Incorporation of these immunologic techniques into the surgical pathology diagnostic arena is the most important advance in diagnostic pathology since the advent of the electron microscope. Electron microscopy still remains a useful and complementary technique, however, immunocytochemical diagnosis is less expensive, less time consuming, and can be performed on routinely fixed and processed biopsies. Given the numerous available monoclonal antibodies directed to cell surface antigens, cytoplasmic antigens, and secretory products, this technique may prove to be more helpful in probing the many facets of unusual neoplasms and malignant tumors that are difficult to classify by conventional techniques.

## TUMOR GRADE

Another major contribution by the pathologist is the evaluation of the histologic characteristics of a neoplasm which relate to the biologic behavior of the tumor. This is known as tumor grading. Tumor grading takes into account a number of histologic and cytologic observations of the neoplasm and the relationship of the tumor to the host stroma. Histologic grading has classically been determined by the degree of differentiation of the malignant neoplasm. The concept of tumor cell grading based on the proportion of the tumor that resembles the normal tissue of origin was first developed by Broders in the 1920's.[6] His four-part grading scale has since been simplified into three grades of poorly, moderately and well differentiated neoplasms by present-day pathologists. For carcinomas, these grades are based primarily on the degree of keratinization, and, to a lesser extent, on nuclear features (nuclear grade) and the number of mitoses. In general, tumors with a high degree of differentiation display prominent keratin production and minor degrees of cytologic atypia. Conversely, poorly differentiated tumors display little evidence of keratin production and marked cellular pleomorphism. Tumors with intermediate features are designated as moderately differentiated. The continued basis for determining the histologic grade of numerous types of neoplasms has been its value in predicting biologic behavior. In general, well-differentiated neoplasms grow in a slow, predictible fashion, and poorly differentiated neoplasms follow a more aggressive course with a higher frequency of early and distant metastasis. However, the value of histologic differentiation in predicting the biologic behavior of squamous cell carcinomas of the upper aerodigestive tract has been disappointing partly because the majority of tumors are in the intermediate group. Isolated correlations with histologic grade and metastatic rate and local recurrence have been observed. Tumor grade does not appear to correlate well with tumor size, and therefore appears to have limited prognostic value in predicting biologic behavior when compared to the combined clinical staging parameters of tumor size and regional lymph node metastasis.

An additional parameter relating to the tumor host-interface is the pattern or mode of stromal invasion. Pattern of invasion reflects tumor organization and cohesion. Tumors with large pushing borders and broad cords of cells have a well defined tumor-stromal interface as demonstrated by very well differentiated carcinomas (Fig. 7.1). Moderately differentiated tumors, however, have thin, irregular less well formed invasive cords of cells. At the far end of the spectrum are poorly differentiated tumors that invade as small aggregates and individual cells in the host stroma (Fig. 7.2). This latter pattern of invasion is almost always a correlate of poorly differentiated

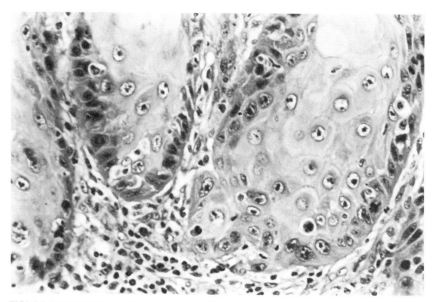

**FIGURE 7.1** Well differentiated squamous cell carcinoma invading as broad cords of cells with well-defined tumorstromal interface (hematoxylin and eosin, ×400).

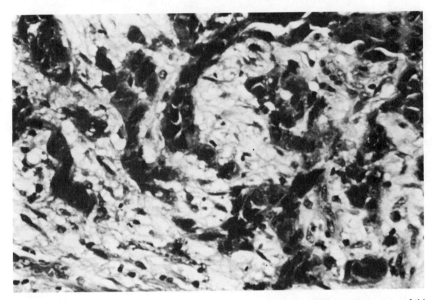

**FIGURE 7.2** Small cell aggregates and individual cells characterize the invasion pattern of this poorly differentiated squamous cell carcinoma (hematoxylin and eosin, X400).

neoplasms and appear to be associated with a greater propensity for the penetration and invasion of blood and lymph-vascular structures.[7] The statistical value of the invasive pattern of squamous cell carcinomas of the head and neck achieves significance in predicting regional lymph node metastasis that is of the same degree of significance as the predictive value of tumor grade for regional lymph node metastasis.[7,8,9] In biopsies of smaller tumors, the pattern of invasion will likely be a significant pathologic finding, as it appears to correlate with other prognostic indicators, i.e., degree of differentiation, and vascular and perineural invasion. In the biopsy evaluation of large tumor masses, however, heterogeneous histologic patterns may be present and this sampling error may detract from the assessment of pattern of invasion in initial biopsies. Other histologic parameters that affect prognosis include the identification of vascular invasion in initial biopsies of head and neck carcinomas. The finding of vascular invasion is associated with regional lymph node metastasis, and is therefore an important predictor of regional metastasis.[10] Another important histologic observation is the finding of carcinoma invading nerves and perineural spaces. This is associated with a poor prognosis and lymph node metastasis as documented for carcinomas of the larynx,[8] the lip,[11] and the oral tongue.[12] The depth of submucosal and soft tissue invasion of carcinomas of the floor of the mouth has been shown to be a significant independent predictor of local recurrence and regional lymph node metastases for T2 tumors of this region.[13] The TNM classification of glottic tumors indirectly assesses depth of invasion by assigning higher T stages to cases with impaired vocal cord mobility or fixation that is usually due to arytenoid muscle infiltration by tumor.[14]

## PATHOLOGIC STAGE

The major objective in the histopathologic evaluation of malignant neoplasms is the pathologist's assessment of predicted biologic behavior of the tumor as reflected in pathologic staging. Pathologic staging relates to the biological progession of the cancer by taking into account tumor size and regional lymph node involvement. This represents pathologic verification of the pretherapeutic clinical parameters in the TNM staging system.[15] In addition, observations regarding tumor relationship to contiguous anatomic structures, assessment of completeness of primary excision, and the evaluation of histologic features such as extranodal tumor spread and location of regional lymph node metastases, are prognostic predictors of subsequent tumor recurrence and metastasis.

In general, larger tumors at presentation correlate with an increased frequency of metastasis. Observations of this nature are reflected in the TNM system of stage groups. In the TNM system, some head and neck sites incorporate the extent of distribution of the neoplasm as well as size in determining the T-stage.[15] Squamous cell carcinomas of the larynx are well characterized with regards to size and extent of tumor. Glottic tumors have been shown to have a progressively increased frequency of lymph node metastasis among 1.9, 16.7, 25 and 65% of patients with regional metastasis associated with T-stages one through four, respectively.[16] The pathologic examination of the specimen refines the clinical impression of involvement of contiguous anatomic structures and depth of invasion. Again, for the larynx, the anatomic distribution of laryngeal tumors into glottic, infraglottic, supraglottic and transglottic areas correlates with increasing frequency of lymph node metastasis of 0, 19, 33 and 52% respectively.[8]

## MARGINS AND COMPLETENESS OF PRIMARY EXCISION

The pathologic evaluation of the completeness of primary excision is an important prognostic parameter. Tumor free margins in the surgical resection have been shown to be a significant parameter that is predictive of non-recurrence of carcinoma.[17] Despite knowledge of the anatomy of the region, tissue changes with fixation may alter the surgical specimen. Close communication between pathologist and the surgeon is necessary, as well as the use of diagrams and markers with sutures within the tissue, for proper orientation and location of previously sampled frozen section margins. Apparent resection margins, especially in fixed specimens, do not always correspond to the true intraoperative surgical margins, so effective communication between both parties cannot be overly stressed. Study of head and neck carcinomas has demonstrated a significant increase in local recurrence and mortality among patients with tumor in the resection margins when compared to those with tumor free margins.[18] The definition of positive margins may vary, and has included tumor within 0.5 cm of the margin, epithelial atypia, and in situ and invasive carcinoma at the margin. With this broad definition of a positive margin, 71% of patients with positive margins have developed local recurrence ranging from 62.5% with stage I disease to 90% with stage IV disease. In comparison, 31.7% of patients with negative margins have developed local recurrence at the primary site, ranging from a low of 14.5% for those with stage I neoplasms to 47.3% for stage IV tumors.[18] The frequency of positive margins appears to correlate with tumor size and increased stage. This in turn may be related to the resectability of the neoplasm and the amount of normal tissue that can be removed by the surgeon. Logically, then, local recurrences are more common in large tumors, and incomplete or close excisions will increase the chance of recurrence.

## MULTIPLE PRIMARIES

The patient with squamous cell cancer of the upper aerodigestive tract is at increased risk for developing second carcinomas. With careful clinical surveillance, there has been an increased frequency of identification of multiple synchronous and metachronous primary squamous cell carcinomas of the head and neck region.[19] Simultaneous primary tumors have been found in over 10% of patients and over 20% of patients eventually develop second neoplasms.[20] A second primary neoplasm has a definite influence on survival; one study has demonstrated an overall 5 year survival of 17% compared to a 35% survival for patients with a single neoplasm of the upper aerodigestive tract.[21]

The histologic criteria and biopsy approaches to multicentric squamous cell carcinoma attempt to verify that its focus is anatomically independent of the presenting carcinoma and is separated by histologically normal intervening mucosa. The demonstration of an in situ mucosal origin is the strongest evidence for a multicentric cancer. A second primary cancer developing at or near the site of an original, previously treated carcinoma can be identified as a second primary in only a limited number of cases and usually represents persisting neoplasm. An intramucosal component may only indicate residual in situ neoplasia remaining at the margins of the previous resection, rather than a newly developed carcinoma.

The histologic diagnosis of persistent squamous cell carcinoma (indicating local treatment failure), rather than a second primary cancer developing in the original treatment field, depends on the fact that most squamous cell carcinomas invade and expand the submucosal tissues. Persistent neoplasm in the submucosal tissues is the usual site of local treatment failure after surgical excision and/or incomplete radiation or chemotherapeutic sterilization. Persistent submucosal tumor often will expand to include the overlying squamous mucosa with subsequent ulceration. In contract to the biopsy approach to an ulcer, the deep submucosal tissues, rather than the firm ulcer edge, may have to be biopsied and re-biopsied to histologically document the deep persistent cancer. These are important clinical and pathologic differential diagnoses. The distinction between an early stage second primary cancer arising from intraepithelial transformation and a persistent deep cancer translates into local therapy for the former and radical salvage therapy for the latter.

## THE FROZEN SECTION

The rapid or frozen section technique for evaluating microscopic portions of tissue is applicable to surgery in the head and neck region for several valid reasons. The first and most commonly utilized is the intraoperative evaluation of resection margins. The margin for frozen section analysis is submitted by the surgeon depending on the operative findings, as opposed to the pathologist's sampling of the total margins of an excised specimen. Knowledge of "positive" margins allows the surgeon to tailor the resection to include all of the identifiable tumor. The gross assessment of mucosal margins by the pathologist is not acceptable, as some oro- and hypopharyngeal carcinomas may invade in small submucosal aggregates that can only be identified by frozen tissue sections.

The histology of a frozen section is less optimal than that of the fixed, paraffin embedded permanent section. However, in experienced hands, errors are kept to a minimum and are usually due to improper or inadvertent tissue sampling. On rare occasions, deeper levels cut into the permanent tissue block may show the presence of carcinoma that was not present on the superficial cut taken at the time of frozen section. However, this tends not to be a problem with experienced surgeons and pathologists who maintain optimum communication.

Preoperative radiation or chemotherapy can alter cellular appearances and cause a degree of inflammation and scarring that contribute to a clinically palpable induration. Such biopsies are more difficult to evaluate histologically at frozen section and are usually the least reliable. Radiation-induced epithelial atypia may be significant and impossible to distinguish from carcinoma in situ. Interpretation should be conservative unless infiltration carcinoma is evident. Therapy may also "melt" away a clinically detected surface carcinoma, yet submucosal disease may persist. Therapy also contributes to uncertainty in histologic interpretation due to the "sterilization" of tumor and the remnants of keratin with foreign body granulomatous reaction. Evaluating the viability of these changes may pose great difficulty at frozen section and is usually resolved more readily on the permanent section. When foci of questionable viability are found near the margin of resection, the conservative approach is to assume that the neoplasm is viable.

Another valid indication for frozen section examination is for primary diagnosis at the time of planned complete excision. This rarely occurs in the diagnosis of head and neck squamous cell carcinoma unless the biopsy is from a relatively inaccessible site. Re-biopsy of a recently biopsied site may prove difficult to interpret on frozen section due to regenerative epithelial atypia and submucosal nests of reactive epithelium.

Biopsies taken for special study—electron microscopic, immunologic, or microbiologic evaluation—may be controlled by frozen section to insure that appropriate tissue is sampled.

The last application of frozen section examination is for the evaluation of tumor extension so that conservation excision may be performed or radical resection deferred. Illustrative cases are: tumor of the larynx in the former, and tumor at the base of the skull in the latter.

## EVALUATION OF RADICAL NECK SPECIMENS

The evaluation of the number and extent of cervical lymph node metastases represents the strongest diagnostic indicator for squamous cell carcinoma of the upper aerodigestive tract. The pathologic evaluation of radical neck dissections is straightforward, since the orientation and anatomic subdivisions of the lymph nodes are usually readily determined. Lymph nodes are segregated into the following anatomic subdivisions that allow the level of lymph node metastases to be documented: (Fig. 7.3)

1. Submental—usually present in the anterior triangle of floor of mouth resections.
2. Submandibular or anterior triangle—the amount of tissue and lymph

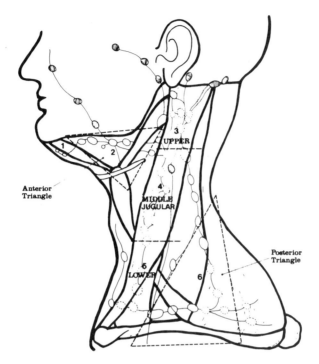

**FIGURE 7.3** Cervical lymph node compartments.

nodes present depends on the origin of the squamous cell carcinoma and the type of surgery performed

3. Subdigastric-upper jugular—arbitrarily the upper perijugular group of lymph nodes just posterior and below the submandibular salivary gland.

4. Mid-jugular—arbitrarily the middle third of the peri-jugular lymph node chain.

5. Low jugular—the lower third of the peri-jugular lymph nodes.

6. Posterior cervical or posterior triangle—the tissue behind the sterno-cleido-mastoid represents the group of lymph nodes posterior to the peri-jugular chain and may be subdivided arbitrarily at levels roughly the same as the jugular chain.

7. Supraclavicular—the lateral supraclavicular fat pad representing the supraclavicular lymph nodes may be designated when it is included in the specimen.

The extent and number of lymph nodes involved, in general, correlate with prognosis. The presence of metastases in the lower levels of the neck results in a marked decrease in survival.[22] Also, for undetected head and neck primaries, the site of adenopathy within the neck may point to the location of the primary. Generally, high neck lymph nodes and posterior cervical triangle lymph nodes drain primary sites in the nasopharynx; upper jugular lymph nodes relate to sites in the oropharynx; mid-jugular nodes reflect sites in the larynx; the lower jugular region drains the hypopharynx; and the supraclavicular lymph nodes correspond to primary sites below the clavicles, usually the lungs or gastrointestinal tract.[23] These are general, but not conclusive, guidelines regarding tumor origin and site of neck node metastases.

In addition to defining the number and site of involved lymph nodes, the pathologist should also comment on the histologic finding of extracapsular spread of squamous cell carcinoma in the lymph nodes of the radical neck dissection. The presence of carcinoma penetrating the lymph node capsule and infiltration of the adjacent soft tissues are prognostic indicators of decreased survival.[24-26] Radical neck dissection specimens usually yield up to 20 lymph nodes, however, fewer lymph nodes, often 6 to 10, may be identified in some specimens because of the lympholytic effect of preoperative radiation or chemotherapy. The sectioning of lymph nodes to detect microscopic metastasis varies from bisection of large nodes to submitting as a whole tiny lymph nodes. Obviously, adequate embedding and sectioning can increase the microscopic yield in the pathologic examination of neck dissections.[27] When lymph nodes from radical neck dissections that were thought to contain tumor or clinical examination were examined histologically, there has been a wide range, from 44 to 88% positivity from numerous studies.[28] In addition, clinically occult cervical metastases have been found in 15 to 60% of patients thought to have clinically negative necks.[29,30] Obviously, there can be a considerable discrepancy between the pathologic staging of necks and the clinical evaluation of palpable lymph nodes.

## FINE NEEDLE ASPIRATION BIOPSY

It has become increasingly popular to sample cervical neck masses by fine needle aspiration biopsy (FNA) technique utilizing "skinny" 22–25 gauge needles. Successful use of this technique requires expertise on the part of the pathologist and close rapport between the pathologist and the clinician. The clinician, in turn, must be capable of communicating an accurate clinical interpretation and working differential diagnosis.

This technique can be useful in the diagnosis of cystic neck masses and inflammatory conditions and in the determination of tissue of origin of neck masses. The main use in Head and Neck Oncology is the documentation of recurrent carcinoma. FNA can be accomplished rapidly and with low morbidity at bedside or on an outpatient basis.[31] Long-term studies do not indicate a significant risk for recurrences of tumor along FNA needle tracks in the head and neck region or other sites as opposed to core biopsy. No tumor recurrences or tract extensions have been noted in a 5 year follow-up of over 600 patients with metastatic carcinoma in neck nodes who underwent FNA.[32] This, and numerous other studies, indicate that needle aspiration biopsy can be dismissed as an important factor in local tumor recurrence.[33]

One drawback of the technique is a significant percentage of false-negative results. The most common cause of false-negative aspirates of known cancer is failure to sample the lesion. Thin needles are utilized (22–25 gauge), for these aspiration biopsies are extremely flexible, and therefore they may also be easily deflected from their course to the tumor by resistance of surrounding tissue, trajectory errors, or patient movements. This is more significant for lesions that are distant from the site of entry such as those in visceral organs, and is less of a factor for the more superficial lesions in the head and neck region. In addition, tumor masses are often partially necrotic with an inflammatory and a desmoplastic stromal component. This may lead to the aspiration of nondiagnostic tissue, even though technically adequate aspiration has been performed. The incidence of false-negative aspirates of this type can be decreased by multiple needle aspirations with slight variation in the approach angle of puncture without withdrawing the needle from the initial skin entry site. Lastly, faulty processing techniques may also contribute to poor cellular preservation and therefore false-negative results. A negative result does not exclude a diagnosis of cancer. When there is a strong clinical suspicion of metastatic neck disease, cases may be pursued by re-aspiration or open biopsy.

The advantage of aspiration biopsy in patients with suspected metastatic cervical carcinoma, especially in those patients who are inoperable or on whom definitive therapy has been performed, is that this select groups of patients may be spared additional neck biopsy and possible cutaneous seeding of tumor. As stated by Klein, "fine needle aspiration biopsy must never be a substitute for clinical judgement or compete with an indicated histopathologic biopsy."[33] The role of fine needle aspiration biopsy in the head and neck region at present is one of aiding evaluation and not the primary histologic diagnosis on which operative decisions are based. With the expertise that time and coordinated efforts produce, FNA may plan a more significant role in the staging and diagnosis of head and neck cancer.

## THE SURGICAL PATHOLOGY REPORT

The surgical pathology report should be a complete but concise communication with pathologic observations sufficient for the clinician to stage the cancer. Lengthy cytologic descriptions of the tenets of neoplasia are superfluous since they translate into histologic grade. The use of diagrams is encouraged. Schematic diagrams utilized in our laboratory for oropharynx/lips, tongue/floor of mouth, base of tongue/supraglottic larynx, posterior oropharynx/hypopharynx, hypopharynx and larynx are reproduced in Figures 7.4–7.9.

The features that should be incorporated into the basic surgical pathology report include:

1. The site and size of the primary carcinoma and any secondary primaries.
2. Histologic evaluation of the grade of differentiation.
3. Extent of infiltration or growth pattern of the neoplasm including the presence of intra-epithelial changes, micro-invasion, angiolymphatic or perineural invasion and massive tumor.
4. Evaluation of the margins of surgical excision with an assessment of the completeness of excision.
5. The site of regional lymph node metastases noting the presence of extra-capsular spread and infiltration of soft tissue.
6. The site of distant metastatic spread.

**FIGURE 7.4** Oropharynx and lips.

**OROPHARYNX AND VERMILLION BORDER OF LIPS**

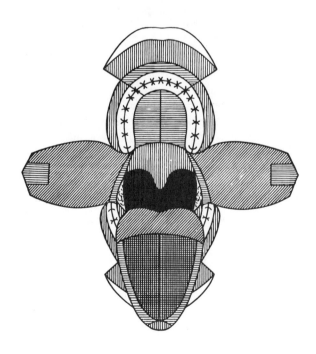

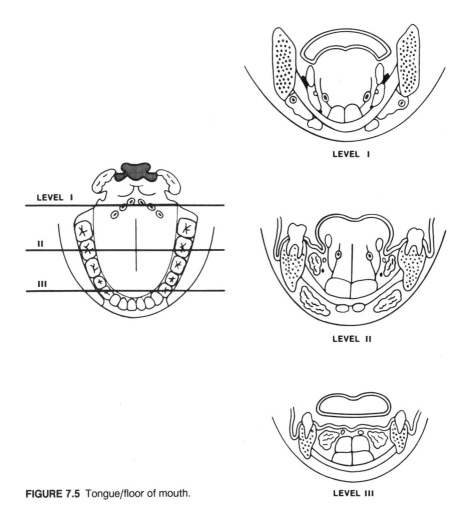

**FIGURE 7.5** Tongue/floor of mouth.

**BASE OF TONGUE AND SUPRAGLOTTIC LARYNX**

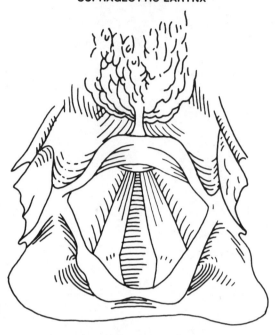

**FIGURE 7.6** Base of tongue and supraglottic larynx.

**FIGURE 7.7** Posterior oropharynx, hypopharynx and larynx.

**POSTERIOR OROPHARYNX, HYPOPHARYNX, LARYNX**

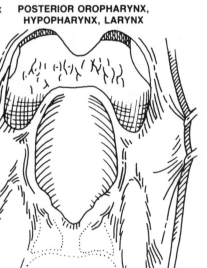

**HYPOPHARYNX**

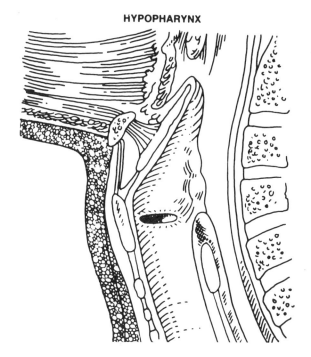

FIGURE 7.8 Hypopharynx.

FIGURE 7.9 Larynx.

**LARYNX**

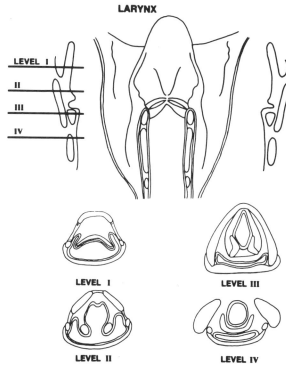

LEVEL I

II

III

IV

LEVEL I

LEVEL III

LEVEL II

LEVEL IV

**95**

# REFERENCES

1. Lin H, Lin C, Yeh S, and Tu S: Fine structure of nasopharyngeal carcinoma with special reference to the anaplastic type. Cancer 1969;23:390–405.
2. Regezi JA, Batsakis JG: Diagnostic electron microscopy of head and neck tumor. Arch Pathol Lab Med 1978;102:8–14.
3. Battifora H: Recent progress in the immunohistochemistry of solid tumors. Sem Diag Path 1984;1:251–271.
4. Moll R, Franke FF, Schiller DL: The catalog of human cytokeratins: Patterns of expression in normal epithelia, tumors and cultured cells. Cell 1982;31:11–24.
5. Nelson WG, Battifora H, Santana H, Sun TT: Specific keratins as molecular markers for neoplasms with a stratified epithelial origin. Cancer Res 1984;44:1600–1603.
6. Broders AC: Carcinoma. Grading and practical application. Arch Pathol 1926;2:376–381.
7. Crissman JD, Liu WY, Gluckman JL, Cummings G: Prognostic value of histopathologic parameters in squamous cell carcinoma of the oropharynx. Cancer 1984;54:2995–3001.
8. McGavran MH, Bauer WC, Ogura JH: The incidence of cervical lymph node metastases from epidermoid carcinoma of the larynx and their relationship to certain characteristics of the primary tumor. A study based on the clinical and pathological findings for 96 patients treated by primary en bloc laryngectomy and radical neck dissection. Cancer 1961;14:55–66.
9. Kashima HK: The characteristics of laryngeal cancer correlating with cervical lymph node metastasis (analysis based on 40 total organ sections), in: Alberti PW, Bryce DP (eds): Centennial Conference on Laryngeal Cancer. New York: Appleton-Century-Crofts, 1976. pp.855–864.
10. Poleksic S, Kalwaic HJ: Prognostic value of vascular invasion in squamous cell carcinoma of the head and neck. Plast Reconstr Surg 1978;61:234–240.
11. Byers RM, O'Brien J, Waxler J: The therapeutic and prognostic implications of nerve invasion in cancer of the lower lip. Int J Radiat Oncol Biol Phys 1978;4:215–217.
12. Carter RL, Tanner NSB, Clifford P, Shaw HJ: Perineural spread in squamous cell carcinomas of the head and neck: a clinicopathologic study. Clin Otolaryngol 1979;4:271–281.
13. Crissman JD, Gluckman J, Whiteley J, Quenelle D: Squamous cell carcinoma of the floor of the mouth. Head Neck Surg 1980;3:2–7.
14. Lesinski SG, Bauer WC, Ogura JH: Hemilaryngectomy for $T_3$ (fixed cord) epidermoid carcinoma of the larynx. Laryngoscope 1976;86:1563–1571.
15. American Joint Committee on Cancer, 2nd ed., in Beahrs OH, Myers MH (eds): Manual for Staging Cancer. Philadelphia: Lippincott, 1983.
16. Skolnick EM, Yee KF, Wheatley MA, Martin LO: Panel discussion on glottic tumors. V. Carcinoma of the laryngeal glottis therapy and end results. Laryngoscope 1975;85:1453–1466.
17. Jacobs JR, Spitznagel EL, Sessions DG: Staging parameters for cancers of the head and neck: A multi-factorial analysis. Laryngoscope 1985;95:1378–1381.
18. Looser KG, Shah JP, Strong EW: The significance of "positive" margins in surgically resected epidermoid carcinomas. Head Neck Surg 1978;1:107–111.
19. Cohn AM, Peppard SB: Multiple primary malignant tumors of the head and neck. Am J Otolaryng 1980;1:411–417.
20. Gluckman JL, Crissman JD, Donegan JO: Multicentric squamous cell carcinoma of the upper aerodigestive tract. Head Neck Surg 1980;3:90–96.
21. Gluckman JL, Crissman JD: Survival rates in 548 patients with multiple neoplasms of the upper aerodigestive tract. Laryngoscope 1983;93:71–74.

22. Platz H, Fries R, Hudec M, Tjoa AM, Wagner RR: The prognostic relevance of various factors at the time of the first admission of the patient. Retrospective DOSAK study of carcinoma of the oral cavity J Max-Fac Surg 1983;11:3–12.
23. Lindberg RD: Distribution of cervical lymph node metastases from squamous cell carcinoma of upper respiratory and digestive tracts. Cancer 1972;29:1446–1449.
24. Johnson JT, Barnes EL, Myers EN et al: The extracapsular spread of tumors in cervical node metastasis. Arch Otolaryngol 1981;107:725–729.
25. Snyderman NL, Johnson JT, Schramm VL Jr, et al: Extracapsular spread of carcinoma in cervical lymph nodes. Impact upon survival in patients with carcinoma of the supraglottic larynx. Cancer 1985;56:1597–1599.
26. Kalnins IK, Leonard AG, Sako K, et al: Correlation between prognosis and degree of lymph node involvement in carcinoma of the oral cavity. Am J Surg 1977;134:450–454.
27. Wilkinson EJ, Haus L: Probability in lymph node sectioning. Cancer 1974;33:1269–1274.
28. Hibbert J, Marks NJ, Winter PJ, Shaheen OH: Prognostic factors in oral squamous carcinoma and their relation to clinical staging. Clin Otolaryngol 1983;8:197–203.
29. Spiro RH, Strong EW: Surgical treatment of cancer of the tongue. Surg Clin NA 1974;54:759–765.
30. Lyall D, Shetlin CF: Cancer of the tongue. Ann Surg 1985;135:489.
31. Frabel WJ, Frable MAS: Thin needle aspiration biopsy. The diagnosis of head and neck tumors revisited. Cancer 1979;43:1541–1548.
32. Engzell U, Jakobsson PA, Sigudson A, Zajicek J: Aspiration biopsy of metastatic carcinoma in lymph nodes of the neck: a review of 1101 consecutive cases. Act Otolaryngol. (Stockh) 1971;72:138–147.
33. Klein TS: Handbook of Fine Needle Aspiration Biopsy Cytology. St. Louis: CV Mosby Company, 1981.

# CHAPTER 8

# The Modified and Radical Neck Dissection for Squamous Cell Carcinoma of the Upper Aerodigestive System

*Lawrence W. DeSanto, MD and*
*Oliver H. Beahrs, MD*

## INTRODUCTION

When cancer from an upper aerodigestive system primary has metastasized to regional lymph nodes, the prognosis is unfavorably altered.[1-9]

The radical or complete neck dissection has been the consummate treatment for actual or probable metastatic carcinoma of the neck from these cancers for most of the twentieth century. The operation is based on the Halstedian principle that adequate treatment of a cancer that has or may have metastasized to regional lymph nodes requires that every cell of cancer from the primary tumor and every lymphatic, node, and lymph nodule in the lymphatic drainage region be removed.

## WHAT IS A RADICAL NECK DISSECTION?

The classic, complete, or radical neck dissection described by Crile removes the following structures from at least one side of the neck: the sternomastoid and omohyoid muscles, anterior and posterior bellies of the digastric muscle, and the styloid hyoid muscle.[10] Also removed are the submaxillary salivary gland, the tail of the parotid gland, the internal jugular vein, the connective tissue of the carotid sheath, and the lymph-bearing tissues of the anterior, posterior triangles, and deep jugular chain, en bloc. Also included are the transverse cervical vessels, the spinal accessory nerve and associated lymphatic chain, and the investing and deep layers of the cervical fascia.

The premise of this operation is that cancer cells, whether spread by embolization or by direct invasion of lymph vessels, will be included in this block of tissue, and that the removal of these cancer cells will contribute to the patient's cure by ending any possibility that cancer will return either to the primary site or to the dissected neck.

## Criticisms of the Radical Neck Dissection

The main problem with this operation is that the promise of cure of metastatic cancer by operation is simplistic. The operation has never cured all metastatic neck disease.[2-9,11,12] Cancer returns in the neck too often after neck dissection.

There are several possible reasons why this occurs: (1) the operation is not done correctly, (2) cancer is left behind in places in the neck not included in the block dissection, (3) cancer cells are sprinkled back into the neck, (4) there is more to curing cancer than just removing cells, and (5) any combination of reasons one to four. The reasons why the operation fails probably vary from case to case. The premise that cancer is cured by separating every malignant cell from the host is either simplistic or impossible.

Since Crile's time, much has been learned about the cervical lymphatic system.[10] The Crile operation and the premise on which it is founded are being reconsidered. Information has been discovered about the anatomy of the lymphatics, the function of the lymph nodes, the effect of operation in general, anesthesia, and node ablation on regional and systemic tumor immunity. We are learning the effects of radiation and various cytotoxic chemicals on cancer cells, lymphatics, and nodes.

Anatomic revelations since Crile's era have shown, for example, that the muscles of the neck do not contain lymphatics.[10] Lymphatics are in the fascia around the muscles.[13,14] The fascial compartment containing the lymphatics and nodes has been described in detail. These findings require revision of the earlier concepts and indicate that removal of the various muscles of the neck adds nothing to the oncologic aspects of the operation. Removal of some of the muscles may make the operation easier to perform.

Another theoretical objection to the block concept is that, by definition, it is compromised by what is left behind. Some structures such as the carotid vessels and the vagus, hypoglossal, phrenic, and lingual nerves are not removed. A true radical neck dissection would remove all of these structures but there are practical reasons not to do so and the concept of the block is compromised from the beginning. Structures that are in proximity to lymphatics and nodes are removed when it is practical and other structures with the same degree of proximity are left behind.

## The Purpose of the Cervical Lymph Nodes

The idea that the cervical lymphatics and nodes are mechanical conduits and passive filters can no longer be sustained. The discovery that all lymphocytes are not the same in origin or purpose was followed by the discovery that there exist whole families of different types of cells with unique but often interrelated purposes, including the modulation of systemic and regional immunity.[15] With the old concept, there were bad lymph nodes (those that contained metastatic cancer) and the others. Now we acknowledge that the regional lymphatic system might have some other purpose that benefits the cancer patient even when one or more of the approximately 300 nodes contain cancer.[16] The loss of the healthy parts of this system may be detrimental.

## Experimental Data

The evidence that the regional nodes are more than passive filters leads to the conjecture that their removal or alteration may contribute to failure to cure cancer in some people.

An inclusive laboratory examination by Schuller of several measurements of regional and systemic immune modulating mechanisms in patients with head and neck primary cancer provides some indication that regional lymph nodes may be stimulated by cancer cells in the area and actually activate a metamorphosis of some species of T-cell lymphocytes into "natural killer lymphocytes" and prompt a regional reaction to tumor that is beneficial.[16] Schuller pointed out that current therapy to neck lymph nodes that tries to eradicate or remove all or most of them can alter or eliminate up to 40% of the body's lymph nodes. He encouraged us to find out what we are doing to regional and systemic immunity by our operations, anesthetic drugs, cytotoxic agents, and radiation.

## The Risk Factors With Neck Metastasis

The conventional risk factors considered important with metastatic disease to the neck are: (1) number of nodes positive for cancer; (2) positive node size; (3) position of the node; (4) extra- or transcapsular extension; (5) tumor invasion into structures that are not removed (e.g., carotid artery); (6) jugular vein invasion; and (7) probably the most important, the presence of metastasis to the nodes or node in the neck.

Of these factors, only the findings of a positive node, node position, and tumor invasion into structures not resected, and invasion of the jugular vein lumen, are consensus risk factors.[5,7-9,12,17-21]

Why the presence of even a single microscopic clump of cancer cells predictably alters prognosis is not understood. There are several possibilities: tumors that metastasize are more aggressive, and the host is immunocompromised and this permits metastasis.

It seems reasonable that the more positive nodes there are in the neck, the greater the risk of failure in the neck or elsewhere, and there is support for this perception.[2,9,22]

There are other data that do not go along with that logic. For example, a recent study of 455 patients by Grandi et al. were unable to correlate the number of positive nodes with prognosis ($0.05 < p < 0.10$).[23] In their report of 242 patients, Schuller et al. could not relate number, percentage, or size of positive nodes with eventual prognosis.[24] It is studies such as these that challenge the basic premise of the end-stage reporting system and the assumptions on which we make basic decisions — particularly whether to use or withhold the use of multimodality therapy in patients with presumed higher risk because of the number or size of nodes.[25]

The latest addition to the list of supposed risk factors is the observation that cancer that has left the lymph node (extracapsular [ECS] or transcapsular spread) is a predictor of a poorer prognosis.[26-29]

There are some problems with this conclusion. To begin with, there is a spectrum of severity of ECS from microscopic to gross cancer that deeply invades surrounding tissue. This spectrum is not defined by our classification scheme. Another problem is that the closer the pathologist looks at the nodes, the higher the incidence of ECS becomes.

Grandi et al.,[23] for example, did their work after this risk factor was popularized and found extracapsular cancer in 12% of clinically negative neck specimens, 46% of single positive node neck specimens, and 66% of cases in which there was more than one positive node and the largest nodes were less than 3 cm. When a positive node was greater than 3 cm, the frequency was 89%. Grandi et al. could not find a difference in neck recurrence rates that was statistically significant when there was ECS.[23] This study used actuarial curves and recurrence in the neck was the end point. Adjusted actuarial survival looked much better than observed survival, indicating that people with head and neck cancer die of causes other than cancer at a greater frequency than their age- and sex-adjusted cohorts. This observation may add to the difficulties in validating our assumptions in studies of the cancer population. Also, patients with the greatest degree of ECS were more likely to have received postoperative radiation. This may have lowered their recurrence rates to approach the recurrence rates of the patients who did not exhibit ECS.

## Functional Problems of the Radical Operation

In the early years of radical operation on the neck nodes, the dissections were done only on the side of palpable adenopathy.[1,10] In the 1950s, Bocca addressed the issue of the high frequency of bilateral metastasis at some point in the treatment of supraglottic and pyriform sinus cancer.[30] He noted:

> In spite of the tremendously high figures [actual or occult bilateral metastasis], many laryngologists maintain that the glands should be left undisturbed except in the cases in which they are manifestly enlarged: otherwise, x-ray therapy should be given to the lateral regions of the neck. (pp. 567 and 568)

He went on to say, "Now, we all know by experience that the therapeutic result of radiation on metastatic lesions is generally poor. And we may add that when clinical metastases have set in, even the result of surgery is poor" (p. 568). Bocca made a case for bilateral neck dissections, therapeutic or elective, depending on the clinical status of the neck.[30] His attitude was, "Limiting it [the dissection] to the side of the prevalent spread of the primary growth would be the equivalent of denying the very principles on which the prophylactic surgery of metastases is based" (p. 568). In raising the level of ablation to both sides of the neck and addressing the issue of elective or prophylactic dissection, the degree of intervention was raised and the issues of morbidity and cost compared with benefit became more germane.

At first, Bocca looked on the consequences of resecting both internal jugular veins and both accessory nerves and muscles as acceptable compared to death from uncontrolled disease.[30] His enormous experience with bilateral radical operations in a staged sequence resulted in few cerebral circulatory consequences in the early postoperative phase or the long term. In fact, he documented only one patient out of 100 with a serious problem. He did recognize that there was room for criticism when only 50% of those with elective operations had any chance of benefiting (those with occult metastasis) but he thought it was better to do 50% "white" operations than to risk failure with metastasis.

A few years later, Bocca and Pignataro questioned the sacrifice of both jugular veins and accessory nerves in the elective operations and later in therapeutic procedures.[31] They described the surgeon's dilemma as "should he run cancerological risks in order to avoid serious functional accidents, or run functional risks in order to avoid serious but less probable cancerological consequences?" (p. 976) The cause of this uncertainty was the conviction at the time that only complete removal of the structures of the lateral neck, with the exception of the carotid artery and vagus nerve, was proper surgical treatment of cancer. Bocca answered this question by accumulating data that documented that, in selected cases, other structures could be preserved when operation was based on the anatomic principles defined by Truffert and the surgical revelations of Suarez.[13,14]

Roy and Beahrs came to the same conclusions regarding the preservation of the accessory nerve.[11] They had performed a substantial number of bilateral simultaneous radical operations and did not observe that the sacrifice of both jugular veins had serious consequences. In the 1950s, Ward and Robben saved accessory nerves without extra risk in selected patients who had composite resection.[32]

During this interval of reconsideration, there were no solid data to intimate that prophylactic dissection was superior for cancer cure to a therapeutic dissection done at the time of obvious clinical disease.

When institutions tried to assess the prophylactic dissection, they arrived at conflicting conclusions. The French school concluded that elective dissection was desirable and Martin's group at the Memorial Hospital decided that it was not.[33,34]

The most recent study on this question was that of Vandenbrouck et al.[28] This was a "controlled and prospective study" that found no evidence of an oncologic value to an elective dissection compared with one done later for clinical metastasis.

The whole notion of prophylactic dissection rests on the intuitive feeling of surgeons that the incidence, degree, and extent of involvement of the neck is less in the elective operation and that the less cancer they are required to remove, the better the prognosis. This may not be true.

## The Spinal Accessory Nerve

There was not much concern about the disability from dividing or resecting the accessory nerve in the radical operation when a single side of the neck was dissected. As prophylactic bilateral operations and bilateral simultaneous or staged therapeutic dissections became more popular, the concerns about shoulder function became more relevant. It is troublesome to do bilateral radical operations on clinically negative sides of the neck that are also pathologically negative and in the process sacrifice both accessory nerves.[6,31] In 1961, Nahum et al. described the "shoulder syndrome" of pain, scapular displacement, and shoulder droop.[35] Almost ten years before, Bocca noted that surgeons were aware of the "inherent disability" of the loss of both accessory nerves and tried to avoid it.[30]

The fascial envelope of the posterior triangle and upper deep jugular area through which the accessory nerve passes is violated by dissection and preservation of the accessory nerve.[10,30,36] Once other functional compromises such as preservation of the vagus nerve were understood to be contrary to the block concept, yet acceptable, it was conceptually easier to add another compromise and preserve the accessory nerve. Surgeons did just that.[5,6,14,31,37,38]

The issue at the beginning of the modified operations that preserved the accessory nerve was oncologic safety. Bocca and Pignataro presented data that survival rates were not altered compared with the radical operation,[31] and Lingeman et al. made the same observation later.[6]

.The question of whether tumor control is better with the radical operation is not totally settled, but if there are differences in neck recurrence rates, they are not large.[4,39] If the number, size, and presence of ECS does not influence neck recurrence rates, then the issue of what kind of dissection is oncologically superior is moot.

A basic assumption of preserving the accessory nerve in some patients is that this provides a benefit of better shoulder function than if the nerve is divided and removed, without a compromise to tumor control.

However, is there a functional benefit to preserving the accessory nerve and, if there is, does every patient enjoy it?

Leipzig et al. compared the functional alterations of the radical and the modified dissections.[40] They found minimal pain and shoulder dysfunction in 40% of patients who had the radical operation and in 65% of those in whom the nerve was preserved. In 14 of 28 patients in whom the nerve was thought to be preserved, there was objective evidence of loss of trapezius muscle function.

Schuller et al. did a prospective analysis of the effect of preserving or sacrificing the accessory nerve on the ability of patients to return to work, their dependence on others, and other practical variables.[36] They could not find a difference in disability when the nerve was preserved. They also noted that those patients who had postoperative radiation were more functionally impaired than those who had only a dissection, regardless of the type. This finding assumes additional importance now as a link evolves between the modified dissection and adjunctive radiation.

There are two new studies of the functional difference of preserving the accessory nerve. Saunders and associates evaluated patients for pain, weakness, stiffness, muscle atrophy, shoulder droop, and abduction after radical and modified operations and an operation in which the nerve was resected and replaced with a graft.[41] Of those in whom the nerve was preserved, 47% had some objective sign of dysfunction and 20% had either no function or severe dysfunction. Of patients in whom the nerve was divided, two-thirds had no function and one-third had altered function. However, only one-third of these had any subjective shoulder-related complaints. Two-thirds of a small number who had the nerve grafted had normal or near normal shoulder function. Sixty-nine percent of those in whom the nerve was preserved had no complaints compared with 50% in whom the nerve was divided. These differences were not statistically significant. All of these procedures were performed by experienced surgeons.

In 1985, Sobol et al. reported on 35 patients who had 44 neck dissections and were studied prospectively.[42] They found no significant difference in the patients' perception of subjective function regardless of the type of dissection. The investigators did observe major differences in objective measurements and electromyographic (EMG) changes between the operations. Patients who had the radical operation had the greatest percentage and the greatest degree of decrease in strength and EMG abnormality. The patients who had a modified operation also had changes in strength and EMG alteration indicating damage to the nerve. There was a tendency toward improvement with time. The authors concluded that all dissections, except those that do not approach the nerve (submaxillary and supraomohyoid), can injure the accessory nerve and that patient complaints do not accurately reflect the degree of nerve injury.

There are practical conclusions that can be drawn from these studies: (1) the neuronanatomy of nerve IX is more complex than we have realized, (2) objective measurements of dysfunction do not always correlate with patients' perceptions of dysfunction, and (3) the anatomic preservation of the accessory nerve is not the same as functional preservation in all cases. This is an observation that we are well aware of, after watching resident physicians pull, poke, squeeze, twitch, devascularize, and otherwise traumatize the nerve in their zeal to save it. In other words, it is easier to do a radical dissection than a modified operation.

## The Sternomastoid Muscle

Another structure that is removed as part of the classic operation is the sternomastoid muscle. The absence of this muscle is tolerated without a serious functional loss in most patients, but some physicians believe there is a cosmetic cost.[22] When preserved, the muscle is stripped of its fascia and deprived of much of its blood supply. The muscle is also usually denervated when the accessory nerve is dissected free. One wonders if a denervated and at least partially devascularized muscle is functional. The cosmetic question is relative. Most patients have a great deal of concern about a tracheostoma or a loss of part of their mandible, face, or an eye but not much concern about the removal of the sternomastoid muscle.

A theoretical advantage of retaining the sternomastoid muscle is carotid protection. Carotid artery exposure is most hazardous when associated with a pharyngocutaneous fistula. When only skin is lost, there are more options. The devascularized sternomastoid muscle lying lateral to the carotid system really does little to protect it when the medial surface of the artery is exposed.

There is little value to preserving the sternomastoid muscle.

## The Internal Jugular Vein

The anatomy of the fascial envelopes popularized by Bocca and Pignataro allows reconsideration of the purpose of removing the internal jugular vein in the neck dissection.[31] When cancer is within nodes, the internal jugular vein is outside of the fascial envelope that contains the nodes, and lymphatics and vein need not be removed for oncologic reasons. The reason for preserving this vein is its role in cerebral circulation. This concern is valid only when both veins are removed. There is abundant clinical and experimental evidence that cerebral and facial venous return is retarded when both veins are absent. The consequences of this are facial swelling, headache, and, at times, alteration of consciousness and papilledema. There have been a few cases of blindness.

The experience of Beahrs and Barber with bilateral simultaneous complete neck dissections and Bocca's work with bilateral staged complete dissections confirm that these complications are rare.[5,30,31] Batson's work on the venous drainage of the head confirms that the cross-sectional area of the paravertebral venous network is greater than that of the jugular system.[43] The concern about the catastrophic risk of removal of both internal jugular veins is overstated.[11,44]

A significant clinical experience with bilateral simultaneous modified dissections led us to wonder if the veins always stay patent after they are preserved. A common experience is gross facial swelling and headache to the same degree as with bilateral simultaneous or staged radical operations after bilateral modified operations.

Nevertheless, the preservation of one internal jugular vein, when possible, makes some theoretical sense. The ritualistic preservation of the internal jugular vein in a unilateral operation is unnecessary. As with the sternomastoid muscle, the removal of the jugular vein makes a tidy dissection easier, faster, and consequently, less expensive.

## The Cervical Plexus

The radical neck dissection divides the sensory nerves of the cervical plexus. This creates numbness of the neck skin and lower ear. This is not a major problem but it is noted by patients. The disability is the same as the sensory changes with parotidectomy.

## Advantages of the Radical Operation

The radical operation is standardized and can be taught easily to residents. This feature cannot be underestimated. When a review of the literature shows neck recurrence rates after dissection for N1 (AJCC) disease that vary from 15% to 60%, one has to ask why.[9,45,46] Either the patients are different or some operations are superior to others. After teaching the neck operations to a large number of residents, we are convinced that all neck dissections are not equal. There is no standard neck dissection as there are standard penicillin pills. For this reason, it is important to master a basic operation and then to learn the modifications.

The classic operation is easier to do. It is important to have a standard operation when working in the difficult neck. Difficult necks are those that are fat, those in patients with neck fixation or kyphosis, and those that have had previous operation, infection, or poorly conceived biopsy incisions.

The occasional surgeon and the physician who is not comfortable with the indications and the subtleties of metastatic neck disease are more likely to perform an operation that is predictable and easy. If one accepts the concept of the neck dissection as a staging procedure that can be therapeutic, and if one is not troubled by doing an operation that may not help when there is no cancer, then more errors are likely to be made by omission of a dissection if it is not important to choose from the menu of modified operations. With so many variations to choose from, there will be confusion about the timing, place, and type of operation. The data are not sufficient to help with these decisions. A significant percentage of head and neck cancer is treated in community hospitals.

Because the modified operations, rightly or wrongly, are linked to postoperative radiation, the dollar cost of the classic operations may, in the composite, be less without any decrease in benefit.

## THE MODIFIED NECK DISSECTIONS
### What Is a Modified Neck Dissection?

The term "modified neck dissection" is used as if there were an operation that satisfied some definition. Today the term is used to describe several different operations that are modified only in that they are not classic or radical operations. Byers recently described six different procedures used by him and his colleagues and called "modified neck dissections" (Table 8.1).[22]

When there are this many different neck operations, various different primary sites, and variations is combined therapy schemes, it becomes clear why we have so few definitive studies of effectiveness in treating head and

TABLE 8.1 Modified Neck Dissections

| Name of Operation | | Structure Removed | | | | | | | |
|---|---|---|---|---|---|---|---|---|---|
| | Nerve IX | Submax. Gland | Int. Jug. Vein | Sternomastoid Muscle | Upper Jug. Nodes | Lower Jug. Nodes | Ant. Jug. Nodes | Post Cervical Nodes |
| Suprahyoid | − | + | − | − | − | − | − | − |
| Supraomohyoid | − | − | − | − | + | − | + | − |
| Anterior modified | − | − | − | − | + | + | + | − |
| Posterior modified | − | − | − | − | + | + | − | + |
| Lower dissection | − | − | − | − | − | + | − | − |
| Functional dissection | − | − | − | + | + | + | + | + |
| Radical dissection | + | + | + | + | + | + | + | + |
| Modified radical dissection* | − | + | + | + | + | + | + | + |

*Used by Byers.[22]

108

neck cancers. Byers reported the seven neck operations that were used to treat tumors from 19 different primary sites, with two combined therapy sequences plus operation alone.[22] This represents 399 different possible combinations of neck operation, primary site, and combined therapy schemes and operation alone.[22]

A practical difference, both anatomically and functionally, between the radical and modified operations centers on the sternomastoid muscle, accessory nerve, and internal jugular vein.

The functional neck dissection, or "Bocca" neck dissection, is the prototype modification and the only one that removes all of the principle nodal groups, with the exception of the submaxillary nodes, but leaves the muscles, internal jugular vein, and accessory nerve. This operation is based on sound anatomic knowledge of the lymphatic compartments. It has been well received because it is understandable, teachable, and reproducible. It is oncologically acceptable because it is effective in the earlier stages of N+ neck disease.[3,6,31,44] The other modifications have not been directly compared with the radical operation.

## Advantages of the Modified Neck Dissection

Bocca developed his ideas because of perceived and intrinsic imperfections of the radical operation in the bilateral and elective situation.[30] The loss of both nerves IX and both internal jugular veins was not worthwhile when there was no cancer in the neck nodes. The bilateral functional operation was an adequate staging procedure that was also therapeutic in the lesser stages of neck disease. The main advantage was the freedom to do bilateral operations with little or no resultant functional disability.

The unilateral modified dissection came later and was the result of the desire to limit surgical morbidity even more, especially in elective or staging operations.[11]

## Criticisms of the Modified Neck Dissection

There are two criticisms of the modifications; the first is functional and the second is oncologic.

The functional criticism is that in the unilateral dissection there is no morbidity to the removal of the internal jugular vein, no cosmetic benefit to saving the sternomastoid muscle, and the accessory nerve does not always function when preserved and it is not often missed when it is resected.

The oncologic issue also involves the accessory nerve. The upper portion of the nerve is in the anterior triangle in close proximity to upper deep jugular nodes. The dissection of the nerve in this portion violates the fascial compartment that contains nodes. Most consider the accessory nerve a posterior triangle structure and because metastases are infrequent in the posterior nodes, it is thought that the nerve can be preserved without oncologic consequences. Schuller et al. clearly demonstrated that this is not so.[47]

Another oncologic issue is the concern that lymph nodes play a role in regional and systemic immunity. If we could be sure which nodes had cancer in them, we could do a true modified dissection that removed only the diseased nodes and leave the rest.

## THE LINK BETWEEN THE MODIFIED NECK DISSECTION AND POSTOPERATIVE RADIATION
### Introduction

The modified neck dissection has been linked with postoperative radiation from the beginning. The literature during the evolution of these operations conveys the sense that "realizing that modifying the neck dissection is yet another compromise, we best add another treatment to adjust the oncologic risk."

Bocca et al. were probably the first to link the modified dissection with combined therapy.[44] They alluded to this in their 1983 paper on supraglottic cancer. They recorded that, in an earlier period, postoperative radiation was almost always used with the functional dissection. They subsequently reconsidered and started that "in the latest decade it is rarely used."

Jesse, it appears, was the force that nearly institutionalized linkage.[48] He was influenced by Strong's observation that 20 Gy delivered preoperatively decreased the neck recurrence rate of patients with multiple nodes suspicious for metastasis from 71% to 37.5% (with no correlative improvement in survival) and his belief that there is no difference in oncologic value between preoperative and postoperative radiation therapy.[45] He championed the modified operation plus radiation after modified dissection in patients with positive nodes. Subsequently, data accumulated in support of this idea and were reported in 1981. The study started with 440 patients but excluded 113 patients who died of other causes within 2 years, 50 patients in whom the primary was never controlled, 27 patients who died of treatment, 33 patients who had a second primary, and 20 patients who were lost to follow-up (a total of 243, or more than half of the data base).[48]

There is little evidence that this exclusion of patients with an unfavorable outcome, if applied in a prospective study, would lead to the salutary conclusion that radiation plus dissection actually is superior to dissection alone.

The use of the modified operations in selected patients would not be contended if the issue were merely radical or modified dissection. If this were all, reasonable judgment would prevail and surgeons would pick and choose between operations, based on the clinical situation. The controversy is because, right or wrong, the modified operation is inexorably linked with postoperative radiation.

## Other Data on the Linkage

We have looked at the linkage issue with both pre- and postoperative radiation and modified dissection as well as radical dissection. The end point of our study was recurrence in the neck. We could find no stage of neck disease with either sequence of radiation or any of the radiation amounts tested (less than or greater than 40 Gy) at which the combined therapy was more effective in decreasing neck recurrence than dissection alone. Although 40 Gy was the cutoff, most patients who had postoperative radiation received 50 Gy or more within 6 weeks of dissection. A special matched-pair analysis was done in addition to the actuarial study in which patients were paired by primary site, date of operation, neck stage (pathologic), age, control of the primary, and all the variables that would be considered in a prospective study. Even with this analysis, we were unable to find a subgroup of patients in which the addition of radiation was of value.[9]

Terz and Lawrence cited 12 different studies in which preoperative radiation was used.[49] In none of these did they find a valid benefit from the radiation in increasing survival.

One observation about all the series available that addresses the combined therapy and linkage issues is that the greater the number of exclusions there are or the smaller the number of patients studied, the more likely the analysis will find some utility of combined therapy.

The much-quoted study by Fletcher and Jesse is illustrative.[50] They started with 344 patients with clinically N+ neck disease and primary sites in the oral cavity, oropharynx, and supraglottic larynx. They excluded 161 patients, nearly one half, because these patients failed to complete the program, had a recurrence of the primary tumor, were thought to have had a "geographic miss" with radiation, received radiation doses they could not calculate, died in less than 2 years, or were lost to follow-up. With these adjustments to the population denominator, they found a positive benefit of radiation after operation.[50]

An example of the influence of sample size is a new study reported by Pearlman et al.[51] Their population was 41 patients in whom modified dissection was followed by radiation. In patients with positive nodes in whom no node was larger than 4 cm, there was an impressive failure rate in the neck of only 8% in patients treated with combined therapy compared with a small control group of four patients who refused radiation. Excluded were 13 patients: five who died in less than 2 years, disease free, and three who "did not respond to radiation." Two of the four controls had neck recurrence. The use of patients who refused treatment as the controls is a statistical manipulation that is misleading.

The prospective randomized study is held out as the standard for data acquisition to resolve these kinds of issues. There are not many of these because they are almost impossible to do. Patients have complications and drop out or are too sick to start radiation. Surgeons are reluctant to randomize treatment because of preconceived notions about the various risk factors. Patients, when asked for their consent, refuse to be assigned to treatment randomly. The few studies that claim to have overcome these difficulties are not impressive in their findings with regard to combined therapy.

The prospective study from the Memorial Hospital in the 1960s studied low-dose preoperative radiation.[45] Another study performed in Boston in the 1970s did the same.[52] Neither could document an increase in survival but they did find some decrease in neck recurrence. The Eastern Oncology Group compared pre- and postoperative high-dose radiation but did not include operation alone.[53] The end point was survival to a point in time with treated supraglottic cancer. The survival rates were about the same whether radiation was before or after operation, and the rates were not impressive.

From the avowed advocates, one gathers that pre- and postoperative radiation have been betrayed every time they are studied by improper doses, wrong fields, imprecise timing, or the wrong particle. They insist that the treatment be judged not by its dismal past but by its radiant future. Common sense advised skepticism. If, after all the time, money, and complications that have accompanied this treatment, all we can show is perhaps a decrease in regional recurrence but no increase in survival, then little has been accomplished. The concern is that there is an increase in distant metastasis rate and treatment deaths and the net result is no increase in survival. The question of whether this is progress in the sense that it is better to die of distant metastasis is a philosophical one. Some think it is.[54] We do not.

There is a clinical and experimental basis for the concern that the combination of operation and radiation may increase the probability of distant metastasis and negate any positive benefit. Fisch did lymphangiographic studies and observed that the injected material bypassed nodes that were radiated and the total number of nodes remaining was less.[55] Engeset demonstrated that the barrier function of lymph nodes in rats was altered after radiation.[56] In 1981, Baker et al. questioned whether distant metastasis rates in humans were increased after radiation, and Lundy et al. asked the same question a few years earlier.[57,58]

A detailed recent study by Wolf et al. addressed this issue specifically in humans with head and neck cancer.[15] They studied T-cell lymphocytes, cells thought to be important in systemic tumor immunity, in patients with upper aerodigestive system cancers treated by both radiation and combined therapy. In both situations, there was a decrease in the absolute number of these cells and also a decrease in the important ratios of cells. The rate of recovery was different. The combined therapy patients showed a continued decrease for a longer period than those treated by radiation alone. This delay in recovery of immune-cell modulators may be a factor in an increased rate of distant metastasis in those treated with combined therapy. Operation plus radiation has a cumulative effect in immunological suppression. Operation depletes the body's response by blood loss, transfusions of lymphocyte-poor blood, depression of nutrition, and the use of certain anesthetic agents. Radiation adds to this by suppressing lymphocyte production.

There are some clinical studies in which conventional combined therapy for some disease yielded poorer results than operation alone.[59,60]

There is a need for more investigation into what our treatments do to the host, and Wolf and associates[1] work points to what needs to be done.[15]

The more the host's role in cancer cure is studied, the more obvious it becomes that our concepts of cancer treatment are simplistic. More may not always be better and no treatment scheme is free of problems. The linkage of the modified neck dissections and postoperative radiation needs to be better thought out. We began the modified operations because the radical operation was imperfect. Then we added another level of therapy, thinking the combination would have superior cure rates. No improvement was forthcoming in cure rates, but maybe there was more local-regional control. We need to ask whether we are adding to the cost, time, and morbidity and in the process altering the host's immune response in a detrimental way. DeFries took this question one step further in asking whether we can treat only those lymph nodes that contain cancer and leave the rest to carry out their business regarding tumor immunity.[3]

## THE LINKAGE ISSUE: THEORETICAL AND PRACTICAL CONSIDERATIONS

The linkage of modified neck dissections and postoperative radiation is based on the theoretical concept of subclinical disease.

After neck dissection, there are recurrences in a predictable proportion of patients. Cancer returns for two reasons: clonogenic clumps of tumor cells are left behind or new cancer develops in the neck that was cleared of all disease and then remetastasizes from a primary site that was not eliminated (this is the concept of "new and old" cancer).

Subclinical disease is disease that you know must be there but you cannot see. This includes microscopic cancer left behind knowingly for some reason such as its invasion into the common or internal carotid artery, vagus nerve, or the margins of the primary tumor such as the pharynx, where the next knife cut would require pharyngeal reconstruction.

Radiobiology experiments indicate that microscopic cancer can range in size up to several millimeters and contain $10^6$ to $10^8$ cancer cells. The death of a cancer cell from radiation is a random event and not intrinsic to being irradiated. The cell must be hit in a critical place. It takes the same amount of radiation to decrease the cell population from $10^8$ to $10^7$ as it does to go from 100 cells to 10 cells. We also know that it takes approximately two and one-half times the amount of radiation to destroy hypoxic cells and there is an upper limit of tolerance of normal tissue to radiation.[61] Clinical experience convinces us that the complication rates with radiation and operation increase as this level is approached.[54]

Theoretically, radiation delivered before neck dissection could destroy microscopic aggregates of cancer within areas not included in the neck dissection and cells that trail out at the periphery of the tumor where oxygenation is better. Theoretically, radiation before operation renders cells less reproducible, decreases the likelihood of throwing cancer cells into the bloodstream, and decreases the chance of spreading cancer cells about in the surgical area.[54]

The clinical reality is that these theoretical benefits are not reflected in increased cure rates. There may actually be an increase in distant metastasis rates and local recurrence.[15,57-60]

In spite of the theoretical advantages of preoperative radiation, this form of combined therapy has pretty much been abandoned because the combination promised more than it delivered and the complication rates were unacceptable.

Postoperative radiation is an old idea and one that was criticized on theoretical grounds in the era of preoperative radiation. It was once said that "if postoperative radiation therapy was indicated, preoperative radiation therapy should have been given" (p. 366).[9] With a rejuvenated theoretical cornerstone of subclinical disease added to the old concept that did not work before, postoperative radiation is back with new promises. Some of the hopes include: (1) decrease of recurrence in the clinically negative neck with treatments alone (this may be the contralateral side of the neck or the ipsilateral undissected neck); (2) decrease in recurrence in the dissected side of the neck; (3) decrease of local recurrence at the primary site; and (4) opportunity to do more conservative resections that remove all "gross disease" but may leave cancer at the margins and on the arteries and nerves as long as it is microscopic. This new dictum suggests to the oncologic surgeon that

> . . . there is no benefit to be derived from trying to remove all microscopic disease, which cannot be done in all patients anyway. The increase in radicalism of the surgical procedure might be counterproductive by increasing the delay for the start of irradiation.[54] (p.1281)

With a lesser operation, "diminished surgical manipulation provides less opportunity for throwing tumor cells into the blood stream" and "there is less scar tissue and, therefore, less possibility of hypoxia of the tumor cells left behind" (p. 1281).[54] When operation is conservative, "the quality of life is better" and, of course, "complications are less."

All of these benefits are theoretical. There is not one bit of substantial evidence that more patients get well and there is some concern that none of these presumed benefits are being experienced by patients. The concept of removing only gross disease ultimately has led to the "debulking" concept. This states that one can leave behind tumor that cannot be seen and "clean it up" with radiation. There is substantial evidence that if known tumor is left behind, even if it is " microscopic," tumor will recur and the patient will die.[17] This "parachute" [authors' quote] concept of postoperative radiation is dangerous. The idea that a modified operation to the neck or a conservative operation to the primary site is quicker and easier with less surgical manipulation is naive. Most of the conservation procedures are technically more difficult, take longer, and require more manipulation. The purpose of operation should not be to get it done quickly so that the real treatment (the radiation) can start, but to do a proper operation so that radiation is not needed. The idea that there is less scar with a conservative operation compared with a complete one is likewise naive. The real problem is that there are no data to verify that combining a modified neck operation with postoperative radiation has any benefit to patients in terms of cure or length of survival.[9,24,53,62-64]

An unmentioned problem with the linkage is cost. Radiation takes weeks and has a dollar cost in itself, plus the cost of time lost. If there are only theoretical benefits in terms of cancer control, marginal functional benefits with a unilateral modified dissection, and the new and serious concern that a combination of operation and radiation may actually have a detrimental effect to regional and systemic immunity in excess of the sum of the effect of each treatment alone, then we should question the entire linkage issue. One other concern is that a gradual accumulation of compromises is occurring, to the point where oncologic principles are being violated. First we leave the accessory nerve, then the jugular vein, then some muscles (none of which in and of itself is essential), and then we start to believe that we can leave a little bit of cancer here and there and clean it up with radiation.

The whole debate over neck dissection, modification, or modification plus radiation has to be more specific to the stage of neck disease being discussed. If the neck is truly negative (i.e., there is no cancer in the neck), then none of the treatments are helpful and the issue becomes: "Which unnecessary treatment is the least harmful?" We think that neck dissection that includes preservation of the accessory nerve without a big fuss over the jugular vein and sternomastoid muscle is the least harmful to the patient who has a clinically negative neck and a primary tumor that has a reasonable possibility of having metastasized. The only value of the dissection is finding out that the cancer has not metastasized. The dissection helps to stage the disease, estimate a prognosis, and settle the issue of combined therapy. It may be reasonable in this situation to do something less, as suggested by deFries, such as sampling the nodes that are at greatest risk so as to take from the neck the least number of lymph nodes and leave the rest to do whatever they do to tumor immunity.[3]

## NECK DISSECTION WITHOUT RADIATION

Not every head and neck oncologist subscribes to the thesis that a modified neck dissection requires postoperative radiation. Linkage is the principal impediment to choosing between the radical and modified dissection in the pathologically N+ neck. This is because of the absence of good data that there is a benefit that justifies the extra cost and morbidity. When the decision of which operation to use is to unencumbered, the choices are easier.

## THE CLINICALLY NEGATIVE NECK

The decision to perform some kind of neck dissection in the clinically negative neck is generally based on a probability estimate of the likelihood of occult metastasis, and the neck is operated on to treat the primary tumor. The decision is also made because of the conviction that removing metastatic disease in its occult stage is a lesser surgical task than waiting for clinical metastasis. This may not be correct.

The probability estimate of metastasis is the key to the elective neck dissection. Large tumors in certain sites are more likely to metastasize than small tumors. There is little need to do any kind of neck dissection, for example, for a glottic cancer of any stage other than the most advanced. In contrast, there is compelling reason to carry out an elective neck dissection for almost any stage of primary cancer of the tongue base and the tonsil area, based on probability of metastasis.

The assumptions that we use to make the decision in the elective situations are: (1) there is no difference in recurrence rates in the elective neck operation that uses a radical neck dissection or a properly performed modified operation if that operation is the functional or Bocca type; (2) the modified operation is technically more difficult but not compellingly so for the experienced surgeon; (3) there is no benefit for the patient from preserving the jugular vein in the unilateral dissection and little benefit from preserving the sternomastoid muscle, even though there is no oncologic benefit for resecting it (taking the muscle merely makes the operation easier); and (4) dissecting out the accessory nerve benefits some patients and can be done more easily when the jugular vein and sternomastoid muscle are removed.

This synthesis permits us and the residents we work with to use a hybrid operation that takes the sternomastoid muscle and internal jugular vein saves the accessory nerve.

In the therapeutic unilateral dissection, the same operation is used except when there are palpable upper deep jugular nodes suspicious for metastasis. In this situation, the accessory nerve is divided and either resected, reanastamosed after completion of the block removal, or, at times, cable-grafted when the upper and lower ends of the accessory nerve can be reconnected. Residents are encouraged to understand that the purpose of the neck dissection is to remove the disease in the neck as cleanly and efficiently as possible, and the fate of the accessory is a secondary issue.

## THE BILATERAL SITUATIONS

Bilateral operations on clinically negative sides of the neck are rarely performed. For primary cancers that have a significant probability of bilateral metastasis, when an operation on the primary is done through the neck, a complete dissection with preservation or repair of the accessory nerve is done on one side. Which side is determined in an unscientific way. If there is a laterality to the primary, then that side is dissected. If there are symptoms such as pain or otalgia on one side, then that side is dissected. The system under which we work provides a frozen-section screening of all nodes while the primary is being resected. If no nodes are involved, the operation is terminated. If metastases are found, a modified operation is done that preserves the internal jugular vein and the accessory nerve on the second side. This sequence is most often followed by supraglottic cancer.

When there is a clinically involved node, the same procedure is followed: a complete dissection with or without preservation of the nerve, a modified operation on the contralateral side, and an attempt to save a jugular vein and the nerve. The only difference is that the dissections are done before removal of the primary tumor.

If both sides of the neck are clinically positive for metastasis, then bilateral complete operation is done in one session. Both jugular veins and both accessory nerves are taken if it seems best to do so. This does not happen often. Bilateral complete dissections need not be avoided at all costs, as the risks are relatively minor and there are no practical alternatives.

## CONCLUSION

The choice between modified and radical neck dissection is not at all clear. There are many unsettled issues, including the most fundamental — is the dissection a valid treatment? The risk factors are not settled and the multimodality questions are ever-changing because of new drugs, radiation techniques, tools, and theories of interaction. These basic issues and others such as elective or therapeutic operations will all be resolved when we understand why some people do better with cancer treatment than others with the same disease and stage. The prevention of these cancers or, at least the ability to find and treat them before neck matastasis, will end this period of uncertainty.

The questions about what is the best treatment for cancer cannot all be answered now. More information is needed about the role of the lymph nodes in immunity and how to identify diseased nodes in a reliable way. The selection of one neck dissection from the menu rests on empirical data and fallible statistical data. We are not ready to abandon many of the old concepts of cancer management, so this debate will continue.

## REFERENCES

1. Okada W: The treatment and prognosis of carcinoma of the larynx. Transactions of the American Laryngological Association 1922;44:162–181.
2. DeSanto LW, Holt JJ, Beahrs OH, O'Fallon WM: Neck dissection: Is it worthwhile? Laryngoscope 1982;92:502–509.
3. deFries HO: Modified neck dissection, in Snow JB Jr (ed): Controversy in Otolaryngology, Philadelphia: WB Saunders, 1980. pp 203–209.
4. Jesse RH, Fletcher GH: Treatment of the neck in patients with squamous cell carcinoma of the head and neck. Cancer 1977;39:868–872.
5. Beahrs OH, Barber KW Jr: The value of radical dissection of structures of the neck in the management of carcinoma of the lip, mouth, and larynx. Arch Surg 1962;85:49–55.
6. Lingeman RH, Helmus C, Stephens R, Ulm J: Neck dissection: radical or conservative. Annals of Otology, Rhinology and Laryngology 1977:86:737–744.

7. Spiro RH, Strong EW: Epidermoid carcinoma of the oral cavity and oropharynx: elective vs therapeutic radical neck dissection as treatment. Arch Surg 1973;107:382–384.

8. Barkley HT Jr, Fletcher FH, Jesse RH, Lindberg RD: Management of cervical lymph node metastases in squamous cell carcinoma of the tonsillar fossa, base of tongue, supraglottic larynx, and hypopharynx. Amer J Surg 1972;124:462–467.

9. DeSanto LW, Beahrs OH, Holt JJ, O'Fallon, WM: Neck dissection and combined therapy: study of effectiveness. Arch Otolaryngology 1985;111:366–370.

10. Crile G: Excision of cancer of the head and neck with special reference to the plan of dissection based on one hundred and thirty-two operations. JAMA 1906;47:1780–1786.

11. Roy PH, Beahrs OH: Spinal accessory nerve in radical neck dissections. Amer J Surg 1969;118:800–804.

12. Jesse RH, Barkley HT Jr, Lindberg RD, Fletcher GH: Cancer of the oral cavity: is elective neck dissection beneficial? Amer J Surg 120 (1970):505–508.

13. Truffert P: *Le cou: anatomie topographique, les aponévroses-les loges.* Paris: L. Arnette, 1922.

14. Suarez O: El problema de las metastasis linfáticas y alejadas del cáncer de laringe e hipofaringe. Revista de Otorrinolaringologia 1963;23:83–99.

15. Wolf GT, Amendola BE, Diaz R, et al: Definite vs adjuvant radiotherapy: comparative effects on lymphocyte subpopulations in patients with head and neck squamous carcinoma. Arch Otolaryngology 1985;111:716–726.

16. Schuller DE: An assessment of neck node immunoreactivity in head and neck cancer. Laryngoscope (94 Suppl) 1984:35:1–35.

17. Stell PM, Dalby JE, Singh SD, Taylor W: The fixed cervical lymph node. Cancer 1984;53:336–341.

18. Santos VB, Strong MS, Vaughan CW Jr, DiTroia JF: Role of surgery in head and neck cancer with fixed nodes. Arch Otolaryngology 1975;101:645–648.

19. Conley JJ: Carotid artery surgery in the treatment of tumors of the neck. Arch Otolaryngology 1957;65:437–446.

20. Petrovich A, Kuisk H, Jose L, et al: Advanced carcinoma of the tonsil: treatment results. Acta Radiologica [Oncology] 1980; 19:425–431.

21. Djalilian M, Weiland LH, Devine KD, Beahrs OH: Significance of jugular vein invasion by metastatic carcinoma in radical neck dissection. Amer J Surg 1973;126:566–569.

22. Byers RM: Modified neck dissection: a study of 967 cases from 1970 to 1980. Amer J Surg 1985;150:414–421.

23. Grandi C, Alloisio M, Moglia D, et al: Prognostic significance of lymphatic spread in head and neck carcinomas: therapeutic implications. Head Neck Surg 1985;8:67–73.

24. Schuller DE, McGuirt WF, Krause CJ, et al: Symposium: adjuvant cancer therapy of head and neck tumors: increased survival with surgery alone vs. combined therapy. Laryngoscope 1979;89:582–594.

25. American Joint Committee on Cancer, 2nd ed.: in Beahrs OH, Myers MH (eds): Manual for Staging of Cancer. Philadelphia: J.B. Lippincott, 1983.

26. Snow GB, Annyas AA, Van Slooten EA, et al: Prognostic factors of neck node metastasis. Clin Otolaryngology 1982;7:185–192.

27. Johnson JT, Barnes ET, Myers EN, et al: The extracapsular spread of tumors in cervical node metastasis. Arch Otolaryngology 1981; 107:725–729.

28. Vandenbrouck C, Sancho-garnier H, Chassagne D, et al: Elective versus therapeutic radical neck dissection in epidermoid carcinoma of the oral cavity: results of a randomized clinical trial. Cancer 1980;46:386–390.

29. Sessions DG: Surgical pathology of cancer of the larynx and hypopharynx. Laryngoscope 1976;86:814–839.

30. Bocca E: Functional problems connected with bilateral radical neck dissection. J Laryngology Otology 1953;67:567–577.
31. Bocca E, Pignataro O: A conservation technique in radical neck dissection. Annals of Otology, Rhinology and Laryngology 1967;76:975–987.
32. Ward GE, Robben JO: A composite operation for radical neck dissection and removal of cancer of the mouth. Cancer 1951;4:98–109.
33. Cachin Y: Valeur pronostique de l'envahissement ganglionnaire cervical dans les carcinomes des voies aéro-digestives supérieures. Can J Otolaryngology 1972;1:116–128.
34. Martin H: Cited by Morfit, HM Discussion. Arch Surg 1962;85:55–56.
35. Nahum AM, Mullally W, Marmor L: A syndrome resulting from radical neck dissection. Arch Otolaryngology 1961;74:424–428.
36. Schuller DE, Reiches NA, Hamaker RC, et al: Analysis of disability resulting from treatment including radical neck dissection of modified neck dissection. Head Neck Surg 1983;6:551–558.
37. Pietrantoni L: Il problema chirurgico delle metastasi linfoghiandolari cervicali del cancro della laringe. *Archivio Italiano di Otologia* (64 Suppl) 1953;14:1–37.
38. Weitz JW, Weitz SL, McElhinney AJ: A technique for preservation of spinal accessory nerve function in radical neck dissection. Head Neck Surg 1982;5:75–78.
39. Brandenburg JH, Lee CYS: The eleventh nerve in radical neck surgery. Laryngoscope 1981;91:1851–1858.
40. Leipzig B, Suen JY, English JL, et al: Functional evaluation of the spinal accessory nerve after neck dissection. Amer J Surg 1983;146:526–530.
41. Saunders JR Jr, Hirata RM, Jaques DA: Considering the spinal accessory nerve in head and neck surgery Amer J Surg 1985;150:491–494.
42. Sobol S, Jensen C, Sawyer W II, et al: Objective comparison of physical dysfunction after neck dissection. Amer J Surg 1985;150:503–509.
43. Batson OV: Anatomical problems concerned in the study of cerebral blood flow. Fed Proc 1944;3:139–144.
44. Bocca E, Pignataro O, Oldini C: Supraglottic Laryngectomy: 30 years of experience. Annals of Otology, Rhinology and Laryngology 1983;92:14–18.
45. Strong EW: Preoperative radiation and radical neck dissection. Surgical Clinics of North America 1969;49:271–276.
46. Spiro RH, Alfonso AE, Farr HW, Strong EW: Cervical node metastasis from epidermoid carcinoma of the oral cavity and oropharynx: a critical assessment of current staging. Amer J Surg 1974;128:562–567.
47. Schuller DE, Platz CE, Krause CJ: Spinal accessory lymph nodes: a prospective study of metastatic involvement. Laryngoscope 1978;88:439–450.
48. Jesse RH: Modified neck dissection with and without radiation, in Kagan AR, Miller JW (eds): Controversies in Cancer Treatment Head and Neck Oncology. Boston, G.K. Hall Medical Publishers, 1981. pp 246–254.
49. Terz JJ, Lawrence W Jr: Ineffectiveness of combined therapy (radiation and surgery) in the management of malignancies of the oral cavity, larynx, and pharynx, in Kagan AR, Miles JW (eds): controversies in cancer treatment Head and Neck Oncology. Boston: G.K. Hall Medical Publishers, 1981. pp 110–125.
50. Fletcher GH, Jesse RH: Interaction of surgery and irradiation in head and neck cancers. Current Problems in Radiology 1971;1:1–37.
51. Pearlman NW, Johnson FB, Kennaugh RC: Modified radical neck dissection and postoperative radiotherapy in squamous cell head and neck cancer. Amer J Surg 1985;150:448–490.

52. Strong MS, Vaughan CW, Kayne HL, et al: A randomized trial of preoperative radiotherapy in cancer of the oropharynx and hypopharynx. Amer J Surg 1978;136:494–500.
53. Snow JB Jr, Gelber RD, Kramer S, et al: Evaluation of randomized preoperative and postoperative radiation therapy for supraglottic carcinoma: preliminary report. Annals of Otology, Rhinology and Laryngology 1978;87:686–691.
54. Fletcher GH: Subclinical disease. Cancer 1984;53:1274–1284.
55. Fisch U: Lymphographische Untersuchungen über das zervikale Lymphsystem. Bibliotheca Oto-Rhino-Laryngologica 1966;14:1–196.
56. Engeset A: Irradiation of lymph nodes and vessels: experiments in rats, with reference to cancer therapy. Acta Radiologica (Suppl 229) 1964:1–125.
57. Baker D, Elkon D, Lim M–L, et al: Does local X-irradiation of a tumor increase the incidence of metastases? Cancer 1981;48:2394–2398.
58. Lundy J, Lovett EJ III, Wolinsky SM, Conran P: Immune impairment and metastatic tumor growth: the need for an immunorestorative drug as an adjunct to surgery. Cancer 1979;43:945–951.
59. Yates A, Crumley RL: Surgical treatment of pyriform sinus cancer: A retrospective study. Laryngoscope 1984;94:1586–1590.
60. Carpenter RJ III, DeSanto LW, Devine KD, Taylor WF: Cancer of the hypopharynx: analysis of treatment and results in 162 patients. Arch Otolaryngology 1976;107:716–721.
61. Cohen L: Theoretical "iso-survival" formulae for fractionated radiation therapy. Brit J Radiology 1968;41:522–528.
62. Vikram B, Strong EW, Shah JP, Spiro R: Failure at distant sites following multimodality treatment for advanced head and neck cancer. Head Neck Surg 1984;6:730–733.
63. Arriagada R, Eschwege F, Cachin Y, Richard JM: The value of combining radiotherapy with surgery in the treatment of hypopharyngeal and laryngeal cancers. Cancer 1983;51:1819–1825.
64. Vikram B, Strong EW, Shah JP, Spiro R: Failure in the neck following multimodality treatment for advanced head and neck cancer. Head Neck Surg 1984;6:724–729.

# CHAPTER 9

# Laser Surgery in the Management of Head and Neck Cancer

*Robert H. Ossoff, DMD, MD and*
*James A. Duncavage, MD, FACS*

Laser is an acronym that means Light Amplification by the Stimulated Emission of Radiation. A laser is an electro-optical device that is usually a gas or crystal. The atoms of this lasing medium typically exist in nature at several different levels across the electromagnetic spectrum. When stimulated by an extrinsic energy source, these atoms emit electromagnetic radiation or photons in a narrow, intense beam. The light emitted from a laser, then, is organized light in direct contrast to the random pattern light that is emitted from the common light bulb. The key to this organization is stimulated emission.

Maiman discovered the first laser, a ruby laser with a wavelength of 0.69 microns (1960).[1] This laser emitted light in short pulses lasting only 1 millisecond or less; however, this discovery generated much interest in the scientific and medical fields and paved the way for the future development of lasers in medicine and surgery. Snitzer discovered the neodymium (Nd)-in-glass laser[2]; its output power surpassed that of the ruby laser (1961).

Interest in the field of medical research was stimulated by the development of these two lasers, especially with regard to the possible application of laser energy to treat and cure cancer. Investigators began to use both of these lasers on various tumor lines implanted in experimental animals, and it was quickly determined that the entire tumor had to be destroyed if a cure was to be achieved. This was relatively difficult with the lowered ruby and Nd-in-glass lasers because of the low absorbtion of these wavelengths in non-pigmented biologic tissue. To facilitate tumor destruction, the investigators

**122**

began to use higher and higher power densities of these two pulsed lasers. This in turn caused mechanical tissue disruption, propelling viable cancer cells elsewhere in the animal and into the laboratory environment (Ketcham 1967).[3] Needless to say, these findings had a significantly negative effect on the use of lasers in cancer research. However, the concept of differential absorption of laser light by biologic tissue was learned from these early experiments and this in turn stimulated the research and development of other lasers.

Interest in the carbon dioxide laser was stimulated by Yahr and Strully when they discovered that they could make a fine incision in skin and also perform a partial liver resection with minimal blood loss (Yahr and Strully 1966).[4] Encouraged by these findings, researchers in the laboratories of the American Optical Corporation developed a carbon dioxide laser system for surgical research.[5] Between 1967 and 1972, numerous concurrent investigations were undertaken in the various surgical specialties using this laser.

The development of an endoscopic delivery system for the carbon dioxide laser by Bredemeier in 1970 advanced the application of carbon dioxide laser energy to the larynx. In 1973, he went on to develop an attachment that coupled the laser beam manipulating arm to an operating microscope which allowed for precise microsurgical techniques in the larynx. This new coupler, called a micromanipulator, was used by Jako in a series of animal experiments and opened the door for clinical trials.[6,7]

The understanding of laser tissue interaction has furthered the use of lasers in head and neck oncology. The tissue effects produced by a laser vary with the wavelength of the laser and the composition of the tissue exposed to the laser beam. The electromagnetic energy of the carbon dioxide laser is absorbed by the tissue and converted to heat. The high water absorption coefficient of the carbon dioxide laser is independent of tissue color and is well absorbed by all soft tissue. When a specific amount of energy is absorbed by the tissue to bring the tissue temperature to 60° to 65°C, denaturation of protein occurs. Blanching of the tissue surface is visible and the deep structural integrity is disturbed. At 100°C, vaporization of intracellular water occurs with resultant vacuolization, cratering, and tissue shrinkage.[8] The high degree of carbon dioxide laser energy absorption in soft tissue with limited lateral thermal damage is the property that makes the carbon dioxide laser a precise surgical instrument for use in vaporizing tissue with a hands-off technique. The hallmark of the carbon dioxide lasers, then, is its surgical precision. The lateral zone of tissue damage extends less than 0.5mm from the impact point with current technology. Because of the precise localization of the carbon dioxide laser beam effect, as well as the sealing effects of the beam, surrounding tissue exhibits minimal edema and scarring.

The laser energy of the carbon dioxide laser cannot presently be passed through a fiber optic system. At present, the laser energy must be reflected via a series of mirrors through an articulating arm to the target tissue. The carbon dioxide laser energy can be used with a focused handpiece for macroscopic surgery, adapted to the operating microscope with a micromanipulator for microlaryngoscopy, or with the use of an endoscopic coupler attached to a rigid bronchoscope

The disadvantages associated with a rigid endoscopic carbon dioxide laser delivery system have prompted the development and use of the Neodymium: Yttrium Aluminum Garnet (Nd : YAG) laser in bronchoscopy. The water absorption of the Nd : YAG laser is low, allowing its energy to be transmitted through clear liquids. The extinction length of Nd : YAG laser energy in tissue is primarily determined by scattering. The energy from the laser beam expands rapidly within the target tissue and much of the energy is scattered both forward and backward through the target tissue. The volume in which the energy is distributed is 100 to 1000 times larger than for a carbon dioxide laser beam of equal spot size. A homogeneous zone of thermal coagulation and necrosis may extend four millimeters from the impact site, making precise tissue destruction impossible.

Argon lasers produce a visible blue-green light. The energy from an argon laser is readily transmitted though clear aqueous tissues. Hemoglobin and pigmented tissues strongly absorb the argon laser beam. The selective absorption of the argon laser energy by melanin and hemoglobin have made this laser an excellent instrument for treating vascular cutaneous lesions. The argon laser is not being used presently in the treatment of head and neck cancers.

The concept of photodynamic therapy has taken on increased emphasis in head and neck oncology with the understanding that laser energy can be absorbed by an injected intracellular photosensitizing drug. The energy from a laser is absorbed by the photosensitizing drug within the malignant cell causing a molecular reaction. This molecular reaction may result in fluorescence of the target tissue or the creation of an irreversible metabolic reaction resulting in the destruction of the cell. An argon pumped dye laser tuned to a specific wavelength of 630 nanometers plus or minus 2 nanometers is used to obtain maximum laser tissue penetration.[9]

## GENERAL REQUIREMENTS FOR LASERS

The carbon dioxide, neodymium: yttrium aluminum garnet, and the argon dye laser all generate heat within the lasing medium. The heat generated by the carbon dioxide laser is dissipated by a closed cooling system within the laser. The Nd : YAG and argon dye laser need an external water source for cooling and a drain for the coolant water runoff. In addition, special electrical adaptors are necessary for the Nd:YAG and argon dye lasers. A dedicated room, preferably within the operating room area, is most suitable for laser oncology. This room should conform to the recommendations of the American National Standards Institute Z136.3 for the Safe Use of Lasers in the Operating Room.

The surgical equipment necessary for laser surgery involves three basic principles. First, the instruments should be nonflammable. Second, the surfaces of the instruments should be nonreflective. Third, there must be a provision for the evacuation of smoke and steam from the operative site.[10]

## ANESTHETIC REQUIREMENTS

The choice of anesthetic technique and safety precautions necessary for laser surgery depend on the operative site and the wavelength of the laser to be used. Therefore, close cooperation between the oncologic surgeon and the anesthesiologist is required for a safe and successful procedure. In general, the oncologic surgeon will require an immobile surgical field with adequate exposure of the lesion. The anesthesiologist will need to provide adequate oxygenation and ventilation of the patient. The patient must have the appropriate depth of anesthesia necessary to accomplsih the surgical procedure.

The selection of an endotracheal tube is determined by the operative site and the wavelength of the laser. The endotracheal tube must be protected from impact by the carbon dioxide laser beam. A silastic or Rusch red rubber endotracheal tube should be wrapped with reflective alumium tape.[11,12] The use of the carbon dioxide laser in the oral cavity may allow for nasal tracheal intubation. In this situation, the endotracheal tube can be used unwrapped. However, it must be completely packed or covered with moistened gauze.

Anesthesia for bronchoscopic laser surgery depends on the surgical technique. Rigid bronchoscopy usually demands general anesthesia, while fiber optic bronchoscopy can be managed with either topical anesthesia and sedation or general anesthesia.[13] Carbon dioxide laser surgery requires rigid bronchoscopy, while the Nd:YAG laser can be used with either technique. However, most surgeons prefer rigid bronchoscopy for all but the smallest lesions.

Adequate precautions must be taken to protect the patient and operating room personnel. The patient's eyes and those of the operating room personnel must be protected with either conventional eyeglasses or clear plastic goggles with the carbon dioxide laser. Special green safety goggles are required for Nd:YAG laser eye protection. The patient's skin and oral region must be protected, and precautions to prevent a fire in the airway are mandatory. Warning signs must be posted for persons entering the operating room.

In as much as combustion may be initiated in the aerodigestive tract at high oxygen saturations or in the presence of methane, the lowest possible concentration of oxygen should be used in laryngotracheal procedures. Mixtures of helium, nitrogen, or room air plus oxygen are commonly used to maintain the $FIO_2$ around but not over 40% and also insure that the patient is adequately oxygenated. Nitrous oxide, like oxygen, is a potent oxidizing gas; therefore, it should not be used in the anesthetic mixture to cut the oxygen concentration.

The use of 100% oxygen during carbon dioxide and Nd:YAG laser bronchoscopy with a general anesthetic seems justified for two reasons. First, with a rigid bronchoscope, there is nothing more flammable than the patient's own tissue which usually provides a sufficient heat sink to prevent ignition. Second, the potent clinical inhalation anesthetics are not flammable in 100% oxygen at clinically useful concentrations.

## MALIGNANCIES OF THE TRACHEOBRONCHIAL TREE

Malignant tumors of the tracheobronchial tree have a distinct tendency to obstruct the major airways, causing obstructive pneumonitis and hypoxia. Surgery, radiation therapy and chemotherapy represent the standard modalities of treatment for these patients. Should their cancers recur, many of these patients will already have received the maximum allowable doses of ionizing radiation and most often their tumors will no longer be responsive to chemotherapy. Here, endoscopic treatment of airway obstruction as a form of palliation to prolong life in selected cases would seem indicated.

The hallmark of the carbon dioxide laser is its ability to precisely vaporize tissue. Because of this precise effect, the surrounding tissue exhibits minimal edema and scarring. Certain limitations are associated with using the carbon dioxide laser for endoscopic palliation of patients with obstructing tracheobronchial tumors.[14] First, the optics of the endoscopic couplers are poor when compared with the newer proximal vision rod lens systems used with the Nd:YAG laser. Second, hemostasis is limited to the microcirculation, vessels of 0.5mm and smaller, which raises difficulty with vascular tracheobronchial neoplasms. Frequently, hemostasis has to be obtained by placing adrenalin saturated pledgets on the tumor or using a bipolar suction cautery. Bronchoscopic carbon dioxide laser surgery is presently limited to a rigid delivery system.

The Nd:YAG laser offers the advantages of tumor coagulation with excellent hemostasis, decreased postoperative edema, excellent healing, and flexibility which would allow it to be directed to an upper lobe bronchus. The characteristics of thermal coagulation make the Nd : YAG laser a crude tool for precise cutting. The use of special sapphire tips on the Nd : YAG fiber may improve the cutting ability.

Airway distress caused by obstructing tracheobronchial tumors was successfully palliated in 19 of 24 patients using the carbon dioxide laser.[15] Tumor bleeding was not reported to be a major problem. In another series of patients with obstructing tracheobronchial malignancies, major intraoperative hemorrhage occurred in 3 of 34 patients treated with the carbon dixode laser bronchoscope.[16]

There is an overlap of use of both the carbon dioxide and Nd : YAG lasers in the tracheobronchial tree. When treating patients with relatively vascular lesions, such as obstructing carcinomas, the Nd : YAG laser is a better choice because of its high penetration and volume absorption.

The selection of patients for laser bronchoscopy is important. Only patients with obstructive intraluminal masses should be considered for palliation. Extrinsic tracheobronchial compression from mediastinal disease or tracheomalacia are contraindications to safe laser bronchoscopy. The Nd : YAG laser should be considered the laser of choice for obstructing malignant lesions of the tracheobronchial tree.[17] The oncologic surgeon should be experienced with both flexible and rigid bronchoscopy. The open rigid ventilating bronchoscope is the delivery system of choice for treating patients with major obstruction of the trachea and proximal bronchi.

Recent interest in employing photodynamic therapy for the management of early and late malignant neoplasms of the tracheobronchial tree has stimulated a long term, multi-institutional study to establish the indications for the use of photodynamic therapy.

## MALIGNANCIES OF THE LARYNX

The carbon dioxide laser is well suited for management of select early vocal cord carcinomas. Endoscopic management of early vocal cord cancers was presented by Lynch (1920).[18] New and Dorton reported a 90% cure rate in ten patients managed with transoral excision and diathermy (1941)[19] Lillie and DeSanto reported on 98 patients who were treated with transoral resection of early glottic carcinomas (1973).[20] Strong reported on 11 patients with early glottic carcinoma (1975).[21] These patients were treated by endoscopic excision with the carbon dioxide laser. Blakeslee used the carbon dioxide laser for excisional biopsy in 103 patients with $T_1$ glottic cancers.[22]

The transoral excision of squamous cell carcinoma of the larynx is an excellent use for the carbon dioxide laser. The advantage of precision, hemostasis, and decreased postoperative edema allow the oncologic surgeon to perform an excisional biopsy of midcordal lesions that may be curative if the surgical margins are negative. The biopsy can also establish the need for further therapy if the margins are positive.

Three distinct roles exist for the use of the carbon dioxide laser in the management of early glottic cancers. First, it is possible to excise bulky cancers, thereby allowing an accurate assessment of the size and depth of invasion of the tumor for purposes of staging. Second, airway re-establishment of the larynx is possible which may avoid the need for a tracheotomy.[23] Third, laser excision of cancer of the vocal cord can be curative if the margins are free of disease.

The anatomic limits of $CO_2$ laser cordectomy have been defined by Davis.[24] These limits can be used to guide the excision of mid true vocal cord lesions. Blakeslee reported in 1983 the evaluation and management of 103 $T_1$ glottic cancers. Their 3-year follow-up on the 103 patients found that the $CO_2$ laser excisional biopsy unequivocally established the diagnosis and stage of the disease. Further, if the margins of resection were free of tumor, the excision was considered curative treatment for the micro and mini squamous cell cancers.

Ossoff reported a 3-year follow-up of 25 patients with selected midcordal squamous cell carcinomas treated by $CO_2$ laser excisional biopsy.[25] They reported that when the biopsy margins were negative for tumor, the 3-year follow-up revealed a disease control rate of 100%.

The management of patients with early cancer confined to the true vocal cords includes an excisional biopsy with the carbon dioxide laser. Supravital staining with toluidine blue is performed as a diagnostic aid prior to biopsy. The surgical specimen must be labeled and oriented prior to frozen section exam. Any questionable margins are controlled by frozen section to the limits of endoscopic cordectomy.

The advantages with carbon dioxide laser excision of patients with early laryngeal cancer include accuracy associated with use of the operating microscope, minimal morbidity, and cost effectiveness if the excisional biopsy is curative. The major advantage of this treatment option is its ability to differentiate deeply invasive early midcordal $T_1$ glottic cancers from those that are truly superficial in nature and establishes the need for further treatment in those cases with deep invasion.

The Nd:YAG laser has not been used to treat cancers of the larynx because of its lack of precision. However, the use of special saphire tips may allow for precise cutting of tissue. The role of photodynamic therapy for early diagnosis and treatment of laryngeal cancer has not been established.

## MALIGNANCIES OF THE ORAL CAVITY

Strong recognized the unique properties of the carbon dioxide laser for management of oral malignancies.[26] They used a carbon dioxide laser coupled to an operating microscope to perform trans-oral tumor resections. They noted the advantages of this modality were its precision, hemostasis, decreased postoperative edema, and pain. They also noted minimal morbidity.

The standard techniques for resecting tumors of the oral cavity all have shortcomings. The use of sharp dissection with a scapel or scissors to remove a tumor from the oral cavity can be difficult due to the highly vascular oral mucous membrane. The troublesome bleeding that occurs makes identification of tumor margins difficult. The degree of tissue handling with this technique to produce adequate visualization can result in significant edema postoperatively. The use of an electrosurgical cutting diathermy unit to remove tumors of the oral cavity has the advantage of controlling the bleeding from the vascular oral mucosa. The degree of lateral heat dissipation to adjacent tissue can be vividly seen when examining specimen margins. This thermal tissue injury is the main disadvantage to the use of this modality in the oral cavity. The damage caused to the surrounding tissues can lead to excessive postoperative edema and pain. The degree of scarring and contracture may be excessive. The ability of the pathologist to read specimen tumor margin control can be compromised due to the heat coagulation of the tissue. The use of cryosurgery for palliative tumor control is cumbersome and precise tumor destruction can be difficult. The amount of postoperative edema can be extensive.

Cancer of the oral cavity represents a broad range of disease. The early diagnosis is dependent on selective accurate tissue examination. The ability to precisely examine those areas of the oral mucosa that appear abnormal under the operating microscope represents a significant advance in the treatment of head and neck cancer. The traditional trans-oral resection of carcinoma of the oral cavity was complicated by lack of adequate visualization.[27] The risk of postoperative edema was high. A tracheotomy to control the airway and allow for working room was frequently a necessity. The introduction of the carbon dioxide laser for the use of excisional biopsies of the oral cavity may lead to the early diagnosis of cancer. The decreased pain and edema make this modality a desirable treatment tool for those patients with multiple areas of dysplastic oral mucosa. The laser can be used repeatedly unlike ionizing radiation which has a limiting tissue tolerance dose.

The necessity of an adequate margin must be maintained even when using the laser for excisional biopsy. The clinical staging of cancers of the oral cavity can at times be difficult because of the inability to judge the extent of deep tumor involvement. Those patients presenting with clinical leukoplakia, erythroplakia, and small invasive cancers are treated with the carbon dioxide laser. The initial biopsy is done in the operating room with either a regional anesthetic block or under general anesthesia depending on the anatomical location and patient tolerance. The laser is coupled to an operating microscope and the patient is placed in the supine position with the neck extended. All cutaneous surfaces of the face are covered with moist surgical towels and the eyes of the patient are covered with moist eyepads. The teeth are protected with moistened telfa strips. The infiltration of a local anesthetic is avoided because of the tissue distortion and increase in tissue fluid content. All lesions are stained with a supravital stain Toluidine blue.[28] The suspicious area is excised with the carbon dioxide laser and the specimen is placed on a saline saturated specimen mount, oriented, and hand carried to the pathologist.

All of the laser excisions of the oral cavity are gently wiped with a saline-soaked sponge to remove the charred carbonaceous debris. This debris will cause a foreign body giant cell reaction.[29]

## SAFETY PRECAUTIONS

Educational programs and qualification procedures must be set up for physicians using the laser, anesthesia personnel, nursing staff and technical support staff. A laser safety committee and laser safety officer have to be appointed. Adequate protective measures for the control of laser hazards should be established and an action plan for the management of a known or suspected laser-related accident should be prepared.[30]

The laser safety committee should appoint the laser safety officer. Additional responsibilities of the laser safety committee include the formulation of a laser safety program and the establishment of qualification requirements. In otolaryngology – head and neck surgery, attendance at a hands-on training course by those members of our specialty not trained in laser surgery during residency would be the minimum requirement. These courses should be 16 to 20 hours in duration with approximately 50% devoted to actual hands-on experience. As additional wavelengths proliferate within our specialty, further hands-on training would be required. Anesthesia personnel, nursing staff and technical support staff must also be trained in laser safety; the nursing staff, in addition, should receive hands-on orientation and training with the laser and its attachments. The committee must keep a list of all physicians approved to use each laser; this list should be available in the operating room or endoscopy suite. Finally, any case involving laser-related morbidity or mortality must be reviewed by the laser safety committee.

The laser safety officer is responsible for the hazard evaluation and classification of each laser installation. Additional responsibilities include the establishment of control measures, implementation of the safety program, initiation of medical surveillance and evaluation of special considerations such as electrical hazards, explosion hazards, optical radiation hazards, fume control, endotracheal tubes, oxygen and flammable gasses, and endoscopes.

To reduce the risk of ocular damage during cases involving the laser, certain precautions should be followed. Protection of the eyes of the patient and surgeon must be addressed; here, the actual protective device will vary according to the wavelength of the laser utilized.

For patients undergoing carbon dioxide laser surgery of the upper aerodigestive tract, a double layer of saline moistened eye pads should be placed over the eyes. All operating room personnel should wear protective glasses with side protectors. When working with the operating microscope, the surgeon need not wear protective glasses; in this case, the optics of the microscope itself provide the necessary protection.

When working with the Nd: YAG laser, all operating room personnel and the patient must wear wavelength specific protective glasses. Special wavelength specific filters are available for the flexible and rigid bronchoscopes; when the filters are in place, the surgeon need not wear protective glasses.

When working with the argon or argon tunable dye laser, all personnel in the operating room including the patient should wear wavelength specific protective glasses which are usually of an amber color. When performing photocoagulation procedures for selected cutaneous vascular lesions of the face, protective metal eye shields rather than protective glasses are usually worn by the patient.

All exposed skin and mucous membranes of the patient outside of the surgical field should be protected by a double layer of saline saturated surgical towels, surgical sponges, or lap pads. When performing microlaryngeal laser surgery, there exists the possibility that the beam might partially reflect off of the proximal rim of the laryngoscope, rather than go down it. For this reason, the patient's face is completely draped with saline saturated surgical towels, exposing only the proximal lumen of the laryngoscope. Great care must be exercised to keep the wet draping from drying out; it should be, therefore, moistened from time to time during the case. Teeth in the operative field also need to be protected; here, saline saturated telfa, surgical sponges, or specially constructed metal dental impression trays can be utilized. Meticulous attention is paid to the protective draping procedures at the beginning of the case; the same compulsive should be displayed for the continued protection of the skin and teeth during the case.

Two separate suction setups should be available for all cases in the upper aerodigestive tract; one provides for adequate smoke and steam evacuation from the operative field, while the second is connected to the surgical suction tip for the aspiration of blood and mucous from the operative wound. When performing laser surgery with a closed anesthetic system, constant suctioning should be used to remove laser-induced smoke from the operating room; this helps to prevent inhalation by the patient, surgeon, or operating room personnel. When the anesthetic system used is an open one, or when working with jet ventilation systems, suctioning should be limited to an intermittent basis to maintain the $FIO_2$ at a safe level. Laryngoscopes, bronchoscopes, operating platforms, mirrors, and anterior commissure and ventricle retractors with built-in smoke evacuating channels facilitate the easy evacuation of smoke from the operative field. Filters in the suction lines should be used to prevent clogging by the black carbonaceous smoke debris created by the carbon dioxide laser.

Optimal anesthetic management of the patient undergoing laser surgery of the upper aerodigestive tract must include attention to the safety of the patient, the requirements of the surgeon, and the hazards of the equipment, including the endotracheal tube. During carbon dioxide laser surgery in the aerodigestive tract (oral cavity, nasopharynx, larynx, or tracheobronchial tree), the endotracheal tube, when used, must be protected. Anesthesia personnel shall use non-flammable endotracheal tubes or red rubber or 100% silicone tubes wrapped circumferentially from the cuff to the top with reflective, metallic tape. The cuff should be inflated with methylene blue-colored saline and neurosurgical cottonoids placed above the cuff in the subglottic larynx. These cottonoids need to be moistened frequently during the procedure. Use of the operating platform is strongly recommended as a further insulation against damage to the cuff. Should the cuff become deflated from an errant hit by the laser beam, the tube should be removed and replaced with a new one.

The Nd : YAG laser has a different interaction with endotracheal tubes than the carbon dioxide laser. In vitro testing of various endotracheal tubes with the Nd : YAG laser has demonstrated that the safest tube to use is a colorless, or white, polyvinyl endotracheal tube or silicone endotracheal tube without any black or dark colored lettering on the tube itself. Also, the tube should not have any lead-lined marking.

## FUTURE DIRECTIONS

The most immediate future application of lasers in head and neck cancer is the concept of photodynamic therapy. Photodynamic therapy is a relatively new modality which utilizes a photosensitizing drup that selectively localizes in tumors and is activated by exposure to light.

The fluorescence of tumors following administration of a photosensitizing drug and exposure to light has been demonstrated in numerous experimental and clinical settings.[31-36] The potential to use the fluorescence to detect lesions that are clinically non-apparent and to determine the extent of tumors has led to multi-institutional investigative studies.

The oral cavity is an excellent area because of its ease of visualization and the propensity for the mucosa to develop early changes suggestive of squamous cell carcinoma. Because of the diffuse nature of these changes and because the macroscopic changes of leukoplakia and erythroplakia are frequently subtle, great difficulty can be encountered in determining whether a suspicious area is benign or malignant.

The use of fluorescence detection to identify those areas of the upper aerodigestive tract that are malignant may represent a significant advance in the early diagnosis of head and neck cancer.

The use of photodynamic therapy to treat patients with early cancers of the head and neck represents another possible advancement. When a photosensitizing drug is injected into a patient, the concentration in tumor at 48 hours is higher than in the surrounding tissues. The absorption of light by the photosensitizing drug hematoporphyrin derivative (HPD) occurs at many wavelengths.[37] The wavelength of 630 nanometers is used because it offers the greatest skin penetration of approximately one centimeter.

The use of sapphire tips for Nd:YAG fibers may be a significant advance for YAG bronchoscopy. The present problems of YAG fiber tips melting or burning off can be overcome by the sapphire contact probe. In addition, it is reported that tissue injury is more precise.

The use of carbon dioxide lasers to excise tumors using short pulse rather than continuous wave may offer more precise tissue cutting with less lateral thermal damage. The introduction of a carbon dioxide laser called a Transverse Electric Atmospheric (TEA) Laser can produce pulse widths as short as 2 picoseconds. This has been reported to result in no visible charring and a zone of thermal damage 50 to 100 microns in width.

Finally, the free-electron laser has many attractive features not simultaneously available with any other laser system. These include broad band tunable operation, high average power, and short pulses. These features could improve the ability to excise or ablate head and neck cancer.

## REFERENCES

1. Maiman TH: Stimulated optical radiation in ruby. Nature 1960;187:493–494.
2. Snitzer E: Optical master action of $Nd^3+$ in Ba crown glass. Phys Rev Lett 1961;7:444.

3. Ketcham AS, Hoye RC, Riggle GC: A surgeon's appraisal of the laser. Surg Clin North Am 1967;47:1249–1263.
4. Yahr WZ, Strully KJ: Blood vessel anastomosis and other biomedical applications. J Assoc Adv Med Inst 1966;1:28–31.
5. Polany TG, Bredemeier HC, David TW, Jr: $CO_2$ laser for surgical research. Med Biol Eng Comput 1970;8:548–558.
6. Jako, GJ: Laser surgery of the vocal cords: an experimental study with carbon dioxide lasers on dogs. Laryngoscope 1972;82:2204–2216.
7. Strong MS, Jako GJ: Laser surgery in the larynx, early clinical experience with continuous $CO_2$ laser. Ann Oto Rhinol Laryngol 1972;81:791–798.
8. Mihashi S, Jako GJ, Incze J, et al: Laser surgery in otolaryngology: interaction of $CO_2$ laser and soft tissue. Ann NY Acad Sci 1976;267:263.
9. Ossoff RH, Pelzer HJ, Atiyah RA, et al: Potential applications of photoradiation therapy in head and neck surgery. Arch Otolaryngol 1984;110:728–730.
10. Ossoff RH, Karlan MS: Safe instrumentation in laser surgery. Otolaryngol Head Neck Surg 1984;92:644.
11. Ossoff RH, Duncavage JA, Eisenman TS et al: Comparison of tracheal damage from laser-ignited endotracheal tube fires. Ann Oto Rhinol Laryngol 1983;92:333–336.
12. Duncavage JA, Ossoff RH, Rouman WC et al: Injuries to the bronchi and lungs caused by laser-ignited endotracheal tube fires. Otolaryngol Head Neck Surg 1984;92:639–643.
13. Eisenman TS, Ossoff RH: Anesthesia for bronchoscopic laser surgery. Otolaryngol Head Neck Surg 1986;94:45–46.
14. Ossoff RH, Duncavage JA, Toohill RJ et al: Limitations of bronchoscopic carbon dioxide laser surgery. Ann Otology Rhinol Laryngol 1985;94:498–501.
15. Ossoff RH, Duncavage JA, Gluckman JL et al: Universal endoscopic coupler for broncho-scopic $CO_2$ laser surgery: A multi-institutional clinical trial. Otolaryngol Head Neck Surg 1985;93:824–830.
16. Shapshay SM, Davis RK, Vaughan CW et al: Palliation of airway obstruction from tra-cheobronchial malignancy: use of the $CO_2$ laser bronchoscope. Otolaryngol Head Neck Surg 1983;91:615–619.
17. Shapshay SM, Dumon JF, Beamis JF: Endoscopic treatment of tracheobronchial malig-nancy: experience with Nd-YAG and $CO_2$ lasers in 506 operations. Otolaryngol Head Neck Surg 1985;93:205–210.
18. Lynch RC: Intrinsic carcinoma of the larynx with a second report of the cases operated on by suspension and dissection. Trans Am Laryngol Assoc 1920;43:119–126.
19. New GU, Dorton HE: Suspension laryngoscopy and the treatment of malignant disease of the hypopharynx and larynx. Mayo Clin Proc 1941;16:411–416.
20. Lille J, DeSanto L: Transoral surgery of early cordal carcinoma. Trans Am Acad Ophthal-mol Otolaryngol 1973;77:92–96.
21. Strong, MS: Laser excision of carcinoma of the larynx. Laryngoscope 1975;85:1286.
22. Blakeslee D, Vaughan CW, Shapshay SM, et al: Excisional biopsy in the selective manage-ment of $T_1$ glottic cancer: a three year follow-up study. Laryngoscope 1984;94:448–494.
23. Davis RK, Shapshay SM, Vaughan CW et al: Pretreatment airway management in ob-structing carcinoma of the larynx. Otolaryngol Head Neck Surg 1981;89:209–214.
24. Davis RK, Jako GJ, Hyams VJ, et al: The anatomic limitations of $CO_2$ laser cordectomy. Laryngoscope 1982;92:980–984.
25. Ossoff RH, Sisson GA, Shapshay SM: Endoscopic management of selected early vocal cord carcinoma. Ann Otology Rhino Laryngo 1985;94:560–564.
26. Strong MS, Vaughan CW, Healy GB, et al: Transoral management of localized carcinoma of the oral cavity using the $CO_2$ laser. Laryngoscope 1979;89:897–905.

27. King GD: Transoral resection for cancer of the oral cavity. Otolaryngol Clin N Am 1972;5:321–325.
28. Vaughan CW: Supravital staining for early diagnosis for carcinoma. Otolaryngol Clin N Am 1972;5:301–302.
29. Durkin GE, Duncavage JA, Toohill RJ, et al: Wound healing of true vocal cord squamous epithelium following $CO_2$ laser ablation and cup forcep stripping. Las Vegas, NV, Presentation, Am Acad of Otolaryngology-Head and Neck Surgery, 1984.
30. Schamm VL, Mattox DE, Stool, SE: Acute management of laser ignited intratracheal explosion. Laryngoscope 1981;91:1417–1425.
31. Auler H, Banzer G: Untersuchungen uber die rolle der prophone bei geschwulstkranken menschen und tieren. *Z Krebforsch* 1942;53:65–68.
32. Figge FHJ, Weiland GS, Manganiello LOJ: Cancer detection and therapy. Affinity of neoplastic embryonic and traumatized regenerating tissues for porphyrins and metalloporphyrins. Proc Soc Exptl Biol Med 1948;68:640–641.
33. Lipson, RL: The photodynamic and flourescent properties of a particular hematoporphyrin derivative and its use in tumor detection. Master's Thesis, University of Minnesota, 1960
34. Hematoporphyrin derivative: a new aid of endoscopic detection of malignant disease. J Thor Cardiovasc Surg 1961;42:623.
35. Gregorie HB, Horger EO, Ward JL, et al: Hematoporphyrin derivative fluorescence in malignant neoplasms. Ann Surg 1968;167:820–827.
36. Lipson RL, Baldes EJ, Olsen AM: A further evaluation of the use of hematoporphyrin derivative as a new aid for the endoscopic detection of malignant disease. Dis Chest 1964;46:676.
37. Dougherty TJ, Potter WR, Weishaupt KR: The structure of the active component of Hematoporphyrin derivative: a new aid of endoscopic detection of malignant disease. J. Thor Cardiovasc Surg 1961;42:623.

# CHAPTER 10

# The Physiologic Basis of Reconstruction of the Head and Neck Cancer Defect

*Martin C. Robson, MD*

The defect resulting from surgical removal of head and neck tumors can cause functional, as well as socially unacceptable, cosmetic deformities. These defects can disrupt the physiology of all, or part, of the anatomical region. The function of the face is to look normal and to provide identity for the patient. It must also encompass the structures which allow the patient to communicate and to eat and breathe normally. Anyone attempting to reconstruct this specialized area must be equipped to perform any of the multiple procedures available today. He must also develop the judgment to choose the appropriate procedure and timing to effect the best reconstruction for his patient. To do this requires a firm foundation in the physiologic bases of reconstructive techniques.

Although timing of reconstruction has been a debatable issue in the past, the overwhelming opinion today is to perform immediate reconstruction. The only absolute contraindication to the immediate repair and/or reconstruction is when it is not technically feasible to perform the reconstruction in one stage. This situation should rarely occur if the extent of the resection is planned ahead and the surgeon has the physiologic understanding and technical ability to perform all possible reconstructive procedures including those using microvascular techniques.

The problem that presents itself too often is that many surgeons today have failed to learn the physiologic bases of the alternatives for head and neck reconstruction. This occurred, I believe, with the discovery of the musculocutaneous flap in 1977,[1,2] and its reported utility in reconstruction of the head and neck in 1979 and 1980.[3-6] The simplicity of the sternocleidomastoid and pectoralis major musculocutaneous flaps yielded an apparent solution to the many complexities presented by the cancer defect. However, the musculocutaneous flaps are not the universal solution. They may give too much bulk, may be limited by pedicles, and in selected circumstances may result in less than an optimal functional and aesthetic result. Total reliance on them may preclude the surgeon from understanding the physiology and utility of the remainder of the reconstructive armamentarium.

To properly approach reconstruction of the head and neck defect, one must outline the goals of the intended reconstruction. The major goals are to provide a means for the patient to breathe as normally as possible, to eat, and to speak. If this is to be achieved, tissue which has been resected needs to be replaced by like tissue. Surface defects are almost always contiguous with body cavity defects, necessitating both lining and covering tissue. The tissue must at times be both pliable and rigid. An important precept which has been overstated is the use of bulk. When intraoral resections were lined with skin grafts, speech and swallowing were a severe problem. Bakamjian pointed out the need for bulk.[7] Unfortunately, the pendulum has swung too far. Often bulky musculocutaneous flaps are used when much less bulky tissue would be optimal. Therefore, another goal is to provide bulk *only* when bulk is needed. Finally, preservation of the patients' "body image" must remain a goal. Simple physiologic maneuvers such as making incisions in Kraissel's lines of minimum tension whenever possible or splitting the lip to preserve normal muscle function can help attain the latter goal.[8,9]

There are many options for reconstruction of the head and neck cancer defect. These include autogenous tissue and alloplastic material. Normal physiology is best maintained with autogenous tissue. Soft tissue defects in the head and neck region, like those elsewhere on the body, can be closed by direct approximation, free skin grafts, pedicled tissue (using local, regional, or distant flaps), or by free flaps transferred by microvascular anastomoses. Skeletal tissue is best provided by living vascularized bone grafts or flaps. Nonvascularized bone grafts or alloplastic material can, on occasion, provide satisfactory bone replacement.

The first consideration in repairing any defect is whether the tissues can be primarily approximated and whether healing by first intention can be effected. Tension is a major problem with primary approximation. This will lead to tissue ischemia and wound disruption. When this occurs in an intraoral closure, it results in a salivary fistula and puts the carotid artery in jeopardy. Even if a tension-free closure can be performed and healing accomplished, it should not be done if it increases the functional and/or aesthetic deformity. Primary closure of the hemiglossectomy defect may result in healing but with a non-mobile tongue which leaves the patient with unintelligible speech. Primary intraoral approximation is often possible following partial mandiblectomy when a rigid structure has been excised. This allows the tissues to collapse somewhat and a tension-free closure can be performed without significant functional disability.

Primary approximation of the external skin is frequently possible in head and neck reconstruction. This is especially true when the pathophysiology of the tumor dictates the resection. Skin should be sacrificed only when involved by tumor. Violation or sacrifice of intact skin only for access is usually unnecessary and is best avoided. As mentioned previously, skin incisions and excisions can be carefully planned and whenever possible placed in lines of minimum tension.

If a defect is too large to allow a tension free closure with adequate functional mobility, the principle of rapid skin expansion can be used. Skin expanders have been quite useful in allowing adjacent skin to be stretched prior to reconstruction. In a relatively short period of time 400–700 cc of expanded volume will allow the overlying stretched skin to reconstruct the defect by direct approximation. The physiology of skin expansion is similar to the surgical "delay" procedure and will be discussed later.

If direct approximation is not possible, either primarily or following skin expansion, a free skin graft can be considered. Skin grafts can be either split-thickness or full-thickness. Intraoral grafts are usually moderate split-thickness. They remain quite useful for lining the defect following a maxillectomy and resurfacing the floor of mouth in the case of field cancerization. Esser's inlay technique, described almost 70 years ago, continues to have applicability in the oral pharynx to recreate the mandibulo-labial sulcus.[10] Skin grafts are also useful for external reconstruction. Full-thickness grafts can give the best color and texture match to the surrounding skin. When the defect is not too large, good results can be obtained using post-auricular or supra-clavicular skin. Larger external defects can be resurfaced with moderately thick split-thickness grafts. Donor sites chosen from cephalad to the nipples give a more satisfactory color and texture match for facial grafts. The scalp can provide an excellent donor site. Its size allows grafts to resurface full aesthetic units and its pore size is particularly suitable for the male face.

Although skin grafts can be useful in selected situations of head and neck reconstruction, they have several disadvantages. Frequently the heavily radiated defect bed will not adequately support graft "take" and survival. The free graft does not inhibit wound infection. A bone graft cannot be placed beneath the skin graft, nor can other secondary procedures be performed beneath the free skin graft.

Pedicled skin flaps, compound flaps, and free flaps are the workhorses of head and neck reconstruction. They can provide bulk when bulk is needed. They can bring needed blood supply to an area to aid healing and eradication of infection. The flaps's blood supply can provide a route to delivery chemotherapy directly to the margins of the resection. Finally, a flap allows future procedures to be done beneath it, such as placement of a bone graft, and a viable flap can provide greater protection to arteries and nerves.

Functional and cosmetic deformities often cannot be avoided without bony reconstruction in addition to soft tissue reconstruction. Several methods of mandibular reconstruction are available. Rib grafts, carved iliac crest grafts, and cancellous bone chips (all from autogenous sources) are the most popular. Regardless of the method of bone grafting used, graft survival varies from 20–90%.[11] Failure is due to some combination of poor blood supply, insufficient cover, fistulae, infection, an avascular graft bed, or inadequate immobilization. Recent attempts at avoiding the problems with free bone grafting for mandibular restoration have been the living osteocutaneous flaps, the musculo-osteocutaneous flaps, and the composite vascularized bone graft transferred by microsurgical vascular anastomoses.[12,13]

Although autogenous tissue appears to be preferable for all phases of head and neck reconstruction, alloplastic appliances continue to be investigated. Alloplastic external cover is never satisfactory to the patient for long term external reconstruction. Although often meeting many of the goals outlined for reconstruction, it usually fails to satisfy the patient's "body image." However, alloplastic external cover may provide temporary cover while the patient undergoes adjuvant therapy or while following the course of an extremely aggressive tumor.

Of all the alternatives discussed briefly above, flaps are the most useful method for head and neck reconstruction. These flaps can be local, regional, pararegional, or from a distant source. They may have a random blood supply from the subdermal vascular plexus, contain a direct axial arteriovenous network, or derive the blood supply from perforating vessels from the underlying muscle. Any of these flaps can be moved into position with their pedicles intact or have their vessel pedicles divided and reanastomosed to an appropriate recipient artery and vein in the defect. A comprehension of the vasular physiology of these flaps is crucial to their utilization.

The cutaneous flap based on a random blood supply from the subdermal plexus has severe limitations in the head and neck area. These flaps must be local in origin and have strict design limitations. Classically, the flap must have a 1 : 1 length : base ratio to assure survival. Being localized to the area of the defect, the vascular supply of the flap may be involved in radiation ports. Kinking or twisting of the flap results in venous obstruction. Despite these drawbacks, random blood supply flaps may be useful in specific situations. Local adjacent tissue can provide the best texture and color match for external reconstruction. Since external reconstruction of the head and neck region generally means the face, some unique features about facial blood supply renders these flaps feasible. Corso has demonstrated that because of the rich blood supply to the face, almost any random flap designed on the face is, in effect, an axial flap containing an arteriovenous network.[14] This removes the dimension limitations of the classical cutaneous or random flap. Therefore, the nasolabial flap, or the Gillies fan flap can be constructed with large length: base ratios and be transferred primarily without requiring "delay" procedures.

The dimensional limitations imposed by the blood supply of a cutaneous or random flap are removed when the flap is based on an axial blood supply from a direct cutaneous artery and vein. The length of such a flap is the length of the specific "watershed"area derived from the artery. The width only need be that necessary to include the artery and vein. Milton and Daniel have demonstrated that the skin bridge is unnecessary at the base of an axial flap.[15,16] This physiologic fact can be used to great advantage in head and neck reconstruction. It means that a bulky pedicle is unnecessary and that paddles of skin can be placed intraorally through small access ports. It also means that venous obstruction due to kinking is less likely to occur than with a random blood supply flap.

The deltopectoral flap is the prototype for axial flaps from the pararegional sources useful in head and neck reconstruction. Although originally designed for replacement of the cervical esophagus, it remains useful for both external cover and internal lining of the oropharyngeal cavity. Based on the perforating intercostal arteries and veins from the internal mammary vessels, a large rectangular-shaped flap can be designed along a variable distance on the shoulder depending on the measured need. An important characteristic of this flap, differentiating it from from most flaps, is its pivot point.[17] Its effective length is measured from the proximal portion of its upper border rather than from its lower border. Therefore, it can be used to reconstruct any defect in an area within a radius no longer than the length of its upper border. Delay procedures are not necessary with this flap, since its base contains the dominant blood supply.

Several other axial flaps deserve mention. The forehead flap and the occipital-based shoulder flap have lost their popularity in head and neck reconstruction. However, they remain useful when primary flaps have failed, in cases of recurrent cancer, and occasionally as a life-saving measure. The total forehead flap based on the temporal and post-auricular arteries remains one of the safest flaps, and one of the easiest quickest flaps to perform in an emergency situation. It can easily resurface the floor of the mouth and separate it from the neck contents. Axial flaps also remain the flaps of choice for nasal reconstruction. Forehead tissue carried on the supratrochlear and/or supraorbital vessels give pliable tissue to reconstruct either a part or all of the nose.

Musculocutaneous flaps are nourished by musculocutaneous perforating vessels from the segmental arteries of muscles. The experimental and clinical recognition of these vessels and their predictable presence between muscle masses and the overlying skin by McCraw, Dibbell, and Caraway is one of the great advances in head and neck reconstruction.[1,2] Ariyan has further demonstrated that musculocutaneous flaps can behave either like random flaps or axial flaps.[12] In the head and neck area, the pectoralis major, trapezius, and latissimus dorsi muscles are flat muscles and have an axial blood supply. Therefore, musculocutaneous flaps based on these muscles can have thin pedicles and can have multiple paddles. Round muscles such as the sternocleidomastoid have only perforating vessels. Therefore, musculocutaneous flaps based on the sternocleidomastoid muscle must include the whole muscle and cannot be split. When attempts are made to split these flaps, one would expect them to become devascularized.

Musculocutaneous flaps have several advantages. First, they provide excellent blood supply to the defect when correctly executed. This is useful in heavily radiated wounds and as Ariyan has demonstrated; in non-radiated wounds, these flaps can tolerate larger doses of postoperative radiation without difficulty.[12] The muscle brings in needed blood supply to eradicate bacteria in a contaminated area. Although this was originally thought to be due to a special property of muscle, it has now been shown to be only due to the musculocutaneous flap's more liberal blood flow. In the face of minimal or moderate wound contamination, the musculocutaneous flaps can decrease the wound bacterial count more effectively than can a similar flap without muscle.[19] In a heavily contaminated wound, no flaps can eradicate the bateria, and placing even a musculocutaneous flap into such a wound is courting disaster and inviting flap necrosis. A final advantage of the musculocutaneous flap is its ability to bring living bone with it to the defect. This has been demonstrated for both the pectoralis major and latissimus dorsi musculocutaneous flaps.[12,13]

The disadvantage of bulky pedicles with all pedicled flaps has been mentioned. In some cases, this may cause a controlled salivary fistula to be created until sectioning of the pedicle. Pedicled flaps also must come from a region not far from the defect. Because of these drawbacks, flaps from a distant source have been devised to be transferred to the head and neck region by division of the pedicles and reanastomosis in the recipient area. These free flaps can be either axial pattern skin flaps, musculocutaneous flaps, or compound flaps containing bone. Large series are now appearing showing the utility of free flap reconstruction. When massive amounts of tissue are needed, free flap reconstruction may become the method of choice. Success rates in excess of 90% make these flaps a necessary part of the armamentarium.

When the vascular physiologic basis of each type of flap available for head and neck reconstruction is understood, specific needs of an individual case can be met. If tissue is simultaneously needed both internally and externally, flaps can be split either longitudinally or tangentially depending on the blood supply.[19] Paddles of skin can be provided whenever necessary if the integrity of the flap vasculature is preserved. Occasionally in non-irradiated facial skin, the blood supply is so rich as to allow skin paddles to survive only on pedicles of subcutaneous tissue. Knowledge of this phenomenon is very useful in using the naso-labial flap for nasal or intraoral reconstruction.

Despite our increasing knowledge of flap physiology, the failing flap remains a devastating complication of head and neck reconstruction. To have a well-designed and well-executed flap slowly necrose at its distal tip renders the flap useless in attaining the goals of reconstruction. Recent knowledge of the pathophysiology of the distal dying flap has allowed progressive necrosis to be prevented and this complication to be minimized. Certain inflammatory mediators, specifically, prostanoid derivatives of archidonic acid, have been implicated in progressive ischemic tissue death in several conditions. Zachary et al and Reus et al. have shown that thromboxane production in the distal flap tip adds to ischemia and cell death.[20-22] Inhibition of the thromboxane can increase the surviving lengths of such flaps. Similarly, administration of exogenus prostacyclin is of benefit in flap salvage. These experimental observations are useful to reverse what appears to be an ischemic insult clinically. Early application of anti-prostanoid drugs can salvage a complex reconstruction. This technique has proved useful in pedicle flaps of all vascular bases as well as in free flaps.

Understanding the role of inflammatory mediators in flap necrosis has yielded useful information in overall flap physiology.[23] Flap elevation produces inflammatory mediators, specifically thromboxane. In a poorly conceived flap, with excess ischemia, this production is significantly high to give more vasoconstriction increasing the ischemia and resulting in flap death. If the initial ischemia is controlled by the flap design, the thromboxane production decreases over time. This explains how surgical "delay" procedures work in random flaps to increase the amount of tissue that can be transferred.[23] Subsequently, elevation of a delayed flap will produce a blunted response in thromboxane production and increase flap survival. With the knowledge that surgical delay procedures are an example of the inflammatory response, pharmacological delay procedures can be achieved.[24] Using these physiological tissue responses, the random or cutaneous flaps may achieve greater usefulness in head and neck reconstruction, since size limitations will decrease. Also the "watershed" area of a given vascular supply of an axial, musculocutaneous, or free flap can theoretically now be increased by pharmacologic delay procedures. This should allow the surgeon to design the size and shape flap necessary to effect the ideal functional and aesthetic reconstruction. These same physiologic principles of inflammation are thought to be active in the expanded skin flap. Rapid skin expansion has been likened to a "delay'" procedure.[25] Tolerance to the inflammatory mediators during the period of expansion are possibly what allows the random flap with much greater dimensions to be successfully transferred.

As greater numbers of patients with head and neck cancer survive because of medical advances, more emphasis must be placed not only on making life more bearable, but worthwhile for those survivors.[26] Bakamjian and Cramer have stated that surgeons have been unwilling and hesitant to perform adequately extensive excisions for advanced cancer because of the fear of producing functional, aesthetic, and social cripples.[27] If this can be prevented by functional and aesthetically acceptable immediate reconstruction, this hesitancy should disappear. Hopefully, having a sound physiologic basis for the reconstruction options will allow this to occur for the benefit of the head and neck cancer patient.

## REFERENCES

1. McCraw JB, Dibbell DG: Experimental definition of independent myocutaneous vascular territories. Plast Reconstr Surg 1977;60:212–220.
2. McCraw JB, Dibbell DG, Carraway JH: Clinical definition of independent myocutaneous vascular territories. Plast Reconstr Surg 1977;60:341–352.
3. Ariyan S: The pectoralis major myocutaneous flap: A versatile flap for reconstruction in the head and neck. Plast Reconstr Surg 1979; 63:73–81.
4. Ariyan S: One-stage reconstruction for defects of the mouth using a sternocleidmastoid myocutaneous flap. Plast Reconstr Surg 1979;63:618–625.
5. Ariyan S: Further experiences with the pectoralis major myocutaneous flap for the immediate repair of defects from excisions of the head and neck. Plast Reconstr Surg 1979;64:605–612.
6. McCraw JB, Magec WP, Kalwaic H: Uses of the trapezius and sternocleidmastoid myocutaneous flaps in head and neck reconstruction. Plast Reconstr Surg 1979;63:49–57.
7. Bakamjian VY: Methods of pharyngoesophageal reconstruction, in Grabb WC, Smith JW (eds): Plastic Surgery – A Concise Guide to Clinical Practice, 1st ed. Boston: Little Brown & Co., 1968. p 363.
8. Kraissel CJ: The selection of appropriate lines for elective surgical incisions. Plast Reconstr Surg 1951;8:1–28.
9. Robson, MC: An easy access incision for the removal of some intraoral malignant tumors. Plast Reconstr Surg 1979;64:834–835.
10. Esser JF: Plastic surgery of the face III. The epidermic inlay. Ann Surg 1917;65:307–321.
11. Bromberg BE, Walden RH, Rubin LR: Mandibular bone graft. A technique in fixation. Plast Reconstr Surg 1963;32:589–599.
12. Ariyan S: Pectoralis major, sternocleidomastoid, and other musculocutaneous flaps for head and neck reconstruction. Clinics Plast Surg 1980;7:89–109.
13. Robson MC, Schmidt DR: One-stage composite reconstruction using the latissimus dorsi musculo-osteo-cutaneous free flap. Am J Surg 1982;144:470–472.

14. Corso PF: Variations of the arterial venous and capillary circulation of the soft tissue of the head by decades as demonstrated by methyl methacrylate injection technique, and their application to the construction of flaps and pedicles. Plast Reconstr Surg 1961;27:160–184.

15. Milton SH: The tubed pedicle flap. Brit J Plast Surg 1969;22:53–59.

16. Daniel RK, Williams HB: Experimental arterial flaps. Surg Forum 1972;23:507–509.

17. McGregor IA, Jackson IT: Extended role of deltopectoral flap, Brit J Plast Surg 1970;23:173–185.

18. Murphy RC, Robson MC, Heggers JP et al: The effect of microbial contamination on musculocutaneous and random flaps. JSR 1986;41:75–80.

19. Krizek TJ, Robson MC: The split-flap in head and neck reconstruction. Am J Surg 1973;126:488–491.

20. Zachary LS, Robson MC, Heggers JP et al: Role of arachidonic acid metabolities in distal dying flap. Surg Forum 1979;30:527–528.

21. Zachary LS, Heggers JP, Robson MC, et al: Effects of exogenous prostacyclin on flap survival. Surg Forum 1982;33:588–589.

22. Reus WP, Murphy RC, Heggers JP, et al: Effect of intraarterial prostacyclin on survival of skin flaps in the pig: Biphasic response, Ann Plast Surg 1984;13:29–33.

23. Murphy RC, Lawrence WT, Robson MC, et al: Surgical delay and archidonic acid metabolities: evidence for an inflammatory mechanisms an experimental study in rats. Brit J Plast Surg 1985;38:272–277.

24. Lawrence WT, Murphy RC, Robson MC, et al: Prostanoid derivatives in experimental flap delay with formic acid. Brit J Plast Surg 1984;37:602–606.

25. Goldwyn RM: Forward, in: Bernstein NR, Robson MC, (eds): Comprehensive Approaches for the Burned Person, New Hyde Park: Med. Exam Publishing Co., 1983.

27. Bakamjian VY, Cramer L: Surgical management of advanced cancer of the tongue, Ann Surg, 1960:152:1058–1066.

# Infections in Patients with Head and Neck Cancer

*Lawrence R. Crane, MD, FACP*

Infection causes about half of the deaths in patients with solid tumor.[1] In an autopsy review of 94 persons with head and neck cancer treated at M.D. Anderson Hospital between 1968–1970, 43 deaths, or 46 percent, were infection related. Pneumonia and bacteremia were the most common infections.[2] Surprisingly, little has been written in the last decade concerning infectious complications of head and neck cancer. In more recent reviews, head and neck cancer patients represented small subpopulations in studies of infections in cancer,[3,4] or in investigations of prophylactic antibiotic regimens for patients undergoing surgery. This chapter details the frequency, possible predisposing factors, clinical features, and outcome of 65 episodes of infection in patients with head and neck cancer seen during a seven and one-half year period at Harper-Grace Hospital.

## METHODOLOGY AND DEFINITIONS

The study was conducted from 1978 to 1985 on patients identified by a review of inpatient Harper-Grace Hospital medical records. Inclusion criteria consisted of histologically proven head and neck cancer and adequate documentation of an infection.

Atelectasis owing to aspiration is common in this population, therefore pneumonia was defined as radiographic documentation of a pulmonary infiltrate persisting 48 hours or longer, with at least one compatible sign (fever, purulent sputum, white count elevation or left shift) and one compatible symptom (chest pain, chills or cough). The microbiologic etiology of pneumonia required either a compatible Gram stain and isolation of a pathogen from expectorated sputum and blood or pleural fluid or compatible Gram stains and recovery of the same pathogen on two consecutive occasions.[6] All other pneumonias were categorized as microbiologically unknown. A patient with bilateral bronchial pneumonia, an acute cold agglutinin titer of 1:64 and a *Mycoplasma pneumoniae* convalescent complement fixation titer of 1:64 was classified as mycoplasma pneumonia. Lastly, new, persisting pulmonary infiltrates appearing at least 72 hours following hospital admission, defined nosocomial pneumonia; all others were defined as community pneumonia.

Wound infections were documented by the presence of purulent material in an incision. The microbiology was based on the Gram stain and culture results. Bacteremia was diagnosed when at least one blood culture yielded at least one organism and the patient had consistent signs and symptoms of a bloodstream infection. Other localized infections were diagnosed by conventional means. Those infections judged to be unrelated to the tumor or its therapy were excluded.[7]

Chang and co-workers' criteria were used for infection to be considered as the major contributor to death.[8] Briefly, bacteremic deaths required either positive blood cultures obtained during the last week of life in patients with clinical evidence of infection, or positive heart-blood cultures at post-mortem examination in those who had shown evidence of severe infection before death. For pneumonia to be considered as a death cause, pathological evidence for extensive pulmonary infection was required.

The primary tumor site was categorized as follows: supraglottic larynx, larynx, base of tongue, oral cavity, paranasal sinus, nasopharynx and salivary. The American Joint Committee staging system was employed to stage tumors.[9] Performance status may influence the outcome of cancer patients with infection. Accordingly, the Eastern Cooperative Oncology Group performance status scoring system were recorded for each patient.[10]

## RESULTS
### Demography, Cancer Therapy, and Outcome

During the 8-year period, 1106 patients with head and neck cancer were admitted 2539 times to Harper Hospital. The attending service listed an infectious complication 100 times. Thirty-one of these admissions were excluded from this review because the infection was not related to the underlying tumor, or its therapy (30 urinary tract infections and 1 uncomplicated herpes zoster).[6] Two admissions coded as pneumonia were excluded because the pulmonary infiltrate disappeared within 24 hours; these cases probably represented atelectasis owing to aspiration of particulate material. Two patients were felt to have osteomyelitis of the mandible. In both cases, radiation therapy preceded radiographic evidence of bone destruction. Bone biopsies were not done, nor was microbiology established. The response to antimicrobial therapy was difficult to assess. Therefore, these patients were also excluded from further analysis. Ten patients were admitted twice for separate infections. The population reviewed, therefore, comprised 55 patients with 65 infections. Their average age was $58 + 15$ years (range $19 - 87$ years); six patients were 49 years old or younger. The sex distribution favored men (male/female sex ratio $= 2.7 : 1$). Most patients were reported as having a history of alcoholism (45/55) and chronic lung disease (37/55). Other associated illnesses included arthritis (4/55), prostatic enlargement (4/55), cirrhosis (4/55), peptic ulcer (3/55), stroke (2/55), myelofibrosis (1/55), and chronic osteomyelitis of the femur (1/55).

Sites and stages of malignancies are shown in Table 11.1. Tumors were observed at the base of the tongue (11 patients), larynx (8 patients), supraglottic larynx (17 patients), and intraoral region, including the tonsil (12 patients). Seven patients had paranasal sinus tumor, two had nasopharynx tumor, and one had a parotid cancer. Twelve patients, or about 22 percent of the total, had early head and neck cancer. One autopsied patient with pneumonia and hepatic failure had a clinically unrecognized stage II supraglottic tumor; this represented the only death in patients with early stage cancer. The remaining 43 patients had advanced cancer, and 33 of these patients died. Thirteen of the 15 patients with metastatic disease died.

The performance status and primary cause of death are listed in Table 11.2. Ten patients were bedridden and moribund (ECOG score 4). No aggressive measures were prescribed. All died; carcinomatosis was considered the cause of death in the three autopsied patients. Infection (seven patients) and pulmonary embolus (one patient) were the primary causes of death in the remaining autopsied patients. Carcinomatosis was considered the cause of death by the attending physician in all non-autopsied patients with ECOG scores of three or four. The clinical cause of death for patients with ECOG performance scores of one or two were: infection 9 patients: carcinomatosis, 3 patients; and myocardial infarction, 1 patient.

The most common treatment was combined modality therapy; 30/55 patients had combined treatment approaches (Table 11.3.). Chemotherapy was the most common treatment employed. Twenty-seven patients had received chemotherapy within 30 days of infection onset. Twenty were given combination chemotherapy consisting of cis-platinum and 5-fluorouracil. Five patients had no treatment; one patient, mentioned earlier, had an early supraglottic cancer found at autopsy. Two patients were lost to follow-up presenting one to two years later with pneumonia or inanition. Lastly, two individuals developed pneumonia during evaluation for newly diagnosed cancer.

**TABLE 11.1** Sites, Stages and Mortality in 55 Head and Neck Cancer Patients with 65 Infections at Harper-Grace Hospitals, 1978–1985

| Site | Early | | | Stage | | | | Total |
|---|---|---|---|---|---|---|---|---|
| | $T_1N_0$ | $T_2N_0$ | $T_{1-2}N_1$ | $T_3N_0$ | $T_3N_1$ | Advanced $T_4N_{0-1}$ | $T_{1-4}N_{2-3}$ | |
| | | | No. patients (No. died) | | | | | |
| Supraglottic | 1 | 4 (1) | 0 | 0 | 1 (1) | 6 (4) | 5 (4) | 17 (10) |
| Base tongue | 0 | 2 | 0 | 1 (1) | 1 | 4 (3) | 3 (2) | 11 (6) |
| Oral cavity | 0 | 1 | 1 | 0 | 0 | 3 (2) | 7 (7) | 12 (9) |
| Larynx | 1 | 0 | 2 | 2 (1) | 0 | 0 | 3 (3) | 8 (4) |
| Paranasal sinus | 0 | 0 | 0 | 1 (1) | 0 | 1 | 2 (2) | 4 (3) |
| Nasopharynx | 0 | 0 | 0 | 0 | 0 | 1 | 1 | 2 (0) |
| Salivary | 0 | 0 | 0 | 0 | 1 (1) | 0 | 0 | 1 (1) |
| Total | 2 | 7 (1) | 3 | 4 (3) | 3 (2) | 15 (9) | 21 (18) | 55 (33) |
| Metastatic disease | 2 | | 3 | 2 | 1 | 3 | 9 | 15 (13) |

**TABLE 11.2** Performance Status, Mortality, and Causes of Death in 55 Head and Neck Cancer Patients with 65 Infections

| | Performance Status Scale[1] | | | | |
| | 1 | 2 | 3 | 4 | Total |
|---|---|---|---|---|---|
| No. of patients | 25 | 26 | 4 | 10 | 65 |
| No. died | 5 | 14 | 4 | 10 | 33 |
| No. autopsied | 2 | 4 | 2 | 3 | 11 |
| Primary cause of death[2]: | | | | | |
|   Infection | 1 | 4 | 2 | | 7 |
|   Carcinomatosis | | | | 3 | 3 |
|   Pulmonary embolus | 1 | | | | 1 |

[1]Eastern Cooperative Oncology Group (ECOG) performance status score (10).
[2]Autopsied patients.

## INFECTIONS IN PATIENTS WITH HEAD AND NECK CANCER

Table 11.4 summarizes the infections that occurred in this population. Pneumonia was the most common infection seen; 44 episodes were documented. Postoperative wound infections, 12 cases, and bacteremias, 7 cases, were the next most common infections. One patient with a supraglottic tumor developed a maxillary sinusitis. Lastly, a patient with a paranasal sinus cancer and an associated cerebrospinal fluid fistula developed a nosocomial pneumococcal meningitis. Fifty infections occurred in the hospital setting. Over two-thirds of the pneumonias were nosocomial. All wound infections occurred postoperatively, and six of the seven bacteremias were hospital-acquired.

**TABLE 11.3** Treatment of Study Population

| Modality | No. of Patients |
|---|---|
| Radiotherapy/chemotherapy/surgery | 10 |
| Chemotherapy | 9 |
| Radiotherapy/chemotherapy | 9 |
| Surgery | 7 |
| Surgery/radiotherapy | 6 |
| Surgery/chemotherapy | 5 |
| Radiotherapy | 4 |
| No treatment | 5 |
| Total | 55 |

**TABLE 11.4** Infections in Patients with Head and Neck Cancer: The Wayne State University Experience; 1978–1985

| | |
|---|---:|
| Pneumonia | 44 |
|   Nosocomial pneumonia | 31 |
|   Community pneumonia | 13 |
| Wound infection | 12 |
| Bacteremia | 7 |
| Maxillary sinusitis | 1 |
| Meningitis | 1 |
| Total infections | 65 |

Twenty percent of infections occurred within one month of diagnosis of cancer. Eighty percent of all infections, occurred within 16 months of diagnosis; of the three most common infections, 38/44 pneumonias, 10/12 wound infections, and 3/7 bacteremias occurred within 16 months after cancer was found.

The 13 patients with community pneumonia were symptomatic for 1–5 days before admission (median: 2 days). Single cases of pneumonia were caused by *Streptococcus pneumoniae, Hemophilus influenzae, Mycoplasma pneumoniae, Staphylococcus aureus,* and Group A *Streptococcus pyogenes.* A microbiologic etiology was not established for the rest (Table 11.5). Four patients with community-acquired pneumonia of unknown etiology died.

**TABLE 11.5** Microbiology and Outcome of Pneumonia in Patients with Head and Neck Cancer: 1978–1985

| Organism | Setting | |
|---|---|---|
| | Community | Nosocomial |
| | (no. died/total) | |
| Anaerobes | | 4/5 |
| *Enterobacteriaceae*[1] | | 5/5 |
| *P. aeruginosa* | | 5/5 |
| *S. pneumoniae* | 0/1 | 1/2 |
| *H. influenzae* | 0/1 | 0/1 |
| *Mycoplasma pneumoniae* | 0/1 | |
| *S. aureus* | 0/1 | |
| *S. pyogenes* | 0/1 | |
| Unknown | 4/8 | 9/13 |
| Total | 4/13 | 24/31 |

[1]*K. pneumoniae*, 3 patients, *E. coli*, 2.

The median day to death was 5.5 days (range 4–17). None of these patients had received chemotherapy or was hospitalized within 30 days of their final admission. One had an autopsy; necrotizing pneumonia was found.

Nosocomial pneumonia occurred 3–93 days following admission (median of 18 hospital days). Etiologic bacteria included: *Pseudomonas aeruginosa*, five cases; other gram negative bacilli, five cases; *S. pneumoniae*, two cases; and *H. influenzae*, one case. Three patients had anaerobic lung abscess and two had anaerobic pneumonitis with empyema; *Bacteroides melaninogenicus* grew in pleural fluids in both. Lastly, 13 patients had pneumonia of unknown etiology (Table 11.5).

Patients with hospital-acquired pneumonia had higher mortality than those with community-acquired cases. Four of the five patients with definite or probable anaerobic pneumonia died, and all with gram negative bacillary pneumonias succumbed. Ten patients had an autopsy. Pneumonia was considered the primary cause of death in seven; the remaining three were considered deaths owing to carcinomatosis. In that regard, the Oncology Service judged that ten patients dying with pneumonia were incurable owing to their cancer. Accordingly, these patients received terminal care only. Eight had nosocomial pneumonias: six of these were pneumonias of unknown etiology, and the other two were *Pseudomonas aeruginosa* pneumonia and *Escherichia coli* pneumonia. Two patients with community pneumonias of unknown etiology had advanced cancer that precluded aggressive clinical measures. The mortality rate, therefore, for potentially salvageable patients with community pneumonia was 18 percent, and for nosocomial pneumonia, was 70 percent.

Table 11.6 details the microbiology and outcome of bacteremic patients. Four patients with bacteremia died. In three of these, sepsis was the cause of death. The cause of death in the patient with the coagulase-negative staphylococcus bacteremia was myocardial infarction. Infected Hickman cannulae caused all gram positive and the *E. coli* bacteremias. The clostridial bacteremia was attributed to tumor infection. All *S. aureus* bacteremias

**TABLE 11.6** Microbiology and Outcome in Patients with Bacteremia and Head and Neck Cancer

| Microorganism | No. Died/Total |
| --- | --- |
| *C. perfringens* | 0/1 |
| coagulase-negative staphylococcus | 1/1 |
| *E. coli* | 1/1 |
| *S. aureus* | 2/4 |
| Total | 4/7 |

**TABLE 11.7** Microbial Isolates from 12 Patients with Wound Infection Following Extensive Resective Therapy for Head and Neck Cancer

|  | No. | Percent |
|---|---|---|
| Aerobic (12 patients cultured) |  |  |
| Streptococcus | 12 | 100 |
| Staphylococcus aureus | 3 | 25 |
| Coagulase-negative staphylococci | 1 | 8 |
| Neisseria sp. | 3 | 25 |
| Enterobacteriaceae | 6 | 50 |
| Pseudomonas aeruginosa | 2 | 17 |
| Candida | 1 | 8 |
| Anaerobic (9 patients cultured) |  |  |
| Peptostreptococcus sp. | 4 | 44 |
| Bacteroides melaninogenicus | 3* | 33 |
| Bacteroides bivius | 2 | 22 |
| Bacteroides sp. | 3 | 33 |
| Fusobacterium sp. | 2* | 22 |
| Veillonella parvula | 1 | 11 |

*One penicillin-resistant strain isolated.

followed recent chemotherapy (0–11 days), but patients were not neutropenic.

*Postoperative wound infections* occurred 3 – 17 days (median: 7 days) following resective surgery. Wound purulence (12/12 patients), and incisional edema (11/12), erythema (11/12) and pain (10/11) were usually noted. Foul odor was documented in seven infections. Nine patients were febrile, and fever lasted 5 – 20 days (median: 8 days). Table 11.7 outlines the microbiology of these infections.

Mixed aerobic and anaerobic isolates were found in all nine patients who had both cultures done. One patient had exclusive growth of *Peptococcus*. In the rest, mixed cultures of *Streptococcus, Peptostreptococcus,* and *Bacteroides* were usually isolated. The mean number of isolates per specimen was 2.9 ± 1.5 aerobes and 1.8 ± 2.0 anaerobes.

Four anaerobic isolates were penicillin-resistant; two were *Bacteroides bivius,* and single strains of penicillinase-producing *Bacteroides melaninogenicus* and *Fusobacterium* were found. In those cases, fever and purulence continued until penicillin was stopped and clindamycin substituted. The average hospital duration was 47 ± 26 days (range: 22 – 127 days). Major complications included fistula formation (8/12 patients) necessitating rehospitalization for repair (7 patients). Total or near-total wound dehiscence occurred in five of these patients. One patient died of pulmonary embolism; the remaining patient survived.

Combined modality therapy, perioperative antimicrobial selection, flap reconstruction, tumor stage and nutritional status are possible risk factors leading to postoperative wound infection in patients undergoing extensive head and neck surgery.[11-13] Table 11.8 lists documented potential risk factors in patients with postoperative wound infection. Eight patients received cefazolin prophylaxis, which may be suboptimal for prevention of anaerobic infection.

## DISCUSSION

In summary, this retrospective review of the Wayne State University experience with infections in patients with head and neck malignancy emphasizes the high mortality rate of non-surgical infections. The overall pneumonia mortality was 64 percent. Even when the terminally ill patient was excluded, every potentially salvageable patient with gram negative bacillary pneumonia died. Pneumonia remains a significant cause of death in persons with head and neck cancer.

The incidence of pneumonia in this series is low, reflecting this review's retrospective nature and case-finding methods. Between 1982 and 1983, the University of Pittsburgh group prospectively surveyed their head and neck cancer patients for pneumonia, reporting a 6% nosocomial pneumonia rate.[14] During 1977, our group reported a 5% prospective nosocomial pneu-

**TABLE 11.8** Post Operative Wound Infections in Patients with Head and Neck Cancer: Possible Risk Factors

| Risk Factor | No. of Patients |
|---|---|
| Cancer stage:[1] | |
| II | 3 |
| III | 5 |
| IV | 4 |
| Prior treatment: | |
| Radiation | 5 (3–20 months) |
| Chemotherapy | 3 (1–7 months) |
| Tracheostomy | 7 |
| Extent of surgery: | |
| Flap | 5 |
| Primary closure | 7 |
| Prophylactic antibiotic: | |
| Cefazolin | 8 |
| Penicillin G | 4 |

[1](Base tongue, 3; larynx, 3; intraoral, 1; supraglottic 5 patients.)

monia rate.[15] On the other hand, prospective surveillance overestimates nosocomial pneumonia rates, particularly in patients who are prone to aspiration. In addition to oropharyngeal bacteria, patients with head and neck cancer aspirate particulate matter, inert fluids, and gastric contents. Rising white blood cell counts, pulmonary infiltrates, and fever, considered clinical and epidemiologic hallmarks of pneumonia, may occur as a result of aspiration of these noninfectious materials.

The issue of differentiating infection from non-infection is clouded further when clinicians consider that infectious complications may follow aspiration of particulate matter or gastric contents. The dilemma of the poor predictive value of clinical and laboratory parameters for the diagnosis of pneumonia is well illustrated by the studies of Andrews and co-workers. The authors correlated the histopathologic and clinical diagnosis of 30 consecutive adults dying of adult respiratory distress syndrome. Sometimes pneumonia was documented at autopsy in patients who were thought to have lung injury. On other occasions, histologic evidence of lung injury was found in patients with clinically diagnosed pneumonia. Nosocomial pneumonia was misdiagnosed 30% of the time.[16]

The respiratory tract's defense system apparatus is complex, involving mechanical, cellular, and humoral components.[17] Table 11.9 lists intrinsic defects of the respiratory tract occurring in patients with head and neck cancer that would either increase the risk of acquiring pneumonia or augment pulmonary infection. Clearly, aspiration is the most important factor causing pneumonia in this setting. An anatomically and physiologically intact epiglottis protects the lower respiratory tract from overwhelming quantities of bacteria-laden secretions. Tumors or intubation that disrupt this barrier result in an increased occurrence of aspiration pneumonia. Surgical procedures may restore the anatomic barrier and reduce aspiration risks. Underlying diseases, and therapy of head and neck cancer may also contribute to the occurrence of severe pneumonia.

Many investigators have reported the appearance of pathogenic gram-negative bacteria in oropharyngeal cultures of critically ill or debilitated patients. Growth of pathogens from upper airway cultures in the absence of pneumonia is termed colonization. Colonization with potential pathogens predisposes to pneumonia in aspirating patients. Most pneumonias in patients with head and neck cancer result from aspiration of bacteria. Adherence of pathogenic bacteria to oropharyngeal mucosal surfaces is a prerequisite for events leading to pneumonia. Adherence involves interaction of the bacterial surface, including specialized organelles that mediate adherence, the epithelial cell, including compounds bound by adhering bacteria, and the mucous layer through which bacteria must traverse before adherence.[18] Adherence barriers are decreased following surgery, and during starvation.[19,20]

**TABLE 11.9** Potential Risk Factors in Patients with Head and Neck Cancer Predisposing to Pneumonia

| Risk Factor | Defect | Potential Infection |
|---|---|---|
| Tumor | Anatomic | Aspiration pneumonia |
| | ?Mucosal adherence | ?Gram-negative pneumonia |
| Associated illnesses: | | |
| Alcoholism | Mucosal adherence | Gram-negative pneumonia |
| | Depressed cough | Aspiration pneumonia |
| | Altered leukocyte migration | Variable pathogens |
| | Complement depletion | *Hemophilus influenza* |
| | T-cell depression | Variable pathogens |
| Chronic lung disease | Mucociliary clearance | Bronchitis, bronchiectasis |
| | Impaired surfactant | Atelectasis, loss opsinic, bactericidal activity. |
| Therapeutic effects: | | |
| Chemotherapy | Polymorphonuclear leukocyte | Gram-negative pneumonia |
| | Cytotoxicity | Drug-induced lung disease |
| | ?Mucosal adherence | ?Gram-negative pneumonia |
| Radiation | Radiation parotitis | Reduced salivary IgA |
| | | Reduced flow saliva |
| | | ?Salivary protease |
| | | ?Reduced salivary lysozyme |
| | ?Mucosal adherence | Gram-negative pneumonia |
| Surgery | Anatomic | Aspiration pneumonia |
| | Bacterial "interference" | Gram-negative, Staphylococcal pneumonia |
| | Mucosal adherence | Gram-negative pneumonia |
| Other | | |
| Nasogastric tubes | Anatomic | Aspiration pneumonia |

The increased incidence of gram-negative colonization in alcoholics suggests a loss of normal adherence barriers.[21] The influence of radiation and chemotherapy on adherence and colonization of respiratory pathogens in head and neck cancer patients requires investigation.

Several salivary components may play a role in defense against pneumonia. Under stress-related conditions, decreased amounts of fibronectin may lower mucosal resistance to adherence of gram-negative bacilli.[22] Fibronectin depletion may be related to increased levels of salivary protease.[23] Radiation of salivary glands results in decreased salivary flow and secretory IgA levels.[24,25] Radiation effects on other potential defense-related salivary constituents, including lysozyme and protease, is not known.

Antimicrobial therapy enhances colonization with potential pathogens. Under ordinary circumstances, normal respiratory flora prevent colonization by potential pathogens including *Staphylococcus aureus* or gram-negative bacteria. Loss of bacterial "interference" occurs rapidly following anti-microbial therapy, including prophylaxis for surgery. Lower respiratory tract defenses include the cough reflex, mucociliary activity, and various humoral and cellular components. Therapy of head and neck cancer, or associated illnesses, may impair some of these defenses. Impaired cough reflex and aspiration may occur in alcoholics or in the post–anaesthesia period. Muco-ciliary clearance and surfactant activity may be decreased or absent in pa-tients with chronic lung disease. Lastly, alcoholism, chemotherapy, and radiation therapy may impair pulmonary humoral and cellular defenses, including polymorphonuclear leukocyte and alveolar macrophage function.

Improved diagnostic techniques are clearly needed for the accurate diagnosis of pneumonia in this notoriously aspiration-prone population. In this review, physicians could not establish a microbiologic diagnosis for almost 40% of pneumonia occurring in possibly curable patients; these pa-tients may not have received appropriate antimicrobial therapy. Invasive diagnostic procedures for culture and histologic examination should be seri-ously considered for potentially salvageable head and neck cancer patients with nosocomial pneumonia. Transtracheal aspiration (TTA) is a logical first consideration in those patients without tracheostomy because there are few contraindications to its use and it is a safe procedure in skilled hands. If TTA cannot be done, more invasive procedures may be considered, includ-ing: shielded fiberoptic bronchoscopic lavage or washings and biopsies; per-cutaneous needle aspiration and/or biopsy; and open lung biopsy. The han-dling of specimens obtained by these procedures should include immediate microscopic examination for bacteria (including *Legionella*), fungi, and parasites including culture for routine, anaerobic, and opportunistic pathogens.[14]

Carefully designed prospectice studies utilizing invasive diagnostic pro-cedures and serologic testing are critically needed to establish the "microbio-logic statistics" of pneumonia in the patient with head and neck cancer. Clearly, in this series, despite broad spectrum coverage of pneumonia of unknown etiology with penicillin and aminoglycosides, many patients died. The frequency of infections caused by fastidious organisms such as *Legion-ella* needs validation.[14] Antibiotic protocols for gram-negative bacillary pneumonia should be developed, and may require combination therapy with beta-lactam antibiotics and high dose aminoglycosides.[26] Beta-lactam combinations may be necessary in order for those patients receiving cis-plat-inum to avoide aminoglycoside-platinum nephrotoxicity.

Specific risk factors must be identified to aid clinicians in the prediction of the pneumonia-prone patient and the probable microbiology. Strategies for prevention need to be developed, and should include: investigations of colonization immunity and the influence of chemotherapy and radiation on the microbial population of the airways; anticolonization vaccine development; and methods to optimally reduce mechanical aspiration of endogenous bacteria.

The prospective identification of risk factors for postoperative wound infection is also clearly needed. The results of ongoing trials should clarify the contribution of preoperative radiation and chemotherapy to wound infection and dehiscence.[11] The anerobic etiology of wound infection in this setting dictates comparative trials of antimicrobial prophylaxis for resective surgery using penicillin or clindamycin rather than cefazolin as the "gold standard." Finally, growth of penicillin-resistant anaerobes in established wound infections in this series raises serious concerns regarding the "drug of choice" for postoperative wound infection. The emergence of penicillin-resistant oral anaerobic bacteria has been well documented in several laboratories, and has been recently reviewed.[27]

## REFERENCES

1. Ketchel SJ, Rodriguez V: Acute Infections in cancer patients. Sem Oncol 1978;5:167–179.
2. Inagaki J, Rodriguez V, Bodey GP: Causes of death in cancer patients. Cancer 1974;33:568–573.
3. Carney DN, Fossieck BE, Parker RH, Minna JD: Bacteremia due to *Staphylococcus aureas* in patients with cancer: report on 45 cases in adults and review of the literature. Rev Infect Dis 1982;4:1–12.
4. Singer C, Kaplan MH, Armstrong D: Bacteremia and fungemia complicating neoplastic disease. A study of 364 cases. Amer J Med 1977;62:731–742.
5. Al-Sarraf M: Chemotherapy strategies in squamous cell carcinoma of the head and neck. CRC Crit Rev Oncology/Hematol 1984;1:323–335.
6. Tillotson JR, Lerner AM: Pneumonias caused by gram-negative bacilli. Medicine 1966;45:65–76.
7. Sen P, Kapila R, Chmel H, et al: Superinfection: another look. Amer J Med 1982; 73:706–718.
8. Chang HY, Rodriguez V, Narboni G, et al: Causes of death in adults with acute leukemia. Medicine 1976;55:259–268.
9. American Joint Committee on Cancer, 2nd ed.: in Beahrs OH, Myers MH (eds): Cancer. Philadelphia: JB Lippincott, 1983, pp 25–54.
10. Stanley KE: Prognostic factors for survival in patients with inoperable lung cancer. J Nat Cancer Inst 1980;65:25–32.
11. Donald PJ: Complications of combined therapy in head and neck carcinomas. Arch Otolaryngol 1978;104:329–332.
12. Johnson JT, Myers EN, Thearle PB, et al: Antimicrobial prophylaxis for contaminated head and neck surgery. Laryngoscope 1984;94:46–51.
13. Johnson JT, Yu VL, Myers EN, et al: Efficacy of two third-generation cephalosporins in prophylaxis for head and neck surgery. Arch Otolaryngol 1984;110:224–227.
14. Johnson JT, Yu VL, Wagner RL, Best MG: Noscomial Legionella pneumonia in a population of head and neck cancer patients. Laryngoscope 1985;95:1468–1471.

15. Crane LR, Emmer DR, Grguras A: Prevention of infection on the oncology unit. Nurs Clin N Amer 1980;15:843–856.
16. Andrews CP, Coalson JJ, Smith JD, Johanson WG Jr: Diagnosis of nosocomial bacterial pneumonia in acute, diffuse lung injury. Chest 1981;80;254–258.
17. Pennington JE: Respiratory tract infections: intrinsic risk factors. Amer J Med 1984; 76 (Supplement 5A):34–41.
18. Schoolnik GK, Lark D, O'Hanley P: Bacterial adherence and anticolonization vaccines, in: Remington JS and Swartz MN (eds): Current Clinical Topics in Infectious Diseases 6. New York: McGraw-Hill 1985, pp 85–102.
19. Johanson WG, Higuchi JH, Chauduri TR, TE Woods: Bacterial adherence to epithelial cells in bacillary colonization of the respiratory tract. Am Rev Respir Dis 1980;121:55–63.
20. Higuchi JH, Johanson WG: The relationship between adherence of *Pseudomonas aeruginosa* to upper respiratory cells in vitro and susceptibility to colonization in vivo. J Lab Clin Med 1980;95:698–705.
21. Smith FE, Palmer DL: Alcoholism, infection, and altered host defenses: a review of clinical and experimental observations. J Chronic Dis 1976;29:35–49.
22. Woods DE, Straus DC, Johanson WG, Bass JA: Role of fibronectin in the prevention of adherence of *Pseudomonas aeruginosa* to buccal cells. J Infect Dis 1981;143:784–790.
23. Woods DE, Straus DC, Johanson WG, Bass JA: Role of salivary protease activity in adherence of gram-negative bacilli to mammalian buccal epithelial cells in vivo. J Clin Invest. 1981;68:1435–1440.
24. Eneroth CM, Henrikson CO, Jakobsson PA: Effect of fractionated radiotherapy on salivary gland function. Cancer 1972;30:1147–1153.
25. Sonis ST: Oral complications of cancer therapy, in: DeVita VT, Hellman S, Rosenberg SA, (eds): Cancer. Principles and Practice of Oncology, 2nd ed. Philadelphia: J. B. Lippencott Co, 1985, pp 2014–2021.
26. Crane LR, Lerner AM: Gram-negative bacillary pneumonias, in Pennington JE, (ed): Respiratory Infections: Diagnosis and Management. New York: Raven Press, 1983, pp 227–250.
27. Bawdon RE, Crane LR, Palchaudhuri S: Antibiotic resistance in anaerobic bacteria: molecular biology and clinical aspects. Rev Infect Dis 1982;4:1075–1095.

# CHAPTER 12

# Overview of Chemotherapeutic Agents with Activity in Cancer of the Head and Neck Region

*Joseph R. Bertino, MD, Dennis Cooper, MD,*
*Yu-Ming Chang, MD, and*
*Laurie Smaldone, MD*

## INTRODUCTION

There has been a substantial amount of progress in the development of effective chemotherapy for patients with carcinoma of the head and neck in the past decade. Most of the requisites for beneficial chemotherapy are in existence, i.e., effective single agents and combination of drugs have been developed, and newer analogs of some of these agents promise to be equally effective with less host toxicity. While definition of the term "effective" is a relative one, by analogy with breast cancer (a disease in which combination chemotherapy is equally or even slightly less effective than treatment of patients with advanced head and neck cancer), combination chemotherapy may be expected to have a beneficial effect when used as adjuvant therapy.

In this manuscript we will review the mechanism of action of four drugs used in the treatment of cancer of the head and neck, as well as briefly discuss promising new analogs of two of these agents, i.e., methotrexate and cisplatin.

### Chemotherapeutic Agents with Activity in Patients with Cancer of the Head and Neck Region

Of the many drugs tested for anti-cancer cavity in head and neck cancer,[1,2] three drugs have demonstrated significant activity; these are methotrexate (MTX), cisplatin (DDP), and bleomycin. Fluorouracil (5FU) and hydrox-

**159**

yurea also have some antitumor activity, but neither of these drugs has been tested extensively.

## Methotrexate

MTX is probably the single most effective chemotherapeutic agent in this disease (30 to 50% response rates), although remissions are usually only partial, and response duration is short.[1,2] MTX has been used in combination with 5FU, bleomycin, and DDP.

*Mechanism of Action.* The major action of MTX is inhibition of the enzyme dihydrofolate reductase (DHFR) (Fig. 12.1). Inhibition of this enzyme activity rapidly leads to depletion of intracellular levels of tetrahydrofolate coenzymes that are essential for thymidylate biosynthesis and for purine synthesis.[3] Recent investigations have shown that MTX is polyglutamylated intracellularly, i.e., additional glutamates (up to four) are added to the molecule via peptide linkage at the -carboxyl of glutamate. This process appears to be an important determinant of MTX cytotoxicity since polyglutamylation allows this drug to be retained intracellularly for long periods of time.[4] It will be important to determine if natural and/or acquired resistance to this antifolate is related to this conversion in patients with head and neck cancer.

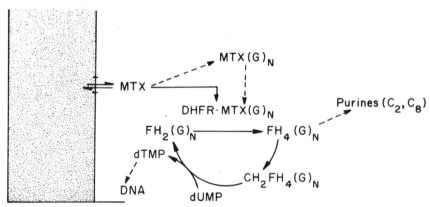

**FIGURE 12.1** MTX enters mammalian cells via a carrier mediated transport process that is utilized by reduced folates for uptake. Once inside the cell, MTX rapidly binds to dihydrofolate reductase (DHFR), "free" MTX is polyglutamylated — a form that also is retained in cells, and is equally as potent an inhibitor of DHFR. As a consequence of inhibition of DHFR, tetrahydrofolate enzymes are not recycled by the thymidylate synthase pathway, and both thymidylate and purine biosynthesis are impaired.

*Resistance to MTX.* MTX is a "cycle active" drug, i.e., it is cytotoxic to cells in S phase, therefore it is perhaps not surprising that the response rate of patients with advanced head and neck cancer is relatively low. In addition, when these tumors are necrotic or have a poor blood supply, in addition to poor perfusion of the drug, many cells are presumably in $G_0$ or $G_1$ phase, and thus are capable of repopulating the tumor mass once MTX levels fall.[5,6] Polyglutamylation, as mentioned above, may be an important element in the treatment outcome following MTX, since these derivatives may not efflux from cells readily.

Acquired resistance, i.e., resistance occurring after a tumor response has been obtained, may be due to one of four mechanisms: impaired uptake of MTX into cells; an increase in the level of the enzyme dihydrofolate reductase; an alteration in this enzyme, so that it binds MTX less well; or decreased polyglutamylation.[7] All of these mechanisms of resistance have been noted in experimental tumor systems, including human squamous cell carcinoma cells grown in vitro.[8] In experimental systems, both gene amplification and impaired transport appear to be commonly observed.[9] Frei et al. have developed squamous cell carcinoma lines resistant to MTX, and have found that low level resistance occurs by more than one mechanism, including decreased MTX uptake and polyglutamylation.[8]

Mechanisms of resistance to MTX in patients with head and neck cancer have not yet been documented, but recent studies in patients with leukemia and small cell cancer indicate that small increases in gene copies of DHFR (2–4) may be associated with MTX resistance.[10-12]

*Recommended Dose of MTX.* Several doses of MTX are employed for the treatment of head and neck cancer, ranging from oral use of 5 to 10 mg/day to weekly or biweekly treatments of 3 to 7 $g/m^2$ with leucovorin (LV) rescue. As a single agent, the two most convenient dosage schedules are 40 to 60 $mg/m^2$ IV weekly without rescue, and 120 to 240 $mg/m^2$ IV weekly with leucovorin rescue, started 24 hours after MTX (Table 12.1). We prefer the latter schedule with rescue because we believe that the toxicity of this regimen is less than with regimens not employing leucovorin, with at least equal efficacy.[13] With higher doses (3 to 7 $g/m^2$), the requirement for hydration and alkalinization and the cost may not be worth the possibly slightly higher response rates noted.[14] The use of high dose MTX (>500 $mg/m^2$) and LV rescue has the theoretical advantage that better premeability and intracellular levels of the drug may be achieved (thus resulting in increased MTX polyglutamylation), and small increases of DHFR and defects in uptake may be overcome. Unfortunately, resistance to these high doses of MTX and LV still occurs rapidly, perhaps due to accumulation and storage of reduced folates, i.e., "rescue" of tumor cells as well as host tissue.

**TABLE 12.1** Commonly Used Dosage Schedules of Methotrexate

| Dose | Schedule | Leucovorin Rescue |
|---|---|---|
| 5–10 mg/day | Daily until toxicity | No |
| 15–25 mg/day × 5 | Every 3–4 weeks | No |
| 30–60 mg/m² | Weekly | No |
| 200–250 mg/m² | Weekly to biweekly | At 24–36 hrs |
| 3–7 g/m² | Weeky to biweekly | At 24 hrs |

Single agent MTX has largely been supplanted by combination chemotherapy, but the principles of administration and monitoring of this drug apply when this drug is used in combination therapy as well.

*Clinical Pharmacology.* MTX absorption is less quantitative as MTX doses are increased,[12] and doses greater than 50 mg should be administered parenterally. The drug is excreted primarily unchanged by the kidney ($t_{1/2}$ = 2.5 hours), although with larger doses, a significant amount of the drug is inactivated by hydroxylation at the 7 position (7-OH MTX).[15]

*Toxic Effects.* The two tissues most susceptible to MTX side effects are the bone marrow and the gastrointestinal epithelium. The oral mucosa and the small intestinal epithelium appear to be more sensitive to the effects of this drug than the large bowel. Marrow suppression results in a circulating WBC and platelet nadir at day nine or ten after a single dose, and recovery by day 14 to 21. Mucositis and diarrhea may occur 4 to 7 days after MTX, and usually improve by day 14.

Nausea and vomiting are relatively uncommon with MTX treatment, even when high doses of the drug are administered. Less common side effects are skin rash (10% of patients), conjunctivitis, serositis (pleural or peritoneal pain), and photosensitivity. Transient liver abnormalities are commonly seen (increased SGOT), but liver fibrosis and cirrhosis are uncommon, and usually seen only in patients with psoriasis treated with this drug for long periods of time.[16]

Renal toxicity, especially with high doses of MTX, can also occur, presumably as a consequence of precipitation of MTX in the kidney tubules. This is a serious event, since the renal impairment results in prolonged high blood levels of the drug, which may lead to pancytopenia.[17] Pretreatment screening of patients with creatinine clearance and the use of hydration and alkalization in patients receiving doses larger than 250 mg/m² have made the use of high dose MTX relatively safe.[18]

In patients with pleural effusions or ascites, MTX may enter these spaces and only slowly be released, thus giving prolonged blood levels. If patients with this "third space" are to be treated, extreme care and careful plasma monitoring of MTX levels should be done. Treatment of patients with MTX at doses of 250 mg/m² or higher should only be carried out in institutions where serum MTX levels are available and can be obtained the same day as drawn. While serum creatinine levels are useful, and toxicity may be predicted when the 24-hour serum creatinine increases to greater than 50 percent of the pretreatment level, one-third of patients with the potential for serious toxicity are not detected with this test alone.[18]

*MTX Analogs.* While not a new analog, dichloromethotrexate (DCM) has been reinvestigated in recent years for use in patients with head and neck cancer (Fig. 12.2). Since this compound is more rapidly metabolized than MTX to the inactive 7-hydroxy derivative, it is therefore an attractive agent for intra-arterial use, since high local concentrations of this potent antifolate may be achieved, and subsequent metabolism by the liver to the 7-hydroxy metabolite prevents systemic toxicity. DCM has also been utilized systemically in combination with cisplatin without the potential for additional renal toxicity noted when MTX and cisplatin are given together. Encouraging results have been obtained in patients with head and neck and bladder cancer.[19,20]

Several new folate analogs are now in clinical trial (Fig. 12.2). CB3711, an antifolate that has as its target thymidylate synthase rather than DHFR, has just completed extensive phase I trials, and antitumor activity has been noted in several tumors.[21] It might be expected that there would not be cross

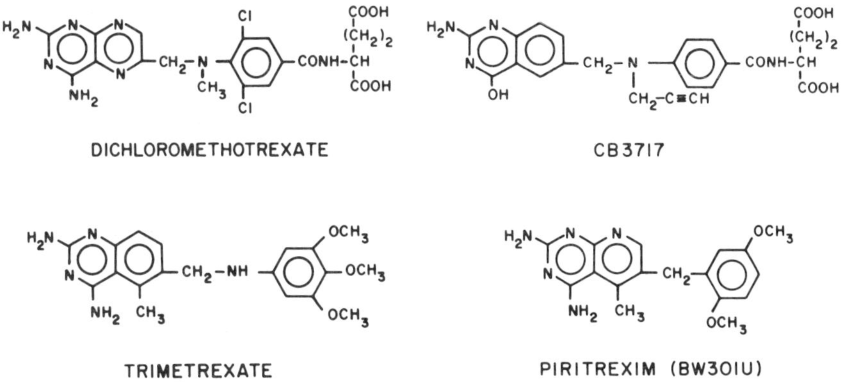

**FIGURE 12.2** Folate analogs in clinical trial.

resistance to MTX in human tumors, since the mechanism of uptake and target are clearly different from MTX.

Phase I trials have also been completed with trimetrexate, and are nearing completion with piritrexim — compounds that have been selected for clinical investigation based on their potency as DHFR inhibitors and their ability to accumulate in tumor cells by a MTX independent transport system.[22-26] In animal tumors, trimetrexate displayed a broader antitumor activity than MTX.[27] The drug is reasonably well tolerated in man, and the limiting toxicity has been hematologic. A phase II trial will be initiated shortly by ECOG, comparing MTX directly with trimetrexate in patients with advanced disease not previously treated with antifolates.

## 5 Fluorouacil (5FU)

Although 5FU does not fulfill the criteria for an "active" drug (i.e., having at least a 20% response rate), recent studies using it as a 4–5 day continuous infusion in combination with cisplatin, or in combination with MTX, have stimulated further interest in this agent. In vitro potency of this agent is markedly increased when the duration of exposure is lengthened to several days. In patients, larger total doses of 5FU may be administered as a 4–5 day infusion than when the drug is given as a bolus. This is a relatively unique occurrence for an antimetabolite (contrast, for example, the opposite results with MTX or 5-fluorodeoxyuridine). In addition, major toxicity becomes gastrointestinal rather than hematologic.[28] Trials comparing 4–5 day infusion therapy of 5FU alone with conventional 5FU schedules have not been reported in head and neck cancer patients; use of 5-day 5FU infusion together with concomitant radiation therapy produced complete remissions in 9 of 12 stage IV patients and one of two stage III patients.[29]

*Combination Therapy with 5FU.* Infusion therapy with cisplatin proved to be more effective than weekly bolus 5 FU in combination with cisplatin.[29-31] A relatively high response rate has also been recently reported using daily x5 pulse doses of 5FU with cisplatin. This combination is clearly a synergistic one, and optimization of the dose schedule may produce more effective treatment as well as a better tolerated program. The basis of this synergistic action is not known.

Similarly, the combination of MTX and 5FU has produced response rates that are additive or perhaps synergistic in most studies reported.[32-34] In trials comparing simultaneous drug administration with a one-hour interval between the drugs (MTX → FU), and in trials in which the MTX → FU sequence was compared with the opposite sequence (1-hour interval), no advantage of the MTX → FU sequence over simultaneous MTX and 5FU could be found.[35,36] Laboratory studies with human cells support the use of a longer interval (7–24 hours) between administration of these drugs.[35]

*Mechanism of Action.* Two, and possibly three, sites of action of 5FU have been identified; inhibition of thymidylate synthase by the nucleotide of 5-FU (namely, 5-fluorodeoxyuridylate); incorporation into RNA as 5-fluorouridylate; or incorporation into DNA.

*Toxicity.* Since 5FU inhibits cell growth in most cells by inhibition of DNA synthesis, its toxicity is similar to that of MTX. Unlike MTX, it causes diarrhea as a common side effect. Less common side effects of 5FU administration are skin rash, photophobia and conjunctivitis, and cerebellar dysfunction. Also like MTX, the drug usually does not cause nausea or vomiting.

Resistance to 5-FU usually occurs by deletion or decreased activity of the enzyme that activates 5FU to the nucleotide form.[36] Since this enzyme activity utilizes phosphoribosyl pyrophosphate (PRPP) as the cofactor, compounds that deplete PRPP stores (e.g., hypoxanthine, allopurinol) lead to decreased 5FU effects, and compounds that cause an increase in PRPP levels (e.g., MTX, 6-mercaptopurine) increase 5FU cytotoxicity.[37]

In cultured human adenocarcinoma cells, cells resistant to 5FU were shown to be lacking the nucleoside transporter; of great interest was the sensitivity of these cells to high doses of MTX along with thymidine.[38,39] This combination was toxic to resistant, but not 5FU-sensitive, cells. The basis of either natural or acquired resistance of squamous cells carcinomas to 5FU is not known.

## Bleomycin

Bleomycin, actually a mixture of bleomycins, is a group of antitumor antibiotics that was first discovered by Umezawa.[40,41] The drug has activity primarily in patients with lymphoma, testicular cancer, and squamous cell cancers. Its role in head and neck cancer is currently limited to its use in combination regimens.

*Mechanism of Action.* Bleomycin has been shown to interact with DNA and cause chain scission. This process appears to require a ferrous iron-oxygen complex.[42] Natural resistance and possibly acquired resistance may occur when inactivating enzymes are present (bleomycin hydrolase).[43]

*Toxic Effects.* Unlike the other agents discussed, bleomycin does not have significant toxicity to marrow stem cells; thus marrow impairment is not a serious problem with this drug. The basis for this lack of marrow toxicity is not clear, but may relate to the presence of bleomycin hydrolase in marrow cells. Thus this drug may be used in full or near full doses in myelo-suppressed patients or in combination with agents whose dose-limiting toxicity is to the bone marrow. The major dose limiting toxicity associated with this drug is pulmonary toxicity.

Mucositis and skin toxicity are commonly noted with this drug, and are a function of intensity of drug treatment and cumulative dose.[44]

## Platinum Compounds

Since the release of cis-diamminedichloroplatinum (II) (NSC-119875, DDP) by the FDA in 1978, it has quickly become established as one of the most versatile drugs in cancer chemotherapy. Used predominantly in combination with other drugs, it has become incorporated into the treatment of a variety of neoplasms. The last several years has seen a reduction in gastrointestinal and renal toxicity despite higher doses of therapy and attempts at exploiting the dose-response curve of many tumors by innovative methods of drug administration. Below we describe the pharmacology of CDDP and of the second generation platinum analogue, carboplatin.

*Mechanism of Action.* Although incompletely understood, the mechanism of action of CDDP appears to be closely related to that of alkylating agents. Cytotoxicity is thought to result from cross-linking of complementary strands of DNA and the establishment of protein-DNA complexes.[45-47] In addition, there is increasing evidence for intrastrand binding that may cause most of the DNA inhibition.[47-49] Inhibition of sublethal and lethal radiation damage may account for synergistic cytotoxicity when combined with radiation.[48] Of greater importance is the ability of CDDP to potentiate the action of several other agents including 5FU, mitomycin-C, VP-16, and Vinblastine. In vitro and in vivo toxicity can be reversed and prevented by several thiol-containing analogues. These compounds are thought to work by binding the active site on the platinum complex, thus interfering with cross-link formation.[49-51]

*Clinical Pharmocology.* The drug is administered intravenously, intra-arterially and most recently, intraperitoneally. The major route of excretion is renal, with 23 – 70% excreted in the first 24 hours.[52,53] Hemodialysis is only partially effective in removing drug due to extensive protein and red blood cell binding.[54] IP administration results in a similar disposition of drug, but results in a two-eight fold increase in drug concentration in tissues lining the peritoneal cavity.[55]

Despite recent attempts to increase the amount of drug that is delivered to a tumor, there is considerable controversy as to whether a dose-response curve exists for CDDP in the treatment of a variety of malignancies. Although laboratory models demonstrate a steep dose-response relationship for many tumors, this effect is clearly exaggerated in tumors that are more responsive to chemotherapy, and is less apparent or absent in inherently less sensitive tumors.[56,57] For example, clinical studies have demonstrated initial response as a function of dose for testicular and ovarian cancer,[58,59] but have failed to demonstrate such a relationship for non-small cell lung, cervical, or relapsed head and neck cancer.[60-62]

*Toxicity.* CDDP will induce moderate to severe nausea and vomiting in virtually all patients soon after administration, and a variable number of patients will experience prolonged anorexia, weight loss, and malaise. Central and peripheral emesis mechanisms are thought to be stimulated by CDDP.[63] A major advance in cancer chemotherapy has occurred with the development of more potent anti-emetic drugs. Metoclopropamide has dramatically reduced the incidence of severe nausea and vomiting and, in general, is well tolerated.[64] Unfortunately, untoward extrapyramidal effects may occur in the younger patient population.[65] A recent study demonstrates that intravenous prochlorperazine may be as effective as high dose metoclopropamide with fewer side effects.[66] Although dexamethasone is an effective anti-emetic agent when used in combination with other drugs, it does not appear to be very effective when used alone in controlling platinum induced emesis.[67] Other drugs which appear to alleviate platinum induced nausea include cannabinoids,[68] and butyrophenones. Patients who receive a prolonged infusion of platinum appear to have less severe nausea and vomiting than patients who receive the drug as a bolus.[69]

Severe renal and G.I. toxicity in phase I studies almost led to the abandonment of CDDP. Approximately one fourth of the patients had significant elevations of BUN after doses of 50 mg/m$^2$. At doses of 100 mg/m$^2$, 61% of the courses were associated with renal injury, with the BUN peaking a mean of four days after therapy. Renal damage was decreased by fractionating the dose over several days, but cumulative toxicity prevented most patients from receiving more than four courses of therapy.[70-72] Renal toxicity can be decreased dramatically by the use of diuretics, mannitol, and most importantly, pretreatment hydration.[73,74] Even with hydration, however, a recent study indicates that the majority of patients will have a decrease in the creatinine clearance of almost 25% despite maintaining a normal serum creatinine.[75] Several investigators have sought to exploit the improved therapeutic-toxicity ratio by escalating the dose of CDDP. Doses of 200 mg/m$^2$ can be safely given when fractionated over 4–5 days and preceded with hypertonic saline.[76-77] The value of hypertonic saline may be less important than the fractionated schedule of drug administration as similar results have been obtained with normal saline.[78]

As adequate hydration has prevented clinically significant renal damage, neurotoxicity has emerged as the most serious end organ damage of chronic CDDP therapy.[79] Although the mechanism of this effect is unclear, central effects such as retrobulbar neuritis and normal pressure hydrocephalus as well as a peripheral sensory neuropathy are similar to the toxicity seen with heavy metal poisoning.[80] Virtually all patients will develop a sensory neuropathy after a cumulative dose of 600 mg/m$^2$ with the earliest changes detected after 300 mg/m$^2$. Often patients will complain of paresthesias and dysethesias and will lack deep tendon reflexes. Motor function appears to be well preserved.[81,82] Neurotoxicity has been especially concerning in studies examining "high dose" CDDP,[76,78,83] however, patient age and pre-existing disease may contribute considerably.[84] For example, much of the literature concerning neurotoxicity and high dose CDDP comes from patients with ovarian cancer, [83] where as many as 40% of the patients may have clinical or physiologic evidence of neurotoxicity prior to therapy.[82] In a recent study examining high dose CDDP in patients with relapsed testicular cancer, neurotoxicity was not dose limiting.[77]

Ototoxicity is related to cumulative dose and appears to be irreversible in most cases.[88] Vestibular dysfunction is rare.[86] Audiometric testing is recommended for patients who are expected to receive a cumulative dose of greater than 400 mg/m$^2$ or who have an underlying sensory neuropathy.[87]

Severe myelosuppression is uncommon, but when used in combination CDDP, may augment the myelotoxicity observed of other agents. Anemia is common after prolonged treatment, and may be related to a direct bone marrow effect, decreased erythropoetin resulting from kidney damage, or immune mediated hemolysis.[88-92.]

## Platinum Analogues

The toxicity of CDDP and the requirement for vigorous pre-treatment hydration have created tremendous enthusiasm for second generation platinum analogues. Carboplatin (JM-8), for example, has undergone extensive phase I studies, and is currently being tested in phase II and III studies, alone and in combination with 5FU.

*Mechanism of Action.* Mechanisms of carboplatin antitumor activity is similar to that of CDDP with the formation of intrastrand and interstrand DNA cross-links.[93] It has also been found that nuclear proteins have become increasingly important targets for nuclear acting cytotoxic drugs. Harrap et al. demonstrated that nuclear protein phosphorylation correlated with cell death.[93] Nuclear protein phosphorylation was more specific for tumor cells than for normal cells with carboplation, whereas cisplatin demonstrated enhanced nuclear protein phosphorylation in both tumorous and normal cells. This selective toxicity of carboplatin towards tumor cells may explain the decreased nephrotoxicity observed with this drug.

*Clinical Pharmacology.* In this first two hours after drug administration, ultrafilterable platinum accounts for 70-80% of total platinum in the plasma.[94] After a 24 hour infusion, 60% of the total platinum remains ultrafilterable.[95] There is a linear relationship between dose and area under the plasma concentration vs. time curve for total platinum over a dose range of 20-520 mg/M². The degree of protein binding has been variably reported. In general, the drug is mostly protein bound which increases with time.[96,97] Carboplatin is primarily excreted by the kidneys and total and renal clearance of free platinum correlates well with the glomerular filtration rate.[98] Renal impairment therefore affects drug clearance and most importantly causes severe thrombocytopenia. This must be taken into account when determining drug dose for patients with renal insufficiency.

*Toxicity.* In contrast to CDDP, dose limiting toxicity is myelosuppression with the greatest effect on platelets. WBC and platelet nadirs are somewhat delayed, occurring approximately three weeks after administration and recovering four to five weeks after treatment.[99-101]

Nausea and vomiting do occur, but are much less severe and protracted as compared to CDDP. Peripheral neuropathy and auditory impairment have not generally been seen, and thus far a small number of patients with renal insufficiency have tolerated treatment without permanent renal damage or prolonged myelosupression.[99,100,107] Studies employing carboplatin in head and neck cancer are underway and potentially hold great promise for the future.

## ACKNOWLEDGMENTS
Supported by Grants CA08341 and CA08010

## REFERENCES

1. Bertino JR, Boston B, Capizzi R: The role of chemotherapy in the management of cancer of the head and neck. A review. Cancer 1975:36:752-758.
2. Mead GM, Jacobs C: The changing role of chemotherapy in the treatment of head and neck cancer. Amer J Med 1982;73:582-595.
3. Bertino JR: Rescue techniques in cancer chemotherapy; use of leucovorin and other rescue agents after methotrexate treatment. Seminars in Oncol. 1977;4:203-215.
4. Galivan J: Evidence for the cytotoxic activity of polyglutamate derivatives of methotrexate. Mol Pharmacol 1980;17:105-110.
5. Neroic C, Badaracco G, Morelli M, Starace G: Cytokinetic evaluation in human head and neck cancer by autoradiography and DNA cytofluorometry. Cancer 1980;45:452-459.
6. Hryniuk WM, Fischer GA, Bertino JR: S-phase cells of rapidly growing and resting populations. Differences in response to methotrexate. Mol Pharmacol 1969;5:557-564.

7. Bertino JR: Toward improved selectivity in cancer chemotherapy: the Richard and Hinda Rosenthal Foundation Award Lecture. Cancer Res. 1979;33:293-304.

8. Cowan KH, Jolivet J: A methotrexate resistant human breast cancer cell line with multiple defect, including diminished formation of methotrexate polyglutamates. J Biol Chem 1984;259:10789-10800.

9. Frei E III, Rosowsky A, Wright JE, et al: Development of methotrexate resistance in a human squamous cell carcinoma of the head and neck in culture. Proc Nat Acad Sci, USA, 1984;81:2873-2877.

10. Carman MD, Schornagel JH, Rivest RS, et al: Clinical resistance to methotrexate due to gent amplification. J Clin Oncol 1984;2:16-20.

11. Horns RC, Dower WJ, Schimke RT: Gene amplification in a patient treated with methotrexate. J Clin Oncol 1984;2:2-7.

12. Curt GA, Carney DN, Cowan KH, et al: Unstable methotrexate resistance in human small cell carcinoma associated with double minute chromosomes. N Engl J Med 1983; 308:199-202.

13. Levitt M, Mosher MB, Deconti RC, et al: Improved therapeutic index of methotrexate with "Leucovorin Rescue." Cancer Res 1973;33:1729-1734.

14. Tattersall MHN, Parker IM, Pitman SW, Frei E III: Clinical pharmacology of high-dose methotrexate. Cancer Chemother Rep 1975;6:25-29.

15. Bleyer WA: The clinical pharmacology of methotrexate: new applications of an old drug. Cancer 1978;41:36-51.

16. Lankelma J, Van der Klein E: The role of 7-hydroxymethotrexate during methotrexate anti-cancer therapy. Cancer Letters 1980;9:133-142.

17. Nyfors A: Benefits and adverse drug experiences during long-term methotrexate treatment of 248 psoriatics. Danish Medical Bulletin 1978;25:208-211.

18. Cleveland JC, Johns DG, Farnham G, Bertino JR: Arterial infusion of dichloromethotrexate in cancer of the head and neck: A clinico-pharmacologic study. Current Topics, in J Surg Res, Zuidema GD, Skinner DB (eds), New York: Academic Press, 1969, pp 113-120.

19. Natale RB, Wheeler RH, Ensminger W, et al: Cisplatin plus dichloromethotrexate: A pharmacologically rational combination with high activity. Proc Amer Assoc Cancer Res 1983;24:166.

20. Wheeler RH, Natale RB, Roshon SG: A phase I-II trial of cisplatin and dichloromethotrexate in squamous cell cancer of the head and neck. J Clin Oncol 1984;2:831-835.

21. Cantwell B, Macauley V, Harris AL, et al: Phase II study of a noval antifolate $N^{10}$ propargyl - 5,8 dideazafolic acid (CB3717) in advanced breast cancer. Proc Amer Soc Clin Oncol 1985;5:63.

22. Lin JT, Cashmore AR, Baker M, et al: Phase I studies with trimetrexate: Clinical pharmacology analytical methodology, and pharmacokinetics. Cancer Res (in press).

23. Donehower RC, Graham ML, Thompson GE, et al: Phase I and pharmacokinetic study of trimetrexate in patients with advanced cancer. Proc Amer Soc Clin Oncol 1985;4:32.

24. Legra S, Tenney D, Ho DH, Krakoff I: Phase I clinical and pharmacology study of trimetrexate. Proc Amer Soc Oncol 1985;4:48.

25. Steward JA, McCormick JJ, Tong W, et al: A phase one study of trimetrexate. Proc Amer Assoc Cancer Res 1985;26:159.

26. Fonucchi M, Fleisher M, Vidal D, et al: Phase I and pharmacologic study of trimetrexate. Proc Amer Assoc Cancer Res. 1985;26:179.

27. Bertino JR, Sawicki WL, Moroson BA, et al: 2,4-diamino-5-methyl-6-[(3,4,5-trimethoxyanilino) methyl] quinazoline (TMQ), a potent non-classical folate antagonist inhibitor--I. Biochem Pharmacol 1979;28:1983-1987.

28. Carlson RN, Sikic BI: Continuous infusion of bolus injection in cancer chemotherapy. Ann Int Med. 1983;99:823–833.

29. Shehata WM, Meyer RL: The enhancement effect of irradiation by methotrexate. Cancer 1980;46:1349–1352.

30. Kish JA, Weaver A, Jacobs J, et al: Cisplatin and 5-fluorouracil infusion in patients with recurrent and disseminated epidermoid cancer of the head and neck. Cancer 1984; 53:1819–1824.

31. Merlano M, Tatarek R, Brimaldi A, et al: Phase I–II trial with cisplatin and 5-FU in recurrent head and neck cancer: an effective outpatient schedule. Cancer Treat Rep 1985;69:961–964.

32. Pitman SW, Kowal CD, Berino JR: Methotrexate and 5-fluorouracil in sequence in squamous head and neck cancer. Semin Oncol 1983;10:15–19.

33. Ringborg U, Evert G, Kinnman J, et al: Sequential methotrexate-5-fluorouracil treatment of squamous cell carcinoma of the head and neck. Cancer, (in press).

34. Jacobs C: Use of methotrexate and 5FU for recurrent head and neck cancer. Cancer Treat Rep 1982;66:1925.

35. Browman GP, Archibald SD, Young JEM, et al: Prospective randomized trial of one-hour sequential versus simultaneous methotrexate plus 5-fluorouracil in advanced and recurrent squamous cell head and neck cancer. J Clin Oncol 1983;1:787–792.

36. Coates AS, Tattersall MHN, Swanson C, et al: Combination chemotherapy with methotrexate and 5-fluorouracil: a prospective randomized clinical trial of order of administration. J Clin Oncol 1984;2:756–761.

37. Benz C, Schoenberg M, Choli M, Cadman F: Schedule-dependent cytotoxicity of methotrexate and 5-fluoruracil in human colon and breast turmor cell lines. J Clin Inv 1980;66:1162–1165.

38. Heidelberger C: Fluorinated pyrimidines and their nucleosides, in: Sartorelli A, Johns D, (eds): Antineoplastic and Immuno Suppressive Agents. New York: Springer-Verlag, 1975, pp 193–231.

39. Buexa-Perez JM, Leyva A, Pinedo HM: Effect of methotrexate on 5-phosphoribosyl 1-pyrophosphate levels in L1210 leukemia cells in vitro. Cancer Res 1980;40:139–283.

40. Sobrero AF, Bertino JR: Sequence dependent synergism between dichloromethotrexate and cisplatin in a human colon carcinoma cell line. Cancer Treat Rep 1985;69:279–283.

41. Sobrero AF, Handschumacher RE, Bertino JR: Highly selective drug combinations for human colon cancer cells resistant in vitro to 5-fluoro-2'-deoxyuridine. Cancer Res 1985;45:3161–3163.

42. Suzuki H, Nagai K, Akutsu E, et al: On the mechanism of action of bleomycin strand scission of DNA caused by bleomycin and its binding to DNA in vitro. J Antibiot 1970;23:473–480.

43. Yagoda A, Mukherji B, Young C, et al: Bleomycin an antitumor antibiotic. Clinical experience in 274 patients. Ann Int Med 1972;77:861.

44. Rudders RA, Hensley GT: Bleomycin pulmonary toxicity. Chest 1973;63:626–628.

45. Roberts JJ: Cisplatin, in Pinedo HM (ed): Cancer Chemother. Amsterdam: Excerpta medica, 1982, pp 95–117.

46. Lippard SJ: New chemistry of an old molecule: cis-(Pt(NH$_3$) Cl). Science 1982; 218:1075–1082.

47. Schabel FM Jr, Trader MW, Laster WR Jr, et al: Cis-dichlorodiammineplatinum (11): combination chemotherapy and cross-resistance studies with tumors of mice. Cancer Treat Rep 1979;63:1459–1473.

48. Carde P, Laval F: Effect of cis-dichlorodiammineplatinum 11 and X rays on mammalian cell survival. Int J Radiat Oncol Biol Phys 1981;7:929–933.

49. Filipski J, Kohn KW, Prather R, Bonner WM: Thiourea reverses crosslinks and restores biological activity in DNA treated with dichlorodiammineplatinum (11). Science 1979;204:181–183.
50. Burchenal JH, Kalaherk Lokys L, Gale G: Studies of cross-resistance synergistic combination and blocking activity of platinum derivatives. Biochimie 1978;60:861–965.
51. Howell SB, Taetle R: Effect of sodium thiosulfate on Cis-dichlorodiammineplatinum(II) toxicity and antitumor activity in L-1210 leukemia. Cancer Treat Rep 1980;64:611–616.
52. Belt RJ, Himmelstein KJ, Patton TF, et al: Pharmacokinetics of non protein bound platinum species following administration of Cis-dichlorodiammineplatinum(II). Cancer Treat Rep 1979;63:1515–1521.
53. Gormley PE, Bull JM, Leroy AF, Cysyk R: Kinetics of Cis-dichlorodiammineplatinum(II). Clin Pharmacol Ther. 1979;25:351–357.
54. Gouyette A, Lemone R, Adhemar JP, et al: Kinetics of cisplatin in an anuric patient undergoing hemofiltration dialysis. Cancer Treat Rep 1981;65:665–668.
55. Pretorius RG, Petrilli ES, Kean C, et al: Comparison of the IV and IP routes of administration of cisplatin in dogs. Cancer Treat Rep 1981;65:1055–1062.
56. Frei E III, Canellos GP: Dose: A critical factor in cancer chemotherapy. Amer J Med 1980;69:585–594.
57. Kaye SB: Intensive chemotherapy for solid tumors—current clinical applications. Cancer Chemother Pharmacol 1982;9:127–133.
58. Samson MK, Rivkin SE, Jones SE, et al: Dose-response and dose-survival for high versus low-dose cisplatin combined with vinblastine and bleomycin in disseminated testicular cancer. Cancer 1984;53:1029–1035.
59. Bruckner HW, Wallach R, Cohen CJ, et al: High-dose platinum for the treatment of refractory ovarian cancer. Gynecol Oncol 1981;12:64–67.
60. Gralla RJ, Casper ES, Kelson DP, et al: Cisplatin and vindesine combination chemotherapy for advanced carcinoma of the lung: A randomized trial investigating two dosage schedules. Ann Int Med 1981;95:414–420.
61. Bonomi P, Blessing JA, Stehman FB, et al: Randomized trial of three cisplatin dose schedules in squamous-cell carcinoma of the cervix: A gynecologic oncology group study. Clin Oncol 1985;3:1079–1085.
62. Tumolo S, Veronese U, Tirelli U, et al: High-dose versus low-dose cis-platinum in advanced head and neck squamous carcinoma. Proc Amer Soc Clin Oncol (abstr) 1983;2:163.
63. Siegel LJ, Longo DL: The control of chemotherapy-induced emesis. Ann Int Med 1981;95:352–359.
64. Gralla RJ, Itri LM, Pisko se, et al: Antiemetic efficacy of high-dose metoclopramide: randomized trials with placebo and prochlorperazine in patients with chemotherapy-induced nausea and vomiting. N Eng J Med 1981;305:905–909.
65. Kris MG, Tyson LB, Gralla RJ, et al: Extrapyramidal reactions with high-dose metoclopramide. N Engl J Med 1983;309:433–444.
66. Carr BI, Bertrand M, Browning S, et al: A comparison of the antiemetic efficacy of prochlorperazine and metoclopramide for the treatment of cisplatin-induced emesis: A prospective, randomized, double-blind study. Clin Oncol 1985;3:1127–1131.
67. D'Olimpio JT, Camacho F, Chandra P, et al: Antiemetic efficacy of high-dose dexamethasone versus placebo in patients receiving cisplatin-based chemotherapy: A randomized double-blind controlled clinical trial. Clin Oncol 1985;3:1133–1135.
68. Vincent BJ, McQuiston DJ, Einhorn LH, et al: Review of cannabinoids and their antiemetic effectiveness. Drugs 1983;25:52–62.

69. Jordan NS, Schauer PK, Schauer A, et al: The effect of administration rate on cisplatin-induced emesis. Clin Oncol 1985;3:559–561.

70. Higby DJ, Wallace HJ Jr, Albert DJ, et al: Diamminedi-cloroplatinum: a phase I study showing responses in testicular and other tumors. Cancer 1974;33:1219–1255.

71. Rossof AH, Slayton RE, Perlia CP: Preliminary clinical experience with cis-diammine-dichloroplatinum(II)(NSC-119875,CACP). Cancer 1972;30:1451–1456.

72. Higby DJ, Wallace HJ Jr, Holland JF: Cis-diamminedichloroplatinum(NSC-119875): a phase one study. Cancer Chemother Rep 1973;57:459.

73. Weiss RB, Poster DS: The renal toxicity of cancer chemotherapeutic agents. Cancer Treat Rep 1982;9:37–56.

74. Comis RL: Cisplatin nephrotoxicity: the effect of dose, schedule and hydration scheme, in Prestayko AW, Crooke ST, Carter SK (eds): Cisplatin: Current status and New Developments. New York: Academic Press, Inc. 1980, pp 485–494.

75. Meiser S, Sleisfer DT, Mulder WH, et al: Some effects of combination chemotherapy with cisplatin on renal function in patients with nonseminatous testicular carcinoma. Cancer 1983;51:2035–2040.

76. Ozols RF, Corden BS, Jacobs J, et al: High-dose cisplatin in hypertonic saline. Ann Int Med 1984;100:19–24.

77. Trump DL, Hortvet L: Etoposide and very high dose cisplatin salvage therapy for patients with advanced germ cell neoplasms. Cancer Treat Rep 1985;69:259–261.

78. Legha SS, Dimery I: High dose Cisplatin administration without hypertonic saline: observation of disabling neurotoxicity. J Clin Oncol 1985;3:1373–1378.

79. Lochrer PJ, Einhorn LH: Cisplatin. Ann Int Med 1984;100:704–713.

80. Von Hoff DD, Schilsky R, Reichert CM, et al: Toxic effects of cis-dichlorodiammineplatinum (II) in man. Cancer Treat Rep 1979;63:1527–1531.

81. Thompson SW, Davis LE, Kornfiled M, et al: Cisplatin neuropathy. Clinical electrophysiologic, morphologic and toxicologic studies. Cancer 1984;54:1269–1275.

82. Roelfs RI, Hrushesky W, Rogin J, Rosenberg L: Peripheral sensory neuropathy and cisplatin chemotherapy. Neurology 1984;34:934–938.

83. Bagley CM Jr, Rudolph RH, Rivkin SE, Yon JL Jr: High-dose cisplatin therapy for cancer of the ovary: neurotoxicity. Ann Int Med, 1985;719.

84. Ozols RF, Young R: (Letter), Ann Int Med, 1985;102:719.

85. Reddel RR, Kefford RF, Grant JM, et al: Ototoxity in patients receiving cisplatin: importance of dose and method of drug administration. Cancer Treat Rep 1982;66:19–23.

86. Schaefer SD, Wright CG, Post JD, Frenkel EP: Cis-platinum vestibular toxicity. Cancer 1981;547:847–849.

87. Schaefer SD, Post SD, Close LG, Wright CG: Ototoxicity of low and moderate-dose cisplatin. Cancer 1985;56:1934–1939.

88. Rothman SA, Weick JK: Cisplatin toxicity for erythroid precursors (Letter). N Eng J Med 1981;304:360.

89. Nowrovsian MR, Schmidt CG: Effects of cisplatin indifferent haemopoetic progenitor cells in mice. Brit J Cancer 1982;46:397–402.

90. Getaz EP, Beckley S, Fitzpatrick S, Dozier A: Cisplatin-induced hemolysis. N Eng J Med 1980;302:334–335.

91. Ngoyen BV, Jaffe N: Cisplatin induced anemia. Cancer Treat Rep 1981;65:1121.

92. Levi A, Aroney RS, Dalley DN: Hemolytic anemia after cisplatin treatment. Brit Med J 1981;282:2003–2004.

93. Harrap KR, et al: Antitumor, toxic and biochemical properties of cisplatin and eight other

platinum complexes in, Cisplatin, current status and new developments. Prestayko AW, Crook ST, Carter SK (eds): 1980, pp 193–211.

94. Egorin MJ, et al: Phase I study and clinical pharmacokinetics of carboplation (LBDCS) CNSC 241240), 4th international symposium on platinum coordination complexes in cancer chemotherapy. (Abstr F15). Burlington: 1983.

95. Curt GA, et al: A phase I and pharmacokinetic study of diammine cyclobutane – dicrobylatoplatinum (NSE 241240), Cancer Res 1983;43:4470–4473.

96. Calvert AH, et al: Early clinical studies with cis-diamine-1-1-cyclobutane-dicarboxylate platinum II, Cancer Chemother Parmacol 1982;9:140–147.

97. Harland SJ, et al: Phase II study of cis-diamine-1-1-cyclobutaine dicarboxylate platinum II (CBDCA, JM8) in carcinoma of the bronchus. 4th international symposium on platinum coordination complexes in cancer chemotherapy, Burlington: (Abstr C17), 1983.

98. Woolley PV, et al: Clinical pharmacokinetics of diamine-1,1-cyclobutane carboxylate platinum (CBDCA). 4th international symposium of platinum coordination complexes in cancer chemotherapy. (Abstr BII) Burlington: , 1983.

99. Leyvras S, Ohnuma T, Lassus M, Holland JF: Phase I study of carboplatin in patients with advanced cancer, intermittent intravenous bolus, and 24-hour infusion. Clin Oncol 1985;3:1385–1392.

100. Koeller JM, Trump DL, Tutsch KD, et al: Phase I clinical trial and pharmacokinetics of carboplatin (BSC 241240) by single monthly 30-minute infusion. Cancer 1986; 57:222–225.

101. Eelto D, Egorin MJ, Whitacre MY, et al: Phase I clinical and pharmacologic trial of carboplatin daily for 5 days. Cancer Treat Rep 1984;8:1103–1114.

# CHAPTER 13

# Curative Chemotherapy of Advanced and Disseminated Solid Tumors of Mice

*Thomas H. Corbett, PhD,*
*Billy J. Roberts, BS,*
*Alfred J. Lawson, PhD, and*
*Wilbur R. Leopold III, PhD*

## INTRODUCTION

Considering the subject matter and intent of this symposium, one would wish to include a review of the progress made in curing transplantable murine squamous cell tumors of the head and neck. In addition, one would wish to focus on the most metastatic murine tumors of this histologic type. Unfortunately, and for a variety of reasons, no transplantable squamous cell tumors of the head and neck have been available for research investigations. Virtually all of the progress that has been made in the treatment of this disease has been made in humans (with drugs discovered in mouse leukemias and combination chemotherapy and combination modality results drawn sparingly from a few animal tumor models; e.g., the discovery of the potentiating combination of 5-FU + CisDDPt).[1]

Thus, this review will be focused primarily on the strategies and principles for curative chemotherapy of advanced staged, highly metastatic murine tumors from other tissues, with the hope that these principles will have a general application to the more difficult-to-treat squamous cell tumors of the head and neck.

**175**

## BIOLOGY OF HIGHLY METASTATIC TUMORS OF MICE

In order to gain an insight into the testing results presented, it is necessary to understand the biologic behavior of non-immunogenic, highly metastatic tumors of mice.

These solid tumors are invariably aggressively invasive and are able to establish new tumor growth with less than $3 \times 10^4$ cells implanted subcutaneously (SC) (Table 13.1).[2] They metastasize to distant organ systems (e.g., lungs) in greater than 80% of the mice before the SC tumor masses reach 1000 mg in size ($1.0 \times 10^9$ cells).[2-6] Most of the tumors have high sensitivity to only a few antitumor agents, and it is rare to find more than four or five agents able to kill greater than $2.0 \log_{10}$ of tumor cells with a single course of treatment.[2-4] Compared with chemotherapy, x-irradiation is able to kill approximately 0.7 to $1.0 \log_{10}$ of tumor cells per 1000 rads delivered to the established tumor masses (Lawson, Leopold, Roberts, and Corbett, unpublished results).

In general, it is a simple matter to cure immunogenic tumors or any tumor that has been implanted at a titer close to the level needed to establish tumor growth.[7] In some cases, it is necessary to implant $5 \times 10^7$ cells to establish growth of relatively non-invasive grade II tumors; e.g., Mam #04/A and Colon #07/A (Table 13.1). Thus, the implantation of this number of cells from one of these relatively non-invasive tumors, followed (within 2 or 3 days) by chemotherapy with an active agent will usually produce a high frequency of cures; giving the illusion of a high tumor cell kill because of the high implant number.[7] Obviously, cure in this setting often represents less than a $1 \log_{10}$ tumor cell kill. In contrast, highly metastatic, highly invasive tumors are difficult to cure in the same experimental design

**TABLE 13.1** Take Rate

| Number of Cells, SC | High Malignancy | | Low Malignancy | |
|---|---|---|---|---|
| | **Mam. 44** | **Colon 26** | **Mam. 04/A** | **Colon 07/A** |
| $10^8$ | — | — | [19/19] | [10/10] |
| $10^7$ | — | — | 17/20 | 6/10 |
| $10^6$ | 10/10 | 10/10 | 10/20 | 1/9 |
| $10^5$ | 10/10 | 10/10 | 0/19 | 0/10 |
| $10^4$ | [10/10] | 9/10 | 0/20 | 0/10 |
| $10^3$ | 9/10 | [10/10] | 0/20 | 0/10 |
| $10^2$ | — | 2/10 | — | — |
| $10^1$ | — | 0/8 | — | — |

Number of mice developing tumors/number of mice implanted.

because of the requirement for a larger $\log^{10}$ cell kill (since these tumors will establish new tumor growth with less than $3 \times 10^4$ cells).

By the time the tumors have reached 300 mg in size ($3 \times 10^8$ cells), it is usually impossible to effect cure with any single chemotherapeutic agent. By the time the tumors have metastasized (400 to 1000 mg size), cure of a high percentage of the mice is usually impossible with any single modality.[2-6] This latter case is the essence of the situation encountered in many head-and-neck patients; i.e., an advanced stage tumor that has become entrenched and disseminated.

Since it is unusual to cure advanced-staged, highly metastatic solid tumors by any single modality, surgical removal of the primary mass is an essential part of the protocol design.[2,4] For these studies, the mice are implanted with 30 to 60 mg size tumor fragments with a trocar on the side midway between the axillary and the inguinal region. The tumors are allowed to grow to the desired size range, culling those animals outside of the desired limits. If chemotherapy is carried out post-surgery, the mice are randomized after surgery to the various treatment and control groups. Given a degree of practice, "en bloc" removal, and the use of a wide excision margin (including the removal of the overlying skin and the first muscle layer beneath the tumor), successful primary site removal is determined by the biologic properties of the tumor as well as the size, location and degree of local extension.[2] For equal size tumors, the ability to effect 100% tumor removal of the SC mass (no primary site regrowth) varies from 60 to 90% of the mice depending on the particular tumor (Fig. 13.1). The number of tumor cells remaining in disseminated sites (or locally) after surgical removal of 400 to 1000 mg size tumors will encompass a very broad range: from 0 (the occasional surgical cure) to $5 \times 10^7$ cells. The median animal will usually harbor between $1 \times 10^4$ and $1 \times 10^5$ cells. Thus, a large improvement in the frequency of cures in a surgery-chemotherapy adjuvant trial represents a relatively large tumor cell kill (since 30 to 50% of the animals harbor $10^5$ to $5 \times 10^7$ cells). The broad range in the number of tumor cells remaining post-surgery is in marked contrast to cell implant experiments (e.g., intravenous implants) in which all the animals within a group will have a relatively uniform number (usually within one $\log_{10}$).

## TYPES OF AGENTS THAT HAVE PRODUCED CURES IN SURGERY-CHEMOTHERAPY ADJUVANT TREATMENT OF HIGHLY METASTATIC MOUSE TUMORS

After examining a wide variety of single agents and combinations (administered as adjuvants to surgery), it was found that curative regimens almost

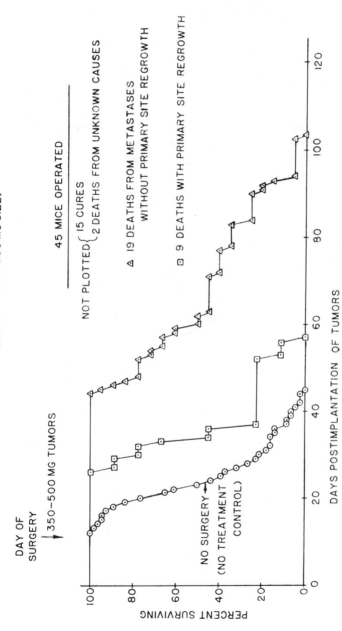

**FIGURE 13.1** Balb/c mice were implanted subcutaneously (midway) between the axillary and inguinal region with 30–60 mg size fragments of colon tumor #26 on day 0. When the tumors reached 350–500 mg in size the tumors were removed (with curative intent). Excision (en bloc) was carried out with wide margins and with removal of the skin over the tumor. If superficial attachment to the body wall was evident, a single muscle layer was removed with the attached tumor. If total removal of the primary tumor could not be accomplished, the mouse was sacrificed immediately and excluded from all data tabulations. Wound closure was effected with clips. The range in the time of death from metastases without primary site regrowth (43–102 days in this trial) is a reflection of the great variation in the number of tumor cells remaining postsurgery among the mice.

invariably contained an *alkylating agent*, a *DNA-binder*, or *both*.[2] Numerous examples can be seen in published reports on a variety of different metastatic tumor models.[2,4-6,8-11] These tumors include: $B_{16}$ melanoma, mammary #44, mammary adenocarcinoma #16/C, colon #26, Dunn osteosarcoma, pancreatic ductal adenocarcinoma #02, and Lewis lung carcinoma. In some cases, the Lewis lung results from the late 1970's and early 1980's are suspect because the NCI Tumor Repository was supplying an aberrant, highly immunogenic subline of the tumor.[7]

## CURABILITY AS A FUNCTION OF TUMOR BURDEN

In the examples shown in Figure 13.2, surgery was performed on mice bearing tumors in two different size ranges (i.e., 250–350 mg size [Fig. 13.2A], and 500–700 mg size [Fig. 13.2B]), followed by an identical chemotherapy regimen. It is evident that the smaller the tumor burden, the greater the frequency of cures attributed to the chemotherapy. Based on previous studies, it was known that both of these alkylating agents were active singly against this tumor (mammary line-44) and the combination was known to be synergistic (based on results of Valeriote).[12]

## INNATE INSENSITIVITY OF A TUMOR FOR A PARTICULAR DRUG

The supposition that any malignant tumor will respond to any anticancer agent if the tumor is optimally treated at a small enough size (favorable growth kinetic status) is clearly not true.[2,3,11] Some tumors are totally unresponsive to agents curative against other tumors.[2,3,4,11] This is not a problem of acquired resistance; i.e., a mutational event.[3] It is simply that the tumor is no more responsive to the drug than rapidly proliferating normal cells of the host (e.g., marrow stem cells or GI epithelium).[3] One highly metastatic tumor has been identified that is unresponsive to 34 different clinically available antitumor agents that encompass all known mechanisms of antitumor action.[3]

Reduction of the tumor burden by surgery, followed by treatment with an agent that is inactive or only marginally active against 60 to 300 mg size masses of the tumor, is not beneficial in the post-surgical adjuvant setting (Fig. 13.3).[4] This same dose of the same drug is curative with surgery in a more sensitive tumor (i.e., mammary 16/C).[4] Other examples of marginally active agents failing to produce improved results with surgery have been published previously.[2,4,11]

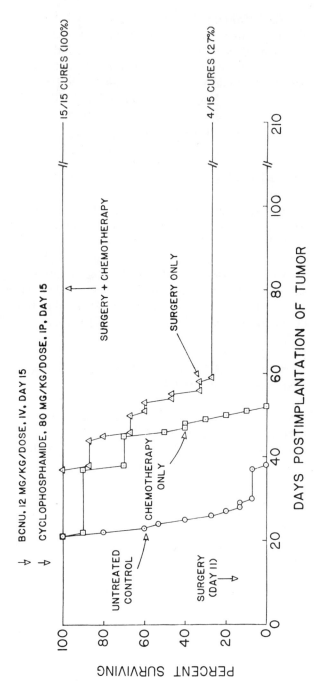

SURGERY + BCNU–CYCLOPHOSPHAMIDE TREATMENT OF MAMMARY TUMORS—LINE 44

EARLY STAGE DISEASE (250–350MG TUMORS)

↓ BCNU, 12 MG/KG/DOSE, IV, DAY 15

↓ CYCLOPHOSPHAMIDE, 80 MG/KG/DOSE, IP, DAY 15

15/15 CURES (100%)

4/15 CURES (27%)

SURGERY + CHEMOTHERAPY

SURGERY ONLY

CHEMOTHERAPY ONLY

UNTREATED CONTROL

SURGERY (DAY II)

PERCENT SURVIVING

DAYS POSTIMPLANTATION OF TUMOR

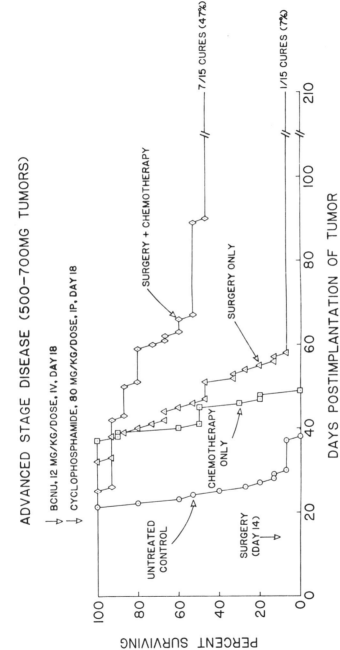

**FIGURE 13.2-A and 13.2-B** Tumor implantation and surgical removal of the primary tumors was carried out as described in Figure 13.1. In this experiment, surgery was carried out at two different times; day 11 postimplant when the tumors were 250–300 mg in size; and day 14, when the tumors were 500–700 mg in size. Chemotherapy with the same dosages of the same agents was administered 4 days post-surgery in each case.

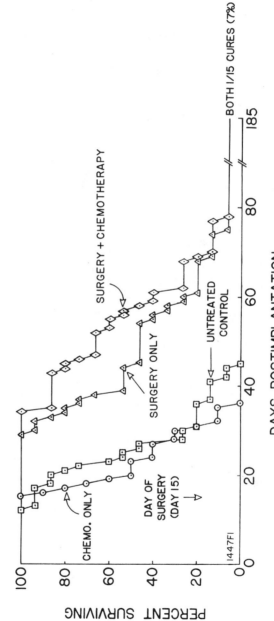

**FIGURE 13.3** Tumor implantation and surgical removal of the primary tumors was carried out as described in Figure 13.1. The tumor (colon #26) at a subcutaneous growth site was known to be only marginally responsive to the agent (Adriamycin). Micrometastatic disease was not signifiantly more responsive (comparing the surgery + Adriamycin treated group with surgery only).

The use of a combination of two agents in which one of the agents is only marginally active or inactive against the tumor has produced results inferior to the optimum post-surgical use of the most active agent alone.[2]

## CURABILITY AS A FUNCTION OF DRUG DOSAGE

The use of higher dosages of agents known to be active against a particular tumor (within the limits of normal tissue toxicity) has invariably produced higher tumor cell kills and a higher frequency of cures.[13,14] One suspects that failure to obtain a meaningful dose-response can usually be attributed to either the inadequate evaluation of lethal toxicity, the use of antigenic tumor models, or the use of inactive or only marginally active regimens.

As expected, curability of metastatic disease after surgical removal of the primary mass is also dose-related (Fig. 13.4)[2]

In humans, considerable variability exists from individual to individual in their ability to tolerate a given $mg/m^2$ dose of a drug.[15] Usually, individualized dosage adjustments are needed to reach a similar degree of normal tissue toxicity within a heterogeneous group of patients. Similar custom treatment is needed for adjuvant chemotherapy,[15] however, escalations (if needed) must be carried out rapidly, or intervals between courses shortened, since cure or lack of cure is decided in the first few courses.[2,8]

## CURABILITY AS A FUNCTION OF SCHEDULE

If chemotherapy is initiated prior to or within a few days after surgery (e.g., less than five), it appears that one to four courses of chemotherapy (at no more than 7 day intervals) are optimum if the regimen has considerable cumulative toxicity. In our experience, all the curative regimens appear to have considerable cumulative toxicity.[2,8] The most extensive series of experiments were carried out in the 1960's by Karrer and Humphreys using Lewis lung carcinoma and cyclophosphamide.[8] In these studies, two or three courses of treatment were clearly optimum for cure. Thus, in the highly metastatic mouse tumors, it appears that all treatments should be included within the first 21 days post-surgery. Given the differences in tumor volume doubling time between the common metastatic human tumors and the metastatic mouse tumors, this would translate to approximately 140 days in the human. Based on the results from mouse trials, chemotherapy after this time would be viewed as palliative in most cases. Clearly, the advent of curative regimens with better host recovery times (than those now available) would lengthen this critical time interval.

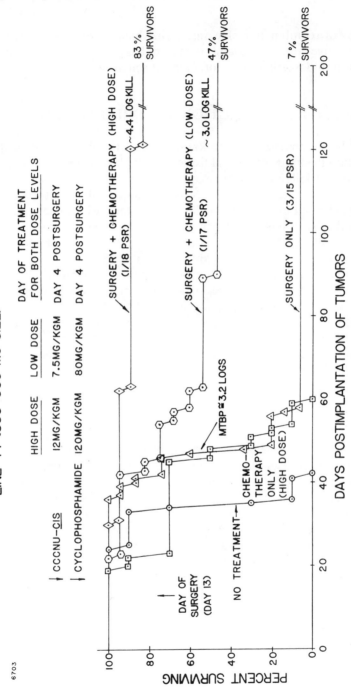

**FIGURE 13.4** Tumor implantation and surgical removal of the primary tumors was carried out as described in Figure 13.1. In this experiment, two different dosages of chemotherapy were compared.

PSR = primary site regrowths.

MTBP = median tumor burden remaining immediately postsurgery.

184

6703

## CURABILITY AS A FUNCTION OF TIMING: CHEMOTHERAPY OR X-IRRADIATION PRE- OR POST-SURGERY

If metastatic disease is known to be present, it would appear that the sooner chemotherapy is initiated, the better. Chemotherapy prior to surgery appears to be more curative than chemotherapy post-surgery (Fig. 13.5, 13.6).[2,4,16] Nissen-Meyer et al have proposed that metastatic spread is frequently caused by the surgical removal of the primary mass.[17] They suggest that chemotherapy should be started the day of surgery and continued several days thereafter. Their results in humans and one trial carried out in mice are consistant with this hypothesis.[2,17] However, the killing of tumor cells in metastatic foci before they can replicate further would also explain the improvements in survival.

The use of x-irradiation prior to surgery has been superior to post-surgical irradiation in reducing the number of primary site regrowths (Table 13.2).[18] Table 13.2 represents pooled results from mice irradiated with a field that included both the primary site and axillary region (a site of metastatic spread for both of these tumors in addition to lung metastasis). The mice bearing the mammary adenocarcinoma #16/C were irradiated with 500 to 1500 rads either 3 days before or 3 days after surgery (non-tumor deaths excluded). A more detailed tabulation of one of the individual experiments is shown in Table 13.3. The mice bearing the mucin producing colon adenocarcinoma #51 were irradiated QDx3 with 590 to 1000 rads/ fraction with a one day rest between surgery and irradiation.

## RATIONALE FOR THE SELECTION OF MULTI-AGENT COMBINATIONS

In general, antitumor agents produce a therapeutic advantage in combination for one or more of the following reasons: (1) There is a lack of overlap in toxicity for vital normal tissues. Therefore, the dosages of the individual agents need not be radically reduced when used in combination. The quantitative expression of the degree of overlap (the Combination Toxicity Index; CTI) has been described.[19,20] Non-overlap in toxicity can be important both in terms of short term toxicities (e.g., leucopenia or thrombocytopenia) and for long term cumulative damage to organs (e.g., heart of kidney); or (2) There is a lack of cross-resistance among the various agents; thus, cells resistant to one agent retain sensitivity to the other agents in the combination. This factor is important in either single course treatment or repeated course therapy in which the total kill exceeds 6 $\log_{10}$. Often, agents are

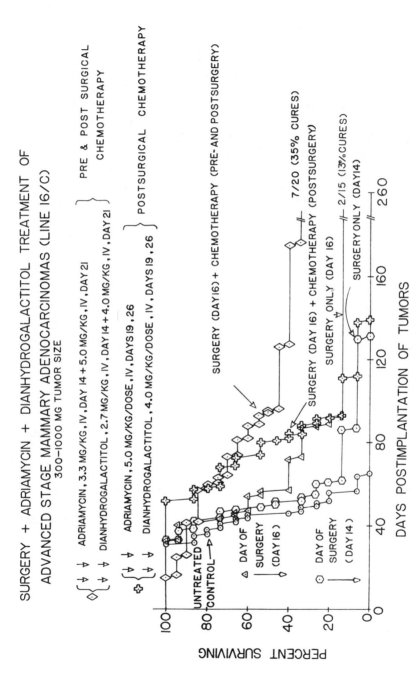

**FIGURE 13.5** Tumor implantation and surgical removal of the primary tumors was carried out as described in Figure 13.1. In this experiment chemotherapy was administered both pre-surgery (day 14) and post-surgery (day 21) (surgery day 16) as well as post surgery only (day 19 and 26) (surgery day 16). Identical dosages and schedule intervals were used.

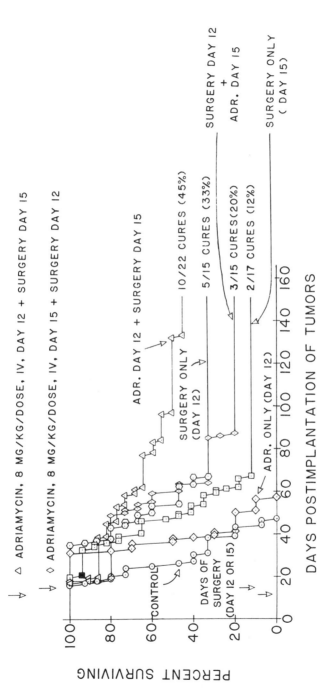

**FIGURE 13.6** Tumor implantation and surgical removal of the primary tumors was carried out as described in Figure 13.1. In this experiment, chemotherapy was administered pre-surgery (day 12) (surgery day 15) or post-surgery (day 15), (surgery day 12).

**TABLE 13.2** Pre- vs. Post-surgical X-Irradiation

| | Primary Site Regrowths (PSR's) | | |
|---|---|---|---|
| | Exp. 1 | Exp. 2 | Total PSR's % Incidence |
| Colon 51 | | | |
| X-Ray Only | 47/47 | 41/41 | 100 |
| Surgery Only | 6/28 | 6/26 | 22 |
| X-Ray before Surgery | 1/24 | 2/22 | 6 |
| X-Ray after Surgery | 7/24 | 2/17 | 22 |
| Mammary 16/C | | | |
| X-Ray Only | — | 46/46 | 100 |
| Surgery Only | 6/8 | 19/26 | 74 |
| X-Ray before Surgery | 2/22 | 7/18 | 22 |
| X-Ray after Surgery | 12/18 | 16/23 | 68 |

selected with different mechanisms of antiproliferative action to avoid overlap in toxicity and cross-resistance behavior. The cross-resistance behavior of a large number of agents has been tabulated[21]; or (3) In some cases there is a biochemical interaction in which the first agent affects a biochemical step or steps in the tumor cell that preferentially render that cell more vulnerable to the action of the second agent than it does for the normal cells of the host. It is important to emphasize the last part of this statement. Frequently, marked increases in cytotoxicity for the tumor cells are exactly paralleled by the same increase in cytotoxicity for vital normal cells.[22] Synergisms due to biochemical interactions appear to be sequence and schedule dependent in many cases.

One of the most useful combinations in the treatment of head and neck is CisDDPt plus 5-FU.[23] This combination was demonstrated to be therapeutically synergistic against tumors of mice.[1] CisDDPt + 5-FU does not totally overlap in normal tissue toxicity (CTI = 1.3 to 1.6) and cross-resistance does not occur.[21] There does not appear to be a marked sequence dependence for the synergism, although the simultaneous use of the two agents appears to be slightly superior (Table 13.4).

Two analogues of CisDDPt (i.e., Carboplatin [CBDCA] and Iproplatin [CHIP]) have recently entered clinical trials. Unfortunately, we could not demonstrate synergism with either of the analogues plus 5-FU against a squamous cell lung tumor (LC-12).[24] Furthermore, the combination of CisDDPt plus 5-FU was slightly superior to both CBDCA plus 5-FU and CHIP plus 5-FU in terms of tumor growth delay against the same tumor

**TABLE 13.3** Comparison of Pre- and Postsurgical Radiation of Mammary Adenocarcinoma 16/C

| Rx | Sched. (Days) | %ILS | Tumor-Free Surv. | Non-Tumor Deaths* | Mets. w/o PSR | Tumor with Mets. | Tumor w/o Mets. | Comment |
|---|---|---|---|---|---|---|---|---|
| **No Rx; MDD = 34 days.** | | | | | | 3/12 | 9/12 | |
| *Radiation After Surgery* | | | | | | | | |
| Surg. | 9 | | 0/12 | 0/12 | — | 3/12 | 9/12 | |
| 1500 R | 12 | −25 | 0/12 | 6/12 | 0/12 | 3/12 | 3/12 | Toxic - 6/12 PSR |
| Surg. | 9 | | | | | | | |
| 800 R | 12 | −14 | 0/12 | 4/12 | 2/12 | 5/12 | 1/12 | Toxic - 6/12 PSR |
| Surg. | 9 | | | | | | | |
| 500 R | 12 | 2 | 2/12 | 2/12 | 2/12 | 3/12 | 3/12 | 6/12 PSR |
| *Radiation Prior to Surgery* | | | | | | | | |
| 1500 R | 9 | | | | | | | |
| Surg. | 12 | −14 | 0/12 | 6/12 | 5/12 | 1/12 | 0/12 | Toxic - 1/12 PSR |
| 800 R | 9 | | | | | | | |
| Surg. | 12 | −6 | 1/12 | 0/12 | 10/12 | 1/12 | 0/12 | Only 1/12 PSR |
| 500 R | 9 | | | | | | | |
| Surg. | 12 | 0 | 2/12 | 3/12 | 6/12 | 1/12 | 0/12 | Only 1/12 PSR |
| *Surgery Control* | | | | | | | | |
| Surg. | 9 | −3 | 0/12 | 4/12 | 2/12 | 3/12 | 3/12 | 6/12 PSR |

*Includes deaths due to surgical and/or radiation trauma, as well as those mice that could not be autopsied due to cannibalism or decomposition of autopsy material, expt. 1724DI.

**189**

**TABLE 13.4** Treatment of Colon Adenocarinoma #38 with 5-FU Plus CisDDPt in BDF$_1$ Male Mice

| Highest Non-Toxic Treatment (LD$_{10}$ or Less) | Time in Days for Median Tumor to Reach 750 mg | Tumor Growth Delay in Days | Log$_{10}$ Cell Kill |
|---|---|---|---|
| *Single Agents* | | | |
| 5-FU, 130 mg/kg/dose, IV, days 4,11,18 | 39 | 22 | 2.7 |
| CisDDPt, 7.5 mg/kg/dose, IV, days 4,11,18 | 27 | 10 | 1.2 |
| *Highest Non-Toxic Combinations (LD$_{10}$ or Less)* Simultaneous Administration | | | |
| 5-FU, 60 mg/kg/dose, IV, days 4,11,18 | | | |
| CisDDPt, 7.5 mg/kg/dose, IV, days 4,11,18 | 48 | 31 | 3.7 |
| Alternating Administration | | | |
| 5-FU, 40 mg/kg/dose, IV, days 4,11,18 | | | |
| CisDDPt, 5 mg/kg/dose, IV, days 6,13,20 | 44 | 27 | 3.2 |
| Untreated Control | 17 | — | — |

There were no tumor free survivors in any of the control or treatment groups.

model (although the number of complete regressions and cures were similar for the three regimens).[24]

## FUTURE ADVANCES

Without a doubt, the largest advancements that have occurred in the treatment of specific malignant diseases have been the discovery of one or more new agents able to produce a large log$_{10}$ cell kill in a high percentage of the tumors. Heretofore, most new agents have been discovered against mouse leukemias, and it is not surprising to find that these agents have high activity and broad activity against leukemias and lymphomas. It is also not too surprising that these same agents have scant or no activity against many solid tumors of mice or humans.[3] It is only recently that the philosophies of drug screening have changed at NCI and elsewhere.[25] With these changes, solid tumors are being used to select new agents.[25-28] One of the most promising new agents discovered is flavone acetic acid (NSC 347512), an agent with broad solid tumor activity but with only scant activity against leukemias.[28,29] As might be expected, this agent does not have marrow toxicity, and is thus unlikely to overlap in normal tissue toxicity with currently used antiproliferative agents. It is likely that agents of this nature, discovered against specific types of solid tumors, will provide the ability to cure advanced stage, disseminated head and neck tumors.

## ACKNOWLEDGMENTS

Supported in part by NIH grant CA-43886, NIH contract NO1 CM-97309, and by the Ben Kasle Trust for Cancer Research.

## REFERENCES

1. Schabel FM Jr, Trader MW, Laster WR Jr et al: Cis-dichloro-diammineplatinum (II): Combination chemotherapy and cross-resistance studies with tumors of mice. Cancer Treat Rep 1979;63:1459–1473.
2. Corbett TH, Griswold DP Jr, Roberts BJ, Schabel FM Jr: Cytotoxic adjuvant therapy and the experimental model, Chapter 10, in Stoll BA (ed): New Aspects of Breast Cancer, Vol 4: Systemic Control of Breast Cancer. London: William Heinemann Medical Books, Ltd., 1981, pp 204–243.
3. Corbett TH, Roberts BJ, Leopold WR et al: Induction and chemotherapeutics response of two transplantable ductal adenocarcinomas of the pancreas in C57B1/6 mice. Cancer Res 1984;44:717–726.
4. Corbett TH, Griswold DP Jr, Roberts BJ et al: Biology and therapeutic response of a mouse mammary adenocarcinoma (16/C) and its potential as a model for surgical adjuvant chemotherapy. Cancer Treat Rep 1978;62:1471–1499.
5. Mayo JG, Laster WR Jr, Andrews CM, Schabel FM Jr: Success and failure in the treatment of solid tumors. III. "Cure" of metastatic Lewis lung carcinoma with methyl-CCNU (NSC 95441) and surgery-chemotherapy. Cancer Chemother Rep 1972;56:183.
6. Griswold DP Jr: The potential for murine tumor models in surgery adjuvant chemotherapy. Cancer Chemother Rep 1975;5:187–204.
7. Corbett TH, Valeriote FA: Rodent models in experimental chemotherapy, in: Kallman RF (ed): The Use of Rodent Tumors in Experimental Cancer Therapy: Conclusions and Recommendations. (in press).
8. Karrer K, Humphreys SR: Continuous and limited courses of cyclophosphamide (NSC 26271) in mice with pulmonary metastasis after surgery. Cancer Chemother Rep 1967;51:439.
9. Hiramoto RN, Ghanta V: Surgical adjuvant chemotherapy of metastatic murine osteosarcoma. Int J Cancer 1980;25:393–397.
10. Schabel FM Jr: Surgical adjuvant chemotherapy of metastatic murine tumors. Cancer 1977;40:558–568.
11. Corbett TH, Griswold DP Jr, Roberts BJ, et al. Evaluation of single agents and combinations of chemotherapeutic agents in mouse colon carcinomas. Cancer 1977;40:2660–2680.
12. Valeriote FA, Bruce WR, Meeker BE: Synergistic action of cyclophosphamide and 1,3-bis(2-chloroethyl)-1-nitrosourea on a transplantable murine lymphoma. J Natl Cancer Inst 1968;40:935–944.
13. Schabel FM Jr: Concepts for treatment of micrometastases developed in murine systems. Amer J Roentgenol Radium Ther Nuclear Med 1976;126:500.

14. Skipper HE: The effect of chemotherapy on the kinetics of leukemia cell behavior. Cancer Res 1965;25:1544.

15. Carpenter JT Jr, Maddox WA, Laws HL, et al: Favorable factors in the adjuvant therapy of breast cancer. Cancer 1982;50:18–23.

16. Pendergrast WR, Drake WP, Mardiney MR: AA proper sequence for the treatment of B16 melanoma: Chemotherapy, surgery, and immunotherapy. J Nat Cancer Inst 1976;57:539.

17. Nissen-Meyer R, Kjellgren K, Malmio K, et al: Surgical adjuvant chemotherapy. Results with one short course with cyclophosphamide after mastectomy for breast cancer. Cancer 1978;41:2088.

18. Lawson AJ, Davis ML, Durant JR, et al: Preoperative vs. postoperative radiation/chemotherapy of the 16/C mammary adenocarcinoma. Radiation Res 1981;87:439.

19. Corbett TH, Roberts BJ, Trader MW, et al: Response of transplantable tumors of mice to anthracenedione derivatives alone and in combination with clinically useful agents. Cancer Treat Rep 1982;66:1187–1200.

20. Skipper HE: Combination therapy: Some concepts and results. Cancer Chemother Rep (Part 2) 1974;4:137–145.

21. Schabel FM Jr, Skipper HE, Trader MW, et al: Establishment of cross-resistance profiles for new agents. Cancer Treat Rep 1983;67:905–922.

22. Corbett TH, Griswold DP Jr, Wolpert MK, et al: Design and evaluation of combination chemotherapy trials in experimental animal tumor systems. Cancer Treat Rep 1979;63:799–801.

23. Al-Sarraf M: Chemotherapeutic strategies in squamous cell carcinoma of the head and neck. CRC Critical Review in Oncology/Hematology 1(4):323–355, 1984.

24. Tapazoglou E, Corbett T, Polin L, et al: Comparison of 5-fluorouracil (5-FU) + cisplatin (CisDDPt) with 5-FU + carboplatin (CBDCA) and 5-Fu + iproplatin (CHIP). Amer Assoc Cancer Res 1986;27:373.

25. Corbett TH, Valeriote, Baker L: Is the P388 murine tumor no longer adequate as a drug discovery model?, Investigational New Drugs 5:3–20, 1987.

26. Corbett TH, Wozniak A, Gerpheide S, Hanka L: A selective two-tumor soft agar assay for drug discovery, in Hanka LJ, Kondo J, White RJ (ed): In Vitro and In Vivo Models for Detection of New Antitumor Drugs; 14th International Congress of Chemotherapy, 1985.

27. Corbett TH: A selective two-tumor soft agar assay for drug discovery. Proc Amer Assn Cancer Res (Abstr #1289) 1984;25:325.

28. Corbett TH, Bissery MC, Wozniak A, et al: Activity of flavone acetic acid (NSC-347512) against solid tumors of mice. Investigational New Drugs 1986;4:207–220.

29. Plowman J, Narayanan VL, Dykes D, et al: Flavone acetic acid: A novel agent with preclinical antitumor activity against Colon Adenocarcinoma 38 in mice. Cancer Treat Rep 1986;70:631–635.

# CHAPTER 14

# Chemotherapy Before Definitive Local Treatment in Previously Untreated Advanced Head and Neck Cancer: A Critical Review

*Steven E. Vogl, MD*

The goal of this review is to provide a sober analysis of what has been achieved in the field of "induction" or "neoadjuvant" chemotherapy of previously untreated head and neck cancer. In addition, we will provide a framework with which the non-chemotherapist can analyze varying chemotherapy trials without concern for the details of treatment, and make suggestions for future areas worthy of research and exploration.

Chemotherapy before surgery or irradiation is quite attractive in head and neck cancer. First, there is abundant documentation that larger and more abundant tumors carry with them a poorer prognosis. Second, there is now a large literature from many continents proving that chemotherapy can substantially shrink tumors in more than half of the patients with metastatic or recurrent disease, and nearly all patients with previously untreated disease. In the latter group, complete clearing of disease has commonly been reported in 20–25% of patients, and in some series as many as 54% of patients. If a smaller tumor is better, and chemotherapy makes a tumor smaller nearly all the time, then chemotherapy should be "good." Furthermore, shrinking a tumor before surgery might allow the surgeon to avoid otherwise necessary mutilation, and might allow him to operate in otherwise "inoperable" situations.

In looking at chemotherapy programs given before local treatment, it makes the most sense to analyze them by their result: partial response, complete response, or complete response with no histologic residual tumor in the surgical specimen. We will not review the extensive literature that shows that while partial response in advanced inoperable tumors is easy to

**193**

achieve with chemotherapy, most such patients relapse despite radical radio-therapy and go on to die of their disease in less than two years, with almost no cures. This was the unfortunate result of the initial Memorial Hospital series using bleomycin and cis-platinum, and also of the subsequent Einstein series using these drugs plus methotrexate, with or without mitomycin.

## PARTIAL RESPONSE TO INDUCTION CHEMOTHERAPY

Unfortunately, partial response before surgery for operable tumors also seems to provide little major, or even detectable, benefit. The largest ran-domized trial of induction chemotherapy in head and neck cancer was the "contract" trial sponsored by the National Cancer Institute. This trial em-ployed a single three week course of bleomycin and cisplatin that pro-duced only a 37% rate of partial remission with only 3% complete remissions evaluated clinically before surgery. Based on the experience of others, a second or third cycle might have doubled the overall response rate and quintupled the complete response rate. In any case, with prolonged follow-up now available, there is no difference in overall survival, or in survival of any subgroup, for those given chemotherapy before surgery and irradiation for operable advanced tumors. Three year survival is 20% for stage IV, 60% for stage III, approximately 55% for N0 and N1, 20% for N2, and 10% for N3. The incidence of histologically positive surgical margins was 16% after sur-gery and 12% after induction chemotherapy and surgery (a non-significant difference).

Overall, 22% had initial relapse in local or regional sites, and 13% had relapse in distant sites. In this trial, half the induction chemotherapy patients were to continue with eight doses of cisplatin at three week intervals after completion of postoperative radiation. About half never started, and only about 12% finished. Nonetheless, the incidence of distant metastases in this group was much lower, especially after the first year. After 2 years, 20% of the control but only 10% of the "maintained" patients had developed distant metastases. Whether or not this marginally effective chemotherapy, which was actually given only to a minority of patients assigned to it, and rarely to a full course even in those who received it, actually reduced the incidence of distant metastases is unclear, since the final paper that describes all the patient characteristics is not yet published. It seems likely that some random variation or quirk in the way the study endpoints were defined and analyzed may be responsible. It can be extraordinarily difficult, in a sick patient, to decide which site of recurrence came first. Further, an apparent decrease in recurrence at some site could reflect a failure to be able to follow that site adequately, or the excess occurrence of intercurrent illness or death in one group.

This trial documented the difficultires of carrying out combined modality trials in a population of heavy smokers and drinkers. Radiation therapy was incomplete in 10% of patients, 4% never came to surgery, and 3% proved unresectable at surgery.

One could argue that a single cycle of chemotherapy producing only 37% remissions does not really test whether partial response before local therapy is of value. Three other series, one of them randomized, also suggest that it is not. First, a group at Walter Reed Army Medical Center employed a chemotherapy program of vinblastine, bleomycin and cisplatin that produced 67% remissions, most of them partial, when given for two cycles. While initial results seemed encouraging, when historical controls were matched for primary site, T and N stage, and subsequent therapy (surgery, radiation or both), survival curves were superimposable in groups of 64 patients each.

Furthermore, a small randomized study of 83 patients at the Medical College of Wisconsin in Milwaukee, in which two cycles of induction chemotherapy with bleomycin, methotrexate, cyclophosphamide and fluorouracil produced 67% remissions (only 5% complete), showed no survival benefit apparent from induction chemotherapy. Of some concern was an apparent deleterious effect upon survival in stage IV patients, perhaps accounted for by a reduced rate of 2-year loco-regional control from 53% to 35% for those treated with primary irradiation along with induction chemotherapy. While this may have been chance event ($p = 0.06$), such an effect could only be determined in a randomized trial, and should be looked for again. A possible explanation could be that chemotherapy resistant cells are also resistant to irradiation, and so pretreatment with chemotherapy could set the stage for failure of radiation to control local tumor. A final analysis of this trial, with a full comparison of all the groups, is still pending.

Finally, in the extensive Wayne State experience with induction chemotherapy, partial response to induction chemotherapy, even if complete response is achieved later with local therapy, augurs a poor prognosis that is not substantially better than that of patients whose tumor does not respond at all to induction chemotherapy. In a collected analysis of three successive trials, median survival was 29 weeks for non-responders, 46 weeks for partial responders, and 136 weeks for complete responders. After 2 years, 94% of partial responders to induction chemotherapy had died.

The group at the Dana-Farber Cancer Institute has gathered data on the value of partial response in the presence of fixed nodal disease in the neck. Overall failure rate in the period of analysis did not decrease when a fixed node or nodes was mobilized by chemotherapy pre-operatively, and neck failure occurred in three out of ten such patients despite further surgery and irradiation.

## COMPLETE REMISSION TO INDUCTION CHEMOTHERAPY

If partial remission on clinical evaluation is of little value, surely one would think complete remission would be of major value. There is one modest-sized randomized trial in which a complete remission rate of 35% with an overall response rate of 75% was realized. This is a Southwest Oncology Group trial, chaired by David Schuller of Ohio State, with 50 patients in each arm. No difference in survival at 2 years has yet been observed in this trial.

The careful analysis of patient populations and results conducted by Al-Sarraf and his colleagues at Wayne State further supports some skepticism as to the ultimate value of induction chemotherapy. Successive studies at this institution (described elsewhere in this volume) have shown increasing complete response rates of up to 54% for induction cisplatin and five-day 5-fluorouracil infusion, with 66% complete remissions for those patients actually completing three such cycles. However, in these trials, better prognosis patients had the better complete remission rates. Such patients with a better prognosis would be expected to live longer and have higher cure rates regardless of whether they were given induction chemotherapy, and regardless of whether or not they responded completely to it. For instance, combining the three trials, complete remission was achieved in 51.5% of stage II or III patients, but only in 38% of those staged IV. Furthermore, among stage IV patients, those staged T4N0 had a 46% complete remission rate versus 25% for those staged T4N3.

Even among patients with complete remissions, many have done poorly, with 60% dying within 3 years. Among 19 complete remissions to induction chemotherapy with positive histology at surgical resection, 17 had relapsed and died within 3 years. Most relapsed tumors were above the clavicles, and most tumors were scattered diffusely in the surgical specimen (J. Jacobs, personal communication). In contrast, among 13 patients without histologically demonstrable tumor in the surgical specimen (10 of whom received the 5-day fluorouracil + cisplatin regimen), none have yet died.

Further evidence that complete response to induction chemotherapy may not be responsible for the improved survival of complete responders comes from a 1983 analysis of the Wayne State experience; complete response to induction had no advantage over either partial or non-response among stage III patients, and there was an approximate 50% survival rate at 2 and 3 years in all groups. Since all stage III patients are truly operable, these data suggest that completely shrinking operable tumor is not really of major benefit.

## CONCLUSIONS

It would not be surprising that induction chemotherapy before surgery would not improve survival or local control if it fails to control the surgical margin, and there is no evidence that it succeeds in this regard. It makes more sense to give chemotherapy before radiation, since radiation generally fails centrally, and since chemotherapy could conceivably improve radiation efficacy by improving central oxygenation and reducing the number of cells potentially radio-resistant. Unfortunately, experience in advanced inoperable head and neck cancers has shown no major advantage for induction chemotherapy—indeed, no truly effective treatment program is available for the vast majority of such patients. Furthermore, there is evidence that chemotherapy and irradiation share cross-resistance. Three American series demonstrate that only 6 to 20% of patients not responding to induction chemotherapy ever achieve even transient local disease control with subsequent radiation.

It may be appropriate now to rethink the strategy of combining chemotherapy with local treatments in head and neck cancer and to use it in a more classical adjuvant setting after completion of local treatment, or at least after surgery. This is being done to some extent in a current national trial in the United States, but only three cycles of treatment are being given before radiation. No data are available to judge whether three cycles are the optimal number.

Major problems of compliance have plagued trials in head and neck cancer in the past, and have been especially severe late in the treatment program, when patients with heavy smoking and drinking histories have been exhausted by two or three different and toxic prior treatment programs. To be effective, any adjuvant program must be accepted by the patient. Programs should be tested in metastatic and recurrent disease to determine if regimens with less subjective toxicity and less intensity given results comparable to the toxic ones now in use. Analogs of cisplatin that are easier to give in terms of hydration and administration, with little nausea, may be very useful in this regard. Reduction in the number of visits, venipunctures, and cost of treatment will all be important. Treatment with small doses at frequent intervals, which can be accompanied by reduced subjective toxicity, should be explored, as they have been in breast cancer. If efficacy can be established, major issues of duration, timing, scheduling, and intensity will need to be worked out, either in the adjuvant setting or in the "model" setting of recurrent or metastatic disease. Concurrent chemotherapy and radiation should be explored further (see Dr. Fu's paper) to reduce the current 22% loco-regional failure rate after postoperative irradiation.

Major research efforts are justified to develop interventional support systems that help patients complete rigorous programs of treatment. Ultimate success will also require efforts to reduce the non-cancer mortality that may affect 25% of these patients over a 2- to 4-year period, to reduce the high incidence of second primary tumors, especially in those who continue to smoke, perhaps by retinoids and other inhibitors of carcinogenesis and precancerous proliferative lesions (see Dr. Weaver's paper), and to curb disease wrought by alcohol and tobacco in the lungs, liver, heart and brain.

In summary, major advantages of induction chemotherapy include prompt shrinkage of tumor with improved swallowing and breathing, less pain, and less deformity. This often allows a period of improved general health prior to rigorous surgery in which nutrition can be improved and medical problems treated while the tumor is shrinking. This can be achieved, as has been emphasized by Lore, with no impairment of wound healing, excellent definition of surgical planes, and no weakening of tissues such as could lead to carotid hemorrhage. Disadvantages include systemic and oral toxicity (with occasional treatment deaths from chemotherapy), added treatment time and complexity, and added cost in terms of drugs, effort, and medical care. To date, no convincing evidence of increased survival is available.

Nonetheless, the reproduceable complete response rate of 40% with the 5-day fluorouracil infusion plus cisplatin program is a major accomplishment, and may lead to improved survival with minor modifications of schedule or timing. The interdisciplinary cooperation and interaction achieved in the head and neck field in the past seven years is unexcelled among solid tumors of adults. The stage is set for a major breakthrough with prompt dissemination throughout the medical community. Hopefully, it will come soon.

# CHAPTER 15

# Recurrent Carcinoma of the Head and Neck: Therapeutic Concepts — 1986

*Julie A. Kish, MD, John F. Ensley, MD,*
*Efstathios Tapazoglou, MD, and*
*Muhyi Al-Sarraf, MD*

## INTRODUCTION

Recurrent head and neck cancer is, by definition, a failure of standard definitive local therapy. The patterns of relapse in these patients are fairly well established. Approximately 40% of the patients treated will recur overall, 20% loco-regionally, 10% with distant disease, and another 10% with both local and distant disease.[1] The majority of patients will relapse within 6–24 months after definitive therapy and have a subsequent median survival of 6 months from diagnosis of recurrence.[1-4] Failure of initial therapy not only signifies a short survival, but also a poor response to subsequent treatment, and underscores the need for the most effective modalities to be used first. Treatment of patients with recurrent carcinoma of the head and neck presents a formidable challenge.

Two important issues are relevant to the discussion of therapy in recurrent carcinoma of the head and neck. First, not all recurrent carcinoma of the head and neck is identical. Second, patients with recurrent head and neck cancer have unique clinical problems that affect their treatment and prognosis.

## STAGING

The generic term recurrent carcinoma of the head and neck encompasses a diverse group of patients. Within this heterogeneous group are patients with minimal local disease with and without lymphangetic skin metastases, patients with systemic disease with and without hypercalcemia, and patients with both local and distant disease. These patients require categorization into various groups to more specifically define therapy. Thus, staging at the time of recurrence becomes important. Proposed staging categories based on tumor burden might include minimal, intermediate, and bulky, with subgroupings based on hypercalcemia and lymphangetic skin involvement. Objective measures, such as the number of lesions and their size, number of organs involved, and the presence and degree of hypercalcemia and lymphangetic skin metastasis would be used. Physical examination would remain the chief assessment tool, but computerized tomography, x-rays, and eventually magnetic resonance imaging (MRI) would be utilized. With an accurate objective assessment of tumor burden, the integration of other modalities such as salvage radiation or surgery with chemotherapy could be accomplished. This would certainly allow for a more aggressive approach as with newly diagnosed disease and possibly increase survival and improve quality of life.

## UNIQUE PROBLEMS OF RECURRENT HEAD AND NECK CANCER PATIENTS

In addition to accurate staging, therapy of recurrent head and neck cancer must consider the unique problems of these patients.

### Second Primary Malignancy

Ten percent of these patients will have a second malignancy in their upper aerodigestive tract either at initial diagnosis or after relapse.[5,6] This issue has been academic in the past; however, the tumor biology and clinical behavior of a new primary in the head and neck area can be significantly different from that of a recurrent lesion. Primary carcinomas in the esophagus or lung can complicate therapy for the head and neck lesion because they behave much differently from head and neck metastases.

### Lung Lesions

Lung lesions in a patient with a head and neck cancer present a complex clinical problem. The approach is affected greatly by the patient's head and neck cancer status. Clearly, biopsy must be performed, if feasible, to establish cell type. The cell type of the lung lesion plus the state of the head and neck cancer together will define therapy. A squamous carcinoma of the lung in a patient with a persistent or recurrent head and neck cancer should be treated as metastatic head and neck cancer. The response to chemotherapy will further define the true nature of the lung lesion. Metastatic disease will respond like the head and neck cancer, a new lung primary usually will not. If the pathology is other than squamous in a patient with an active head and neck cancer, there is no standard approach. With an inactive head and neck cancer, the lung lesion, despite cell type, should be approached as a lung primary with local therapy, if appropriate. The dilemma of the lung lesion in a patient with head and neck cancer will be increasing in prevalance as our therapies for the primary improve.

## Other Medical Problems Affecting Therapy

This group of patients has a high incidence of life-style related problems (such as chronic obstructive pulmonary disease and ethanol abuse) that substantially affect our ability to deliver full doses of chemotherapy such as bleomycin, cis-platinum and methotrexate. They also suffer with typical age-related diseases such as hypertension, cardiac problems and diabetes mellitus. Again, these seriously affect their ability to tolerate drugs — specifically 5-fluorouracil (5-FU), and cis-platinum. Of particular importance is the bone marrow suppressant effect of chronic ethanol exposure. Bone marrow biopsy and aspiration should be done early in a head and neck cancer patient who is persistently leukopenic or thrombocytopenic after appropriate nutrition and vitamin supplementation has been initiated to establish bone marrow reserve. A serverely depleted bone marrow will obviously effect doses of chemotherapy.

## Nutrition

The importance of nutrition in these patients cannot be overemphasized. One of the major negative influences on treatment of recurrent head and neck cancer is malnutrition, secondary to tumor and often alcohol. Provision for adequate caloric and vitamin intake must be established at the outset of treatment, e.g., Dobhoff tube or a gastrostomy. Additionally, reversal of a positive nutritional state to a negative one — (weight loss, hypoalbuminemia) should be regarded as a poor prognostic indicator.

## Hypercalcemia

Of particular significance and increasing prevalance in head and neck cancer is hypercalcemia with and without bone disease. When seen as part of the initial presentation of head and neck cancer, the hypercalcemia is more responsive to treatment and does not portend ill, as it does in recurrent disease. A retrospective study at Wayne State University disclosed a median survival of one month in patients with recurrent disease.[7] Hypercalcemia in these patients usually requires fairly aggressive fluid and furosemide treatment and occasionally steroids and mithramycin. Treatment of the underlying malignancy is essential, but the serum calcium should be lowered and the patient adequately hydrated before cis-platinum can be safely administered. The serum calcium can then be used as a therapeutic marker.

## Meningeal Carcinomatoses

As our therapies improve, patients are living longer and developing new problems previously not described. As the locally recurrent tumors progress and advance inward toward the base of the skull, cranial nerves are sequentially affected and meningeal invasion occurs. Lumbar puncture is required for diagnosis. A CT scan to rule out intracranial involvement and mid-line shift must be performed before the lumbar puncture is attempted. Evaluation of CSF glucose and protein levels and CSF cytology are essential. Once the diagnosis is made, intrathecal methotrexate alone with systemic therapy is indicated. Placement of an Omaya reservoir is advantageous for prolonged intrathecal therapy. The use of leucovorin is recommended with the intrathreal therapy.

## Infection

Aspiration pneumonia and local wound cellulitis complicate the treatment of recurrent head and neck cancer. Delays of chemotherapy occur as sepsis and fevers resolve and antibiotic courses are completed. Less serious infections can be handled often with concommitant chemotherapy and antibiotics. A significant threat to successful chemotherapy of recurrent head and neck cancer is the use of nephrotoxic antibiotics. Every effort must be made to avoid these agents because the nephrotoxicity of platinum often becomes a reality after drugs like gentamycin.

## Hemorrhage

Carotid hemorrhage or small vessel bleeding can produce a major obstacle to therapy since the nausea and vomiting associated with chemotherapy can aggrevate bleeding. Local fulgaration, or occasional carotid embolization, have been used to control bleeding.

## Previous Therapy

The presence or absence of previous exposure to chemotherapy and/or radiotherapy can alter a patient's ability to tolerate further bone marrow suppressive therapy.

## CHEMOTHERAPY OF RECURRENT HEAD AND NECK CANCER

The treatment of the broad category of recurrent cancer of the head and neck has been palliative and primarily based on chemotherapy. Historically, as with other malignancies, single agents were used initially, followed by combination chemotherapy. The following is a brief review of chemotherapy through 1986.

The "gold standard" single agent has been methotrexate, administered in a weekly dose of 40 mg/M$^2$. Escalating the dose with leucovorin rescue has not had significant impact on response rate and/or survival. The response rate for methotrexate is 30%. Other important single agents utilized were bleomycin and cis-platinum, with response rates of 20% and 28% respectively.[8] Prior to cis-platinum, overall response to a variety of combinations was 50%, and median duration of response was 6 months. Table 15.1 de-

**TABLE 15.1** Recurrent Head and Neck Cancer Combination Chemotherapy Excluding Cis-Platinum and 5-FU Infusion 1983–1986

| Authors | Drugs | Evaluable Patients | Response | Median Duration (Mos) |
|---------|-------|--------------------|----------|------------------------|
| Britan (9) | CYT, A | 26 | 46% | 6.5 |
| Dimery (10) | MTX, 5FU, CACP | 46 | 21% | 3 |
| Gonzalez (11) | Bleo + CACP alternating with MTX, VLB | 31 | 45% | 6.5 |
| Hill (12) | VCR, Bleo, MTX 5FU, steroids | 63 | 41% | 11 |
| Panasci (13) | CACP + Bleo alternate MTX + 5FU | 30 | 33% | 3 |
| Pitman (14) | MTX with Leucovorin, 5FU | | | |
| Sandler (15) | CYT, A | 36 | 30% | 4 |
| Sridhar (16) | MTX-Leucovorin Bleo, CACP | 45 | 22% | 2.5 |

MTX: Methotrexate; CYT: Cytoxan; CACP: Cis-platinum; A: Adriamycin.

scribes the 1983–1986 experience reported in the literature with combination chemotherapy without cis-platinum and 5-FU infusion.

Current chemotherapy for head and neck cancer is based on the "platinum" standard. Cis-platinum alone produces response rates comparable to methotrexate alone, i.e., approximately 30%. Cis-platinum has been combined with methotrexate, bleomycin, and, most effectively, with 5-fluorouracil. The cis-platinum + 5-fluorouracil infusion has become one of the most active and commonly used regimens for head and neck cancer. Table 15.2 reviews several reports of this combination in recurrent disease. When a cis-platinum dosage of 100 mg/M$^2$ (day one) and 5-fluorouracil dosage of 1000 mg/M$^2$/dx4 are used, an overall response rate of 70% can be expected. Authors reporting significantly lower responses have altered doses and schedules, except in Creagen's study, which uses identical doses and achieves a response of only 25%.[17] The complete response rate in these studies ranges from 0–27%. All of these studies were single institution studies.

Clinical trials of phase II agents have been part of the saga of chemotherapy for recurrent head and neck cancer. Their role has become increasingly more important since cis-platinum cannot be used indefinitely in responding patients because of serious neurotoxicity and often nephrotoxicity. The list of phase II agents is seen in Table 15.3. There is a glimmer of optimism with the platinum analogues particularly carboplatin (CBDCA). This agent is now entering clinical trial with 5-fluorouracil infusion vs. cis-platinum and 5-fluorouracil vs. methotrexate in the Southwest Oncology Group (SWOG). The search for other effective safer drugs must continue as we improve existing therapies.

Few randomized chemotherapy trials exist exclusively for recurrent disease. Most include patients with advanced, previously untreated disease.

**TABLE 15.2** Combination Chemotherapy Recurrent Head and Neck Carcinoma 5-FU + CACP 1983–1986

| Author | Number of Evaluable Patients | % Response Rate |
|---|---|---|
| Creagen (17) | 20 | 25 |
| Dashampatra (18) | 18 | 11 (only 2 courses) |
| Fosser (19) | 21 | 62 |
| Kish (20) | 30 | 70 |
| Merlano (21) | 27 | 59 |
| Raymond (22) | 16 | 75 |
| Rowland (23) | 28 | 71 |
| Sridhar (24) | 20 | 72 |

**TABLE 15.3** Recurrent Head and Neck Cancer Phase II Agents

| Authors | Agent | No. Patients | % Response Rate |
|---|---|---|---|
| Abellí, et al (25) | Doxifluridine | 20 | 15 |
| Aapró (26) | Mitoxantrone | 13 | 0 |
| Carugati, et al (27) | Aclacinomycin | 21 | 0 |
| Conix, et al (28) | Methyl-GAG | 20 | 0 |
| Creagan, et al (29) | AZQ | 17 | 0 |
| Decker, et al (30) | Gallium Nitrate | 21 | 0 |
| DeJager, et al (31) | Mitoxantrone | 39 | 5 |
| Demenge & Richard (32) | Vindesine | 14 | 21 |
| Dimery, et al (33) | PCNU | 30 | 0 |
| Forastiere, et al (34) | Bisantrene | 26 | 4 |
| Gad-El-Mowla, et al (35) | Hexamethylmelamine | 20 | 15 |
| Grohn, et al (36) | Prospiden | 22 | 18 |
| Haas, et al (37) | Vindesine | 24 | 0 |
| Hornedo-Muguiro, et al (38) | CBDCA | 32 | 18 |
| Kish, Al-Sarraf (39) | Aclacinomycin | 18 | 6 |
| Kish, et al (40) | CBDCA | 9 | 56 |
| Kish, et al (40) | CHIP | 6 | 33 |
| Krasnow, et al (41) | Traizinate | 26 | 8 |
| Luedke, et al (42) | Methyl-GAG | 38 | 8 |
| Mattox, et al (43) | Flutamide | 9 | 33 |
| Megee, et al (44) | Epidoxorubicin | 25 | 12 |
| Sledge, et al (45) | Vindesine | 15 | 13 |
| Szpirglas, et al (46) | Vindesine | 36 | 14 |
| Thongprasert, et al (47) | Methyl-GAG | 27 | 11 |
| Wheeler, et al (48) | ICRF-18 | 25 | 8 |
| Witherspoon, et al (49) | m-AMSA | 34 | 4 |
| Williams, et al (50) | Mitoxantrone | 53 | 2 |
| Vogl, et al (51) | Dibromodulcitol | 34 | 0 |
| Vogl, et al (51) | Mitoxantrone | 21 | 5 |
| Vogl, et al (52) | Vindesine | 25 | 8 |

Table 15.4 delineates various combinations as single agents and combination vs. other combinations. The best non-platinum regimen to date is 5-fluorouracil + methotrexate. 5-FU infusion + cis-platinum produces the highest overall response rate. Given all the available data and conflicting reports, a new randomized trial that compared the old and new standards of chemotherapy and phase II agents was needed. SWOG has undertaken a three arm randomized trial for recurrent head and neck cancer that encompasses these concepts. Patients are randomized between methotrexate alone vs. cis-platinum + 5-FU infusion vs. carboplatinum (CBDCA) + 5-FU infusion. This protocol is designed to test several hypotheses: (1) efficacy of the

**TABLE 15.4** Randomized Chemotherapy Trials in Recurrent Head and Neck Cancer

| Author | Drugs | Number of Patients | % Response |
|--------|-------|:---:|:---:|
| Al-Sarraf (8) | MTX | 51 | 33 |
| | vs. | | |
| | CACP, Onc, Bleo | | 40 |
| Browman (53) | MTX-5FU-Sequential | 72 | 38 |
| | vs. | | |
| | MTX + 5FU | | 62 |
| Davis (54) | CACP | 57 | 13 |
| | vs. | | |
| | CACP + MTX + Bleo | | 11 |
| DeConti (55) | MTX | 237 | 26 |
| | MTX + Leucovorin | | 24 |
| | MTX + Leucovorin + Cytoxan + ARA-C | | 18 |
| Grose (56) | MTX | 100 | 16 |
| | CACP | | 8 |
| Hong (57) | CACP | 44 | 28 |
| | vs. | | |
| | MTX | | 23 |
| Jacobs (58) | CACP | 80 | 18 |
| | vs. | | |
| | CACP + MTX | | 33 |
| Kish (59) | CACP + 5FU (infusion) | 38 | 72 |
| | CACP + 5FU (bolus) | | 20 |
| Taylor (60) | MTX + Leucovorin | 47 | 32 |
| | vs. | | |
| | MTX alone | | 22 |
| Vogl (61) | MTX | 163 | 35 |
| | CACP, Bleo, MTX | | 48 |
| Williams (62) | MTX | 190 | 16 |
| | CACP, Velban, MTX | | 24 |

MTX: Methotrexate; CACP: Cis-platinum; Bleo: Bleomycin.

single agent MTX ("gold standard") against 5-FU infusion + cis-platinum combination ("platinum standard"), and (2) efficacy of the new combination carboplatin (CBDCA) + 5-FU infusion vs. cis-platinum + 5-FU infusion vs. MTX. The results of this trial should have a major impact on treatment of head and neck cancer.

The answer is not clear yet. In the past, a chemotherapy regimen was judged by its overall response with the anticipation that this would translate into improved survival time. A randomized pilot study was done at Wayne State University for recurrent disease comparing 5-FU infusion + cis-platinum vs. 5-FU bolus + cis-platinum. Although the response rate for infusion was higher, the overall survival was not appreciably different from bolus patients (Fig. 15.1). The goal of treatment must be the production of the highest histologic complete response rate. Those patients who achieve this survive longer with a better quality of life than those who do not.[63] These patients represent the tail of the survival curve, and as the numbers of these patients increase, the median survival should improve.

The actual drugs utilized are not the only issue. How many courses are appropriate? We have seen in the past that increasing therapy from two to three courses of the combination 5-fluorouracil (5-FU) infusion + cis-platinum increased the complete response rate dramatically from 24% to 50%.[64] How long should chemotherapy continue once a complete response is obtained? If chemotherapy is to be prolonged for greater than the standard three courses, side effects must be scrupulously monitored. More convenient methods of administration and scheduling need to be established. With the current emphasis on hospital bed utilization, decreasing in-patient days is certainly a consideration. When should other therapies such as salvage surgery or radiation be used — before, after, or concomitantly with chemotherapy? All of these treatment related issues will have an impact on the patient's acceptance of therapy and compliance.

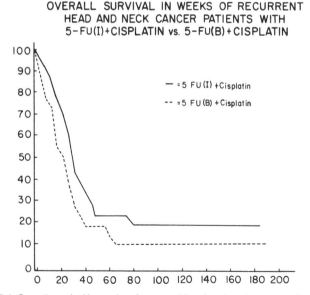

**FIGURE 15.1** Overall survival in weeks of recurrent head and neck cancer patients with 5-FU (infusion) + cis-platinum vs. 5-FU (bolus) + cis-platinum.

## CONCLUSION

The treatment of recurrent carcinoma of the head and neck is challenging. The vagaries of the illness and the patient require complex maneuvering in a mire of clinical problems. The only way we are going to conquer this disease is to utilize an innovative and organized approach. The mentality of only "palliative therapy" for recurrent carcinoma of the head and neck is a hindrance and must be discarded. Accurate specific staging at time of recurrence needs to occur. Identification of the chemotherapy regimen with the highest therapeutic efficacy and lowest risk/benefit ratio must become reality. Achieving the highest histologically complete response must be the goal of therapy. Compulsive prompt attention to the unique medical problems of these patients cannot be ignored, and finally, skilled planned integration of all therapeutic modalities—surgery and radiation with chemotherapy—must be attempted within the limits of the patient's previous treatment.

## REFERENCES

1. Bromer R, Hong W, Vaughan R, et al: Patterns of relapse in advanced head and neck cancer patients who achieved complete remission after combined modality therapy. Proc Amer Soc Clin Oncol 1983;2:629.
2. Luna MA, Dimiery IW: Causes of death in head and neck squamous carcinoma. Proc Internatl Conf Head Neck Cancer 1984;73:196.
3. Glick JH, Tayla SG: Integration of chemotherapy into a combined modality treatment plan for head and neck cancer: A review. Internatl Radiation Oncol Biol Phys 1981;7:229–242.
4. Wittes RE: Combination chemotherapy of head and neck cancer in the United States. Recent Results Cancer Res 1981;76:276–286.
5. Atkinson D, Fleming S, Weaver A: Triple endoscopy, A valuable procedure in head and neck surgery. Amer J Surg 1982;144:415–419.
6. Wikram B, Shong E, Shat T, et al: Second malignant neoplasms in patients successfully treated with multimodality treatment for advanced head and neck cancer. Head Neck Surg 1984;6:734–737.
7. Won C, Decker D, Drelichman A, et al: Hypercalcemia in head and neck carcinoma, incidence procedure in head and neck surgery. Cancer 1983;52:2261–2263.
8. Al-Sarraf M: Chemotherapy strategies in squamous cell cancer of the head and neck. CRC Critical Review in Oncology/Hematology, 1984;1:323–355.
9. Bitran JD, Goldman M: A phase II trial of cyclophosphamide and adriamycin in refractory squamous carcinoma of the head and neck. An effective salvage regimen. Amer J Clin Oncol 1985;8(1):61–64.
10. Dimery C, Legha S, Goepfert H: Phase II trial of MTX, 5-FU and cisplatin in recurrent head and neck squamous cancer. Proc Amer Soc Clin Oncol 1984;3:184.
11. Gonzalez MF, Valdiverso JG, Sarliano G: Combined intravenous infusion combination chemotherapy for head and neck squamous cell cancer. Oncology 1984;41(6):377–382.
12. Hill BT, Sharro HJ, Dalley VM, et al: 24 Combination chemotherapy without cisplatin in

patients with recurrent or metastatic head and neck cancer. Amer J Clin Oncol 1984;7(4):335–340.

13. Panasci L, Gravenor D, Black M, et al: Alternating combination chemotherapy using cisplatin-bleomycin with sequential MTX-5-FU with leucovorin rescue in patients with head and neck cancer. Cancer Treat Rep 1985;69(9):1015–1017.

14. Pitman S, Fischer D, Kowal C, et al: Sequential methotrexate – 5-fluorouracil (M–F) in squamous head and neck cancer. Prolonged survival in patients with recurrent disease. Proc Amer Soc Clin Oncol 1983;2:650.

15. Sandler S, Bonomi P, Taylor B, et al: Doxorubicin and cisplatin for recurrent or metastatic squamous cancer of the head and neck. Cancer Treat Rep 1984;68(9):1163–1165.

16. Sridhar KS, Oknuma T, Beller H: Combination chemotherapy with high dose methotrexate, bleomycin and cisplatin in management of head and neck squamous cell carcinoma. Amer J Clin Oncol 1985;8(1):55–60.

17. Creagan ET, Ingle JN, Schult AF, et al: A Phase II study of cis-diaminodichloroplatinum and 5-fluorouracil in advanced upper aerodigestive neoplasms. Head Neck Surg 1984;6:1020–1023.

18. Dasmhapatra KS, Yee R, Hill GJ, et al: 5-FU and cisplatin in advanced squamous cell head and neck cancer. Proc Amer Soc Clin Oncol 1985;4:132.

19. Fosser VP, Paccagnella A, Degli A, et al: Cisplatin and 5-fluorouracil 120 hour infusion in patients with recurrent head and neck cancer. Proc Amer Soc Clin Oncol 1985;4:150.

20. Kish JA, Weaver A, Jacobs J, et al: Cisplatin and 5-FU infusion in patients with recurrent and disseminated epidermoid cancer of the head and neck. Cancer 1984;53(9):1819–1824.

21. Merlano M, Talarek R, Grimaldi A, et al: Phase II trial with cisplatin and 5-FU in recurrent head and neck Cancer II: An effective outpatient schedule. Cancer Treat Rep 1985;69(9):961–964.

22. Raymond MG, Lyman GH: Treatment of unresectable/recurrent epidermoid cancer of the head and neck with cisplatin + 5-FU infusion. Proc Amer Soc Clin Oncol 1985;4:133.

23. Rowland KM, Taylor SG, O'Donnell MR, et al: Cisplatin and 5-FU infusion in advanced/recurrent cancer of the head and neck. ECOG pilot. Proc Amer Soc Clin Oncol 1984;1(3):184.

24. Sridhar KS, Hirsch K, Tountziles G, et al: Sequential cisplatin and 5-FU in advanced squamous cell head and neck cancer. Proc Amer Assn Cancer Res 1984;25:1980.

25. Abelli R, Kaplan E, Grossenbacher R, et al: Phase II study of doxifluridine in advanced squamous cell carcinoma of the head and neck. Eur J Cancer Clin Oncol 1984;20:333.

26. Aapro MS, and Alberts DS: Phase II trial of mitoxantrone in head and neck cancer. Investigative new drugs 1984;2:329.

27. Carugati A, Olivari A, Campos D, et al: A phase II comparison of aclacinomycin A and methotrexate in advanced squamous cell carcinoma of the head and neck. Proc Amer Soc Clin Oncol 1985;4:145.

28. Conix P, Nasca S, Jazckora D, et al: Phase II trial of mitoguazone in patients with recurrent head and neck cancer. Bull Cancer 1985;72:153.

29. Creagan ET, Long MJ, Kvols LK et al: Phase II trial of diaziquone in advanced upper aerodigestive cancer. Cancer Treat Rep, 1985;69:141.

30. Decker DA, Costanzi JJ, McCracken JD, Baker LH: Evaluation of gallium nitrate in metastatic or locally recurrent squamous cell carcinoma of the head and neck. A southwest oncology group study. Cancer Treat Rep 1984;68:1047.

31. DeJager R, Cappelaeare P, Armand JP, et al: An EROTC phase II study of mitoxantrone in solid tumors and lymphomas. Eur J Cancer Clin Oncol 1984;20:1369.

32. Demenge C, Richard JM: Chimiotherapie des carcinomas des voies aerodigestives par le sulfate de vindisine. Essai therapeutique phase II. Ann Otolaryngol 1984;101:119.

33. Dimery IW, Legha SS, Murphy WR, et al: Phase II study of PCNU in the treatment of head and neck carcinoma. Cancer Treat Rep 1984;68:437.
34. Forastiere AA, Crain SM, Garbino C, et al: Phase II trial of bisantrene in advanced epidermoid carcinoma of the head and neck. Cancer Treat Rep 1984;68:687.
35. Gad-El-Mowla N, MacDonald JS, Khaled H: Hexamethylmelamine in advanced head and neck cancer. A phase II study. Amer J Clin Oncol 1984;68:427.
36. Grohn P. Heinonem E, Appelgvist P, et al: Prospidin chemotherapy in recurrent head and neck carcinoma: A phase II Study. Cancer Treat Rep 1984;68:915–917.
37. Haas CD, Fabian CJ, Stephens RL, Kish J: Vindesine in head and neck Cancer. A Southwest Oncology Group phase II pilot study. Investigative New Drugs 1984;1:339.
38. Hornedo-Muguiro J, So M, Spaulding MB, et al: Phase II trial of carboplatin (CBDCA) in aerodigestive malignancies. Proc Amer Soc Clin Oncol, 1986;4:136.
39. Kish JA, Al-Sarraf M: Aclacinomycin: Phase II evaluation in advanced squamous carcinoma of the head and neck. Amer J Clin Oncol 1984;7:535.
40. Kish J, Ensley J, Al-Sarraf M, et al: Activity of CHIP and CBDCA (platinum analogs) in recurrent epidermoid cancer of the head and neck (HNC). Proc Amer Soc Clin Oncol 1985;4:130.
41. Krasnow S, Eisenberger M, Green M, et al: Phase I–II study of triazinate for advanced head and neck cancer. Proc Amer Assn Cancer Res 1985;26:172.
42. Leudka D, Maddoz BR, Schlueter J: Phase II trial of methyl glyoxal bis (guanylhydrazone) (MGBG) in advanced head and neck squamous cell carcinoma. Proc Amer Soc Clin Oncol 1985;4:130.
43. Mattox DE, VonHoff DD, McGuire WL: Androgen receptors and antiandrogen therapy for laryngeal carcinoma. Arch Otolaryngol 1984;110:721.
44. Megee MJ, Howard Bosl GJ, Wittes RE: Phase II trial of 4'epidoxorubicin in advanced carcinoma of head and neck origin. Cancer Treat Rep 1985;69:125–126.
45. Sledge GW Jr, Clark GM, Griffin C, et al: Phase II trial of vindesine in patients with squamous cell cancer of the head and neck. Amer J Clin Oncol 1984;7:209.
46. Szpirglas H, Marneur M, Vailant JM: La vindesine dans les cancers stomatologiques. La Presse Med 1985;14:405.
47. Thongprasert S, Bosl GJ, Geller NL, Wittes RE: Phase II trial of mitoguanzone in patients with advanced head and neck cancer. Cancer Treat Rep 1984;68:1301.
48. Wheeler RM, Bricker LJ, Natale RB, Baker SR: Phase II trial of ICRF-187 in squamous cell carcinoma of the head and neck. Cancer Treat Rep 1984;68:427.
49. Witherspoon RP, Legha SS, Reimer RR, et al: Phase II trial of amsacrine in metastatic or locally recurrent squamous cell carcinoma of the head and neck primaries: A Southwest Oncology Group study. Cancer Treat Rep 1984;68:435.
50. Williams SD, Birch R, Velez-Garcia E, Games R: Phase II study of mitoxantrone in advanced squamous cell carcinoma of the head and neck. A Southeastern Cancer Group trial. Investigative New Drugs 1985;3:311.
51. Vogl SE, Ryan L, Wernz J, Kaplan BH: Ineffective agents in the chemotherapy of head and neck cancer: mitoxantrone, dibromodulcitol and vinblastin. The Earthern Cooperative Oncology Group Experience. Proc Amer Assn Cancer Res 1985;26:711.
52. Vogl SE, Carnacho FJ, Kaplan BM, O'Donnel MR: Phase II trial of vindesine in advanced squamous cell cancer of the head and neck. Cancer Treat Rep 1984;68:559–560.
53. Browman GD, Archiblad SD, Young JE, et al: Prospective randomized trial of sequential vs. simultaneous MTX and 5-FU in advanced and recurrent head and neck cancer. J Clin Oncol 1983;1(12):789–792.
54. Davis S, Kessler W: Randomized comparison of cis-platinum versus cis-platinum, bleo-

mycin and methotrexate in recurrent squamous cell carcinoma of the head and neck. Cancer Chemother Pharmacol 1979;3:57–59.

55. DeConti RC, Schoenfeld D: A randomized prospective comparison of intermittent methotrexate with leucovorin and a methotrexate combination in head and neck cancer. Cancer 1981;48:1061–1072.

56. Grose WE, Lehane DE, Dixon DO, et al: Comparison of methotrexate and cisplatin for patients with advanced squamous cell carcinoma of the head and neck region: A Southwest Oncology Group study. Cancer Treat Rep 1985;69:577–581.

57. Hong WK, Schaefer S, Issell B, et al: A prospective randomized trial of methotrexate versus cisplatin in treatment of recurrent squamous cancer of the head and neck. Cancer 1982;52(2):206–210.

58. Jacobs C, Meyers F, Hendricksen C, et al: Randomized phase III study of cisplatin with or without MTX for recurrent squamous cancer of head and neck. Northern California Oncology Group study. Cancer 1982;52(9):1563–1569.

59. Kish JA, Ensley JF, Jacobs J, et al: A randomized trial of cisplatin (CACP) and 5-fluorouracil (5-FU) infusion and CACP + 5-FU Bolus for recurrent and advanced head and neck cancer. Cancer 1979;43:2202–2206.

60. Taylor SG, McGuire WP, Hauck WW, et al: A randomized comparison of high dose infusion MTX versus standard dose weekly therapy in head and neck squamous cancer. J Clin Oncol 1984;2(9):1006–1011.

61. Vogl SE, Schoenfeld DA, Kaplan BH, et al: A randomized prospective comparison of methotrexate with a combination of methotrexate, bleomycin and cisplatin in head and neck cancer Cancer; 1985,56:432–442.

62. Williams SD, Velez-Garcia E, Essessee I, et al: Chemotherapy for head and neck cancer. Comparison of cisplatin + vinblastin + bleomycin versus methotrexate. Cancer 1986; 57:18–23.

63. Al-Kourainy K, Kish J, Ensley J, et al: Achievement of superior survival for histologically negative vs. histologically posterior clinically complete responders vs. cis-platinum combination in patients with locally advanced head and neck Cancer. Cancer (in press).

64. Rooney M, Kish J, Jacobs J, et al: Improved complete remission rate and survival in advanced head and neck cancer after three course induction therapy with 120 hour 5-FU infusion and cisplatin. Cancer 1985;55:1123.

# CHAPTER 16

# Involvement of Polypeptide Growth Factors and Their Receptors in the Neoplastic Process

*Toshiaki Kawakami, MD, PhD,*
*Marc S.C. Cheah, Fernando Leal, PhD,*
*Hisanaga Igarashi, PhD,*
*Claire Y. Pennington, MS, and*
*Keith C. Robbins, PhD*

## INTRODUCTION

Investigations to uncover the molecular events involved in conversion of normal cells to malignant ones have recently focused on a small set of normal cellular genes, designated proto-oncogenes. The identification of these genes was made possible by the study of certain retroviruses which are capable of rapidly inducing malignant tumors when injected into experimental animals. Components required for the tumorigenic activity of these viruses lie within sequences termed *onc* genes that are derived from the host genome. However, retrovirus *onc* genes invariably represent altered versions of their proto-oncogene progenitors. Thus, certain normal cellular genes possess the potential to become oncogenic when incorporated as *onc* genes within retrovirus genomes.

Other evidence has suggested that proto-oncogenes might also be activated as oncogenes in a manner independent of retroviruses. A number of genetically aberrant proto-oncogenes have been isolated from certain human and animal tumor cells because of their ability to induce foci of transformation when incorporated into cultured cells. In addition, specific chromosomal aberrations associated with certain types of human cancers have been shown to interfere with the structural integrity of other proto-oncogenes. These and other findings have suggested that alterations affecting proto-oncogenes may contribute to the naturally occurring malignant process.

Important properties of proto-oncogenes include their unique representation within the normal cell and their high degree of conservation in an evolutionary sense. The most striking example of this point comes from studies of the *ras* proto-oncogenes, first identified in rat cells. Genes of the *ras* family are also present in humans, fruit flies, and even yeast. Evidence such as this has strongly suggested that proto-oncogenes must play critically important roles in normal cellular processes such as growth and development. Thus, understanding the functions of proto-oncogenes would likely provide great insight into the process of carcinogenesis.

Very recently, molecular dissection of the oncogene in simian sarcoma virus (SSV), combined with independent investigations of platelet proteins capable of stimulating normal cell growth, have together led to the discovery that the SSV oncogene, v-*sis*, encodes a potent growth-inducing polypeptide. These and subsequent finding have provided the basis for the current hypothesis that growth factors and their proliferative pathways are involved in the neoplastic process.

## THE LINK BETWEEN ONCOGENES AND GROWTH FACTORS

Simian sarcoma virus (SSV) was isolated from a naturally occurring woolly monkey fibrosarcoma, and represents the only acute transforming retrovirus isolated from a primate species. Upon inoculation, this virus induces malignant fibrosarcomas and glioblastomas in experimental animals. After developing an appropriate biologic system to study SSV in tissue culture,[1] the SSV genome was isolated using recombinant DNA techniques, and its cell-derived transforming gene, v-*sis*, was identified.[2] The complete nucleotide sequence of v-*sis* made it possible to predict the structure of its gene produce and to attempt detection of this putative v-*sis*-coded protein.[3] By immunizing animals with small synthetic peptides that mimicked regions of the predicted protein, we obtained antibodies that were used to identify the v-*sis* gene product, designated p28$^{sis}$.[4]

The intensive investigations of oncogenes and their encoded proteins were paralleled by studies of polypeptides that stimulated normal cell growth. One such molecule, human platelet-derived growth factor (PDGF), is a potent mitogen for connective tissue cells. PDGF is a heat-stable, cationic protein normally stored in secretory granules of platelets, and is thought to play a major role to the process of wound healing. Its biologically active forms are disulfide bonded and range in size from 28,000–35,000 daltons. Upon reduction, the molecule loses biologic activity, yielding two distinct polypeptides (designated PDGF-1 and PDGF-2), each of which is around 18,000 daltons in size.

Antoniades and Hunkapiller, working on the structure of human PDGF, had purified this molecule and reported a partial amino acid sequence for each of its polypeptide chains.[5] Upon entering these newly published sequences into his computer bank of amino acid sequences, Doolittle made the startling observation that the amino acid sequence of PDGF-2 matched very closely with a stretch of the v-*sis* coded transforming protein, p28*sis*.[6] Studies by another group working on PDGF structure led to similar conclusions concerning the relationship of these two proteins.[7] These findings provided the first link between an oncogene and a known normal cellular function.

## STRUCTURAL RELATIONSHIP OF p28*SIS* AND PDGF

The amino acid sequence determined for both PDGF polypeptide chains, as well as that predicted for p28*sis*, is shown in Figure 16.1. Approximately half of the amino acids present in PDGF-1 are also found at identical positions within the PDGF-2 sequence, defining a 50% homology between these two proteins. An even greater degree of homology (87%) exists between PDGF-2

```
p28sis   1   M T L T W Q G D P I P E E L Y K M L S G H S I R S F D D L Q R L L Q G D S G K E D G A E L D L N M T   50

p28sis  51   A S H S G G E L E S L A R G K R S L G S L S V A E P A M I A E C K T R T E V F E I S R R L I D R T N   100
PDGF-2   1                               S L G S L T I A E P A M I A E C K T R E V F C I I C R R L T D R ? ?    34
PDGF-1   1                                     S T E E A V P A V C K T N T V I Y E I I S R R E L D I ? ?    28

p28sis 101   A N F L V W P P C V E V Q R C S G C C N R S V Q C R P T Q V Q L R P V Q V R K I E V V R K K P I F  100
PDGF-2  35   ? ? ? ? ? ? I P P C V E V K A C T G C C N A N V K C A P S Q V Q L A I ? Q V A K I E L V A K L      80
PDGF-1  29   A N F L L                                                                                      32

p28sis 151   K K A T V T L E D H L A C K C E I V A A A R A V T R S P G T S Q E Q R A K T T Q S R V T I R T V R V  200
PDGF-2
PDGF-1

p28sis 201   R R P P K G K H A K C K H T H D K T A L K E T L G A                                              226
PDGF-2                                                           ]
PDGF-1                                                           ]
```

A, alanine; C, cysteine; D, aspartic acid; E, glutamic acid; F, phenylalanine; G, glycine; H, histidine; I, isoleucine; K, lysine; L, leucine; M, methionine; N, asparagine; P, proline; Q, glutamine; R, arginine; S, serine; T, threonine; V, valine; W, tryptophan; Y, tyrosine.

**FIGURE 16.1** Sequence relationship between p28*sis* and human PDGF. Amino acid identities between p28*sis* and both PDGF polypeptide chains are boxed.[3,5] A question mark indicates that no amino acid assignment had been made for that position.[6] Amino acids are shown by their single letter designations.

and the v-*sis*-coded protein starting at position 67 of p28$^{sis}$. Moreover, differences in the PDGF-2 sequence with respect to p28$^{sis}$ could be accounted for on evolutionary terms since the PDGF used for analysis was of human origin, whereas p28$^{sis}$ was the product of a "new world" primate gene. In addition, a proteolytic cleavage signal within p28$^{sis}$ immediately proceeded the region of PDGF-2 homology. Examination of SSV transformed cells revealed that p28$^{sis}$ was cleaved at or near this proteolytic site,[8] providing direct experimental evidence that p28$^{sis}$ was a precursor for primate PDGF-2.

The fact that PDGF is biologically active only in a disulfide linked form implied that transformation by p28$^{sis}$ might require this molecule to assume a similar dimeric configuration. To test this hypothesis, p28$^{sis}$ was examined in SSV transformed cells for evidence of dimer formation. As shown in Figure 16.2, under electrophoretic conditions which do not break disulfide bonds, p28$^{sis}$ migrated as a dimer. Furthermore, the disulfide linked form of this molecule, designated gp56$^{sis}$, was also specifically recognized by antiserum prepared against PDGF. These findings demonstrated that the v-*sis* gene product assumed a conformational structure in vivo similar to that of biologically active PDGF, and established an antigenic relatedness between the v-*sis* transforming protein and human PDGF.

## BIOSYNTHETIC PATHWAY OF p28$^{SIS}$

PDGF exerts a stimulatory effect only on certain cell types, such as glial cells, fibroblasts, and smooth muscle cells, all of which possess surface receptors capable of specifically binding this ligand. Once PDGF binds its cellular receptor, a growth-promoting signal is sent to the affected cell. Although the nature of this signal is not completely understood, it is known that the activated receptor molecule is immediately but transiently phosphorylated on a tryosine residue located within the cytoplasmic portion of the receptor protein. Thus, in an effort to learn where the v-*sis*/PDGF-2 protein might interact with its cellular targets, we investigated the p28$^{sis}$ biosynthetic pathway in SSV transformed cells.[9] Findings from these studies, summarized in Figure 16.3, document the biosynthetic pathway of the v-*sis* coded transforming protein. This molecule is synthesized as a glycosylated precursor which dimerizes rapidly within the lumen of the endoplasmic reticulum to yield gp56$^{sis}$. The unprocessed precursor then passes through the Golgi apparatus where its N-linked oligosaccharides are modified. After reaching a distal membrane location, processing of its amino and then its carboxy termini occurs, leading finally to p24$^{sis}$, a primate PDGF-2 dimer. Further localization studies reveal that approximately 10% of total cellular v-*sis*-

coded protein is detectable on the cell surface, but that less than 1% is secreted from the transformed cell. Thus, the v-*sis* gene product is not quantitatively secreted from transformed cells.[9]

Little is presently known about normal PDGF biosynthesis, except that the growth factor is stored within platelet secretory granules. Current understanding indicates that the Golgi apparatus is the site at which newly synthesized proteins are sorted for packaging or release. Our findings suggest that

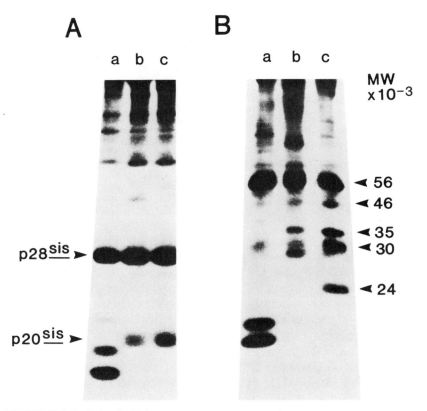

**FIGURE 16.2** Analysis of p28[sis] under reducing or nonreducing conditions. Protein was extracted from SSV transformed cells that had been metabolically labeled with [35]S-cysteine and methionine. Extracts were immunoprecipitated with sera that recognize the amino (Lanes a) or carboxy (Lanes b) terminus of p28[sis] or human PDGF (Lanes c). Immune complexes were examined by sodium dodecyl sulfate polyacrylamide gel electrophoresis in the presence (Panel A) or absence (Panel B) of reducing agent. Molecular weights of proteins detected are also shown.

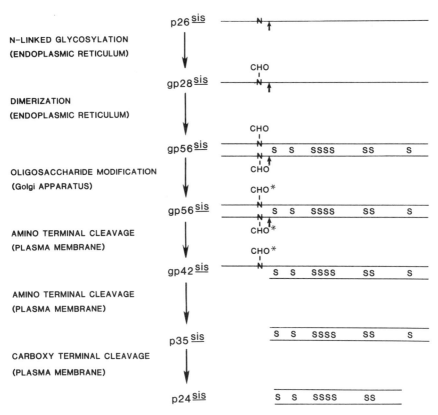

**FIGURE 16.3** Summary of p28^sis biosynthetic pathway. Solid lines represent single polypeptide chains. N or S represent asparagine or cysteine residues, respectively, present in the primary v-*sis* transitional product. CHO and CHO* represent N-linked carbohydrate and modified N-linked carbohydrate, respectively.

biosynthesis of the SSV transforming protein closely parallels that predicted for PDGF at least up to the point at which PDGF is packaged into granules. The peripheral membrane accumulation of the v-*sis* gene products in SSV-transformed fibroblasts may reflect the fact that fibroblasts lack differentiated functions required for storage of the protein in granules.

As much as 10% of the steady-state levels of the v-*sis* gene product is detectable in physical association with the outer surface of the SSV-transformed cell membrane. Our findings also indicate that some of the unprocessed p56$^{sis}$ dimer reaches an extracellular location. Thus, it is possible that some *sis* protein is nonspecifically extruded or released from the transformed cell and immediately sequestered at the cell surface by the PDGF receptor. Another hypothesis is derived from the novel synthesis of both the growth factor (*sis*/PDGF-2) and its receptor by the same cell. Known receptors for growth factors typically are synthesized in the endoplasmic reticulum and pass through the Golgi apparatus as they travel to the cell surface. Since the v-*sis* gene product exhibits this same biosynthetic pathway, the v-*sis*/PDGF-2 protein may bind the PDGF receptor at a common intracellular location, with some of the complex reaching the cell surface. This later possibility might account for the observation that PDGF does not possess transforming activity, whereas synthesis of the v-*sis* coded protein within a cell readily induces its morphologic transformation.

## THE V-*SIS* GENE PRODUCT SHARES BIOLOGIC PROPERTIES WITH PDGF

Utilizing SSV-transformed cell membranes as the source of v-*sis*-coded protein, we devised a means of functionally characterizing cell-associated molecules that could be unequivocally identified as products of the v-*sis* gene.[10] As shown in Table 16.1, it was possible to demonstrate that v-*sis* translational products synthesized by and associated with SSV transformed cells specifically induced DNA synthesis in quiescent fibroblasts. Moreover, v-*sis* coded proteins possessed the capacity to bind PDGF receptors and induce tyrosine phosphorylation of PDGF receptors. In each case, the v-*sis* coded nature of these activities was established by specific inhibition with antibodies directed against different regions of the v-*sis* translational product, p28$^{sis}$. These findings demonstrated that the SSV transforming protein possessed all of the growth stimulatory properties known for PDGF.

## EVIDENCE THAT SSV TRANSFORMING ACTIVITY IS MEDIATED BY THE PDGF RECEPTOR

If transformation by SSV were directly mediated by the interaction of v-*sis* translational products with cellular PDGF receptors, one should expect to observe a strict correlation between target cells susceptible to SSV transformation and cell types possessing PDGF receptors. To address this question,

**TABLE 16.1** SSV Transforming Gene Product Possesses Fibroblast-Specific Mitogenic Activity

| Mitogen | Protein added $\mu$g) | Inhibiting Peptice Antibody¶ | [³H]-Thymidine Incorporation† | |
|---|---|---|---|---|
| | | | BALB/MK | NIH/3T3 |
| None | — | — | 2,840 | 26,641 |
| | — | sis-N | N.T. | 29,125 |
| | — | sis-N* | N.T. | 27,555 |
| SSV transformed cell membrane | 20 | — | 2,976 | 497,111 |
| protein | 20 | sis-N | 2,676 | 244,023 |
| | 20 | sis N* | 2,702 | 484,275 |
| | 20 | sis-C | 2,462 | 110,260 |
| | 20 | sis C* | 2,814 | 486,970 |
| Uninfected cell membrane protein | 20 | — | 2,898 | 28,868 |
| PDGF | 0.003 | — | 2,485 | 255,621 |
| EGF | 0.001 | — | 195,320 | 362,514 |

*Indicates that antibodies were incubated with homologous peptide prior to inhibition study.

¶The amount of antibody required to precipitate all of the sis gene product recognized in membrane preparations was determined in parallel immunoprecipitation experiments using [³⁵S]-labeled HF/SSV cells as the source of membrane protein. The antibody concentration utilized was in two-fold excess.

†BALB/MK or NIH/3T3 cells were plated in 96 well culture dishes and grown to confluence without media changing. Sixteen hours after test samples were added, medium was supplemented with $2\mu$Ci[³H]-thymidine (New England Nuclear; specific activity 20 Ci/mmol) per well and incubated an additional five hours. Trichloroacetic acid insoluble material was measured by scintillation counting. EGF and PDGF receptor grades were purchased from Collaborative Research. Raw counts without substraction of background are shown.

N.T., not tested.

we investigated the ability of SSV to transform a variety of cells in culture. We analyzed those cell types shown to possess PDGF receptors, including fibroblasts and smooth muscle cells, as well as cultures of epithelial or endothelial cells that lacked PDGF receptors. As a control, the transforming activity of SSV was compared with that of another acute transforming retrovirus, Kirsten-MSV, rescued by the same helper virus.

As shown in Table 16.2, Kirsten-MSV efficiently transformed each of the target cells analyzed. In contrast, SSV showed a more restricted pattern. We observed high titered SSV transforming activity for fibroblasts and smooth muscle cells. However, there was no discernible morphologic or detectable growth alteration of either epithelial or endothelial cells in response to SSV infection. The complete correlation between those assay cells susceptible to SSV transformation and those possessing PDGF receptors

**TABLE 16.2** Susceptibility of Cell Types Which Possess or Lack PDGF Receptors to SSV Transformation

| Cell Type | Presence of Surface PDGF Receptors | Transforming Activity | |
|---|---|---|---|
| | | SSV | Ki-MSV |
| *Fibroblast* | | | |
| Mouse (NIH/3T3) | + | + | + |
| Human skin | + | + | + |
| *Smooth muscle* | | | |
| Bovine | + | + | + |
| *Endothelial* | | | |
| Bovine aorta | − | − | + |
| *Epithelial* | | | |
| Mink (MvILu) | − | − | + |

Biologic activity of rescued transforming virus was determined by direct focus or soft agar colony-forming assays. Foci or colonies were scored at 14–21 days following infection.

strongly implied that SSV transforming activity was mediated by the obligatory interaction of its *sis* gene product with the PDGF receptor.[10] Thus, our findings demonstrate that coexpression of a growth factor and its cognate receptor can lead cells to the transformed state.

## THE HUMAN *SIS* PROTO-ONCOGENE ENCODES PDGF POLYPEPTIDE CHAIN 2

In view of the striking structural and functional similarities between human PDGF and the v-*sis* oncogene product, we have explored, at the molecular level, the possible role of the human *sis* proto-oncogene in human malignancies. In order to characterize the human *sis*/PDGF-2 locus, we isolated v-*sis*-related sequences from normal human DNA using recombinant DNA technology.[11] The DNA clones identified represented a contiguous stretch of approximately 30 kbp of human DNA. By molecular hybridization with a v-*sis* probe, five v-*sis*-related gene segments, or exons, were identified and could be localized within a 15-kbp region. Nucleotide sequence analysis of these v-*sis*-related stretches demonstrated that a protein coding sequence was contained within the first five human c-*sis* exons. When this predicted coding sequence was compared with the amino acid sequence determined for human PDGF-2, there was essentially complete identity.[11-13] These findings demonstrated that the human *sis* proto-oncogene was the structural gene for PDGF-2.

## IDENTIFICATION OF AN ADDITIONAL C-*SIS*/PDGF-2 CODING EXON

Cell-derived sequences present within oncogenic retroviruses invariably represent only a portion of the proto-oncogene from which they arise. Thus, expression of retrovirus *onc* genes requires viral regulatory signals for their transcription and often for the initiation and termination of translation. Nucleotide sequence analysis of the human *sis* proto-oncogene demonstrated that v-*sis* was an incomplete version of the human c-*sis*/PDGF-2 gene since its 5' most v-*sis*-related exon lacked a translation initiation codon.[14] This conclusion was further supported by the observation that v-*sis* was 1 kbp in length, whereas the human c-*sis*/PDGF-2 transcript was a 4.2 kb mRNA.[15]

In order to search for additional upstream exons of the c-*sis*/PDGF-2 gene, cloned human DNA segments residing 5' of the v-*sis*-related region were used as probes in attempts to detect the 4.2 kb c-*sis*/PDGF-2 mRNA. One DNA segment located 10 kbp upstream of the 5' most v-*sis* related exon was identified by this approach. This DNA clone, designated pc-*sis* 1, did not detect v-*sis* RNA, and thus represented an exon of the c-*sis*/PDGF-2 gene not captured during the genesis of SSV. Nucleotide sequence analysis of pc-*sis* 1 revealed a methionine codon followed by a short open reading frame that was in phase with the remainder of the c-*sis*/PDGF-2 gene.[14] Confirmation that pc-*sis* 1 contained the codon for initiation of PDGF-2 synthesis was subsequently obtained by comparing its sequence with that of DNA clones representing the 4.2 kb c-*sis*/PDGF-2 mRNA.[16,17]

## ACTIVATION OF THE NORMAL HUMAN C-*SIS*/PDGF-2 GENE AS AN ONCOGENE

Our strategy for assessing the transforming potential of the normal c-*sis*/PDGF-2 proto-oncogene involved introduction of PDGF-2 coding sequences into a cell that was susceptible to SSV-induced malignant transformation. As shown in Figure 16.4, transfection of NIH/3T3 cells with the entire PDGF-2 coding sequence had no effect on the morphology or growth of these cells. However, when the normal PDGF-2 coding sequence was positioned downstream of a retroviral transcriptional promoter capable of inducing mRNA expression, the molecular construct transformed NIH/3T3 cells at a level of activity comparable to that of SSV DNA (Fig. 16.4).

Transformants induced by the activated human *sis*/PDGF-2 coding sequence contained two major *sis*/PDGF-2 related species of 52,000 and

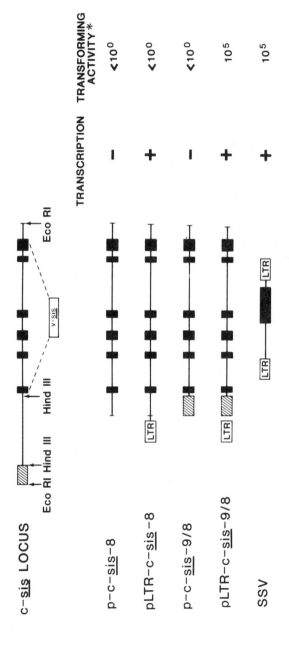

**FIGURE 16.4** Expression of the normal PDGF-2 coding sequence induces morphologic transformation of mouse fibroblasts. Genomic DNA molecules cloned in plasmid vectors were transfected onto NIH/3T3 cells and tested for transcriptional activation and transforming activity. Filled boxes indicate c-sis/PDGF-2 exons which are related to v-sis; hatched boxes indicate the upstream c-sis/PDGF-2 exon not related to v-sis; LTR, retrovirus long terminal repeat.

*Focus-forming units per pmol of PDGF-2 coding sequences

35,000 daltons, which were detected using anti-*sis* peptide sera. Moreover, a 26,000 dalton species, presumed to be the PDGF-2 monomeric precursor, was also observed. We conclude from all of these findings that transcriptional activation of the normal human *sis*/PDGF-2 gene under conditions leading to PDGF-2 dimer synthesis is sufficient to cause morphologic transformation of susceptible cells.

These findings established that derepression of a normal human growth factor gene can cause it to acquire oncogenic properties. Moreover, when captured by a retrovirus, the v-*sis*/PDGF-2 transforming gene has been shown to induce fibro-sarcomas and glioblastomas,[18,19] the very same types of human tumors known to express *sis*/PDGF-2 transcripts.[15] Thus, transcriptional activation of this gene in a cell susceptible to the growth promoting action of PDGF may be an important step in the induction of naturally occurring tumors. If so, it will be critical to gain more detailed knowledge of the mechanisms that normally control expression of the human *sis* proto-oncogene.

## ONCOGENES AND PATHWAYS OF GROWTH CONTROL

The discovery that the v-*sis* oncogene was derived from a normal growth factor gene represented the first link between a transforming gene and a known cellular fuction. More recently, two additional retrovirus *onc* genes have been shown to be altered versions of normal cellular genes encoding cell surface receptors for other growth factors, namely epidermal growth factor (EGF) and colony stimulating factor-1 (CSF-1).[20-22] Taken together, these findings have strongly implicated the constitutive activation of growth factor-mediated stimulatory pathways in the malignant process.

One of the first clues regarding *onc* gene function was provided by the observation that one *onc* gene, v-*src*, encoded a relatively rare enzymatic activity that catalyzed phosphorylation of tyrosine residues (see Ref. no. 23). Moreover, receptors for normal growth factors such as EGF, insulin, and PDGF all respond to ligand binding by autophosphorylation of tryosine residues present in their cytoplasmic domains. Thus, it is thought that tyrosine phosphorylation may be intimately associated with transmitting a proliferative signal to cells exposed to these growth factors. The fact that roughly half of the 20 or so oncogenes isolated to date encode tyrosine kinases suggests that additional links between oncogenes and growth factor mediated proliferative pathways will be discovered.

## THE FGR ONCOGENE ENCODES A TRYOSINE KINASE

Gardner-Rasheed feline sarcoma virus (GR-FeSV) is a sarcomagenic retrovirus initially isolated from a cat fibrosarcoma.[24] The transforming protein of GR-FeSV is a 70,000 dalton molecule that possesses a kinase activity with specificity for tyrosine residues.[25] Nucleotide sequence analysis of GR-FeSV DNA has revealed that its transforming gene arose as a result of genetic recombination involving two distinct cellular genes, one encoding the cytoskeletal structural protein actin and the other a tyrosine-specific protein kinase.[26] The molecular structure of this transforming gene, as well as the protein it specifies, are shown in Figure 16.5.

The presence of actin sequences near the amino terminal region of this transforming protein raises interesting questions. Actin is a highly conserved and abundant structural protein present in all eukaryotic cells. Six actin isoforms are known in vertebrates: four muscle types and two nonmuscle types. Each muscle-type actin is functionally involved in muscle contraction and is expressed only in particular muscle tissues. Conversely, cytoplasmic actins participate in a variety of functions, such as cell motility, mitosis, and maintenance of the cytoskeleton, and are expressed in all cell types. Stable alterations of cell shape and motility have been considered as one of the

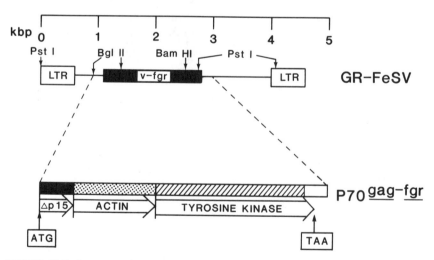

**FIGURE 16.5.** Summary of the major structural features of the GR-FeSV genome and its translational product, P70$^{gag\text{-}fgr}$. Translation initiation (ATG) and termination (TAA) codons are shown. Regions of P70$^{gag\text{-}fgr}$ related to feline retrovirus p15, $\gamma$-actin and other tyrosine-specific protein kinases are also indicated. LTR, retrovirus long terminal repeat; kbp, kilobase pairs.

phenotypic characteristics of transformed cells. There also appears to be some correlation between the presence of the variant actins and increased ability of these cells to produce tumors in nude mice. It is therefore possible that the GR-FeSV transforming protein P70$^{gag-fgr}$, which contains 134 out of actin's 375 amino acids, represents an aberrant form of actin that interferes with the formation of proper cytoskeletal structure in cells transformed by GR-FeSV. Alternatively, the actin moiety of P70$^{gag-fgr}$ may serve to direct its tyrosine kinase to a limited set of cytoskeletal targets that would not normally be accessible for phosphorylation. Further investigation will be required to determine how the actin sequence relates to the oncogenic activity of this virus.

The other GR-FeSV cell-derived gene, designated v-*fgr*, was shown to specify a protein highly related to previously described *onc* gene coded tyrosine kinases. By computer analysis, it was determined that the v-*fgr* gene product was 80% and 74% related in amino acid sequence to proteins specified by v-*yes* and v-*src* genes, respectively.[26] The highly conserved nature of the predicted products of feline-derived v-*fgr* and avian-derived v-*src* and v-*yes* raised the possibility that the *fgr* proto-oncogene was the cat homologue of either c-*src* or c-*yes* chicken proto-oncogenes. To address this question, human DNA was analyzed with v-*fgr*, v-*src* and v-*yes* probes. Although each probe detected related sequences in restriction enzyme treated DNA, none of the human DNA fragments hybridized by v-*src* or v-*yes* probes corresponded to those detected with *fgr* probes. Thus, the human genome must contain distinct proto-oncogenes related to each of these tyrosine kinase-encoding *onc* genes. These findings have implied a strong envolutionary pressure to conserve a similar structure and kinase function at three different human loci.

Detection of the *fgr* proto-oncogene in human DNA made it possible to isolate and characterize this sequence utilizing recombinant DNA techniques.[27] A small portion of the human *fgr* proto-oncogene sequence was then used to locate this gene within the human genome. As shown in Figure 16.6, the human *fgr* proto-oncogen was localized by *in situ* hybridization techniques to chromosome 1 at p36.1–36.2. Previous studies have shown that many forms of cancer, including solid and hematopoietic tumors,[28,29] display alterations affecting chromosome 1.[30,34] This chromosome is also known to contain a number of other genes that affect cell growth, including the oncogenes B-*lym* (p32) and N-*ras* (p11–p13).[35,36–39] as well as the gene encoding nerve growth factor (p21–p22).[40] Specific deletions involving lp31–36 have been described in certain neuroblastomas and result in monosomies of the terminal region of lp.[30–34] Studies are in progress to determine whether *fgr* proto-oncogene structure and/or expression is perturbed in human tumors possessing chromosome 1 alterations.

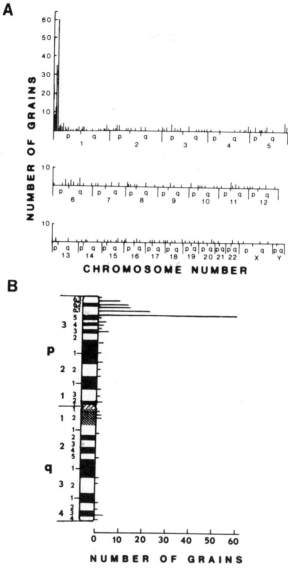

**FIGURE 16.6** Localization of the human *fgr* proto-oncogene by in situ hybridization. Human lymphocyte chromosomes were hybridized with a human *fgr* probe, G-banded and scored. (A) Histogram of silver grain distribution in 102 metaphases based on localization to a 400-band ideogram. (B) Distribution of silver grains of chromosome 1.

## EXPRESSION OF FGR PROTO-ONCOGENE mRNA IN NORMAL AND MALIGNANT CELLS

To investigate whether the *fgr* proto-oncogene was expressed in human tumor cells, RNAs were prepared from selected cell lines that represented a diverse spectrum of human cancers. After selection on oligo dT columns, poly(A)$^+$ RNAs were examined for the presence of *fgr* proto-oncogene mRNA by the Northern hybridization technique. Such transcripts were detected in 6 of 11 cell lines derived from myelo- or lymphoproliferative disorders and in one of seven sarcomas, but not in any of the nine carcinoma cell lines examined. An experiment representative of these findings, shown in Figure 16.7, also revealed that the size of *fgr* proto-oncogene mRNA was 3 kb.[41]

Because our initial survey had indicated the presence of human *fgr* proto-oncogene mRNA in cell lines derived from lymphoproliferative disorders, our analysis was extended to include various B cell lines derived from African and American undifferentiated lymphomas of the Burkitt's and non-Burkitt's types. The c-*fgr* transcript was detected in approximately one half of the Burkitt's lymphoma cell lines tested. Further examination revealed that only those cell lines infected with Epstein-Barr virus expressed detectable *fgr* mRNA. The single exception, DS179, was derived from a non-Burkitt's lymphoma. Neither specific chromosomal rearrangements associated with the Burkitt's lymphoma cell lines nor their geographic origin had any bearing on this correlation. Thus, detection of *fgr* proto-oncogene mRNA was specifically associated with Burkitt's lymphoma cells which had been naturally infected with Epstein-Barr virus.

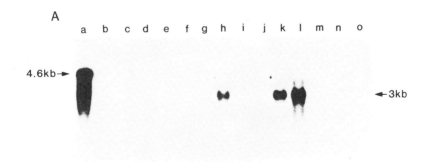

**FIGURE 16.7** Survey of human tumor cell lines for *fgr* proto-oncogene expression. RNA was prepared from human tumor cell lines and fractionated by agarose gel electrophoresis. RNA was transferred to nitrocellulose filters and hybridized with a v-*fgr*-specific probe. Cell lines derived from carcinomas (Lanes b-g), lymphomas (Lanes h-l) or sarcomas (Lanes m-o) were examined. RNA from GR-FeSV-transformed mink cells (Lane a) was used as a control.

The correlation of increased *fgr* proto-oncogene expression with Epstein-Barr virus infection of transformed lymphocytes was nearly absolute. Increased levels of c-*fgr* mRNA were detected in Burkitt's lymphoma cells whether infected naturally or deliberately in tissue culture. In addition, umbilical cord or peripheral blood lymphocyte cell lines established by EBV infection also expressed detectable c-*fgr* mRNA. Increases in the levels of transcripts related to other mammalian-derived tyrosine kinase coding *onc* genes were also detected in some EBV infected Burkitt's lymphoma cell lines. However, such RNAs were not consistently detected in EBV infected lines and were, in some cases, also detectable in noninfected cell lines. Taken together, these findings established a specific relationship between EBV infection and expression of the *fgr* proto-oncogene.

Evidence from several fields of investigation suggests that Burkitt's lymphoma results from a multi-step process which might involve the alteration of several genetic elements.[42] Epidemiologic data show that EBV plays an important role in the etiology of African Burkitt's lymphomas.[43] Furthermore, molecular studies have strongly implicated alterations of *myc* proto-oncogene expression in the process leading to American as well as African Burkitt's malignancies.[44,45] However, there is no evidence to indicate that such genetic alterations are the only changes required to achieve lymphoid cell transformation. From our investigation of human *fgr* proto-oncogene expression, we concluded that increased levels of c-*fgr* mRNA are not alone sufficient to induce malignant transformation of normal lymphocytes or even to immortalize them as continuous cell lines. Moreover, there was no direct evidence that EBV-induced immortalization involved c-*fgr*. Nevertheless, our findings demonstrated for the first time the induction of a proto-oncogene mRNA in response to infection by a DNA tumor virus and suggested the possibility that one step in EBV induced B cell immortalization might involve transcriptional activation of the *fgr* proto-oncogene.

## C-SLK, A NOVEL HUMAN TYROSINE KINASE GENE

The prototype tyrosine kinase gene, v-*src*,[23] and its close relatives, v-*yes* and v-*fgr*,[46,26] were each identified initially within oncogenic retroviruses as components derived from distinct cellular genes.[11] In an effort to search for new *fgr*-related genes within the human genome, we have taken a more general approach not reliant upon the identification of novel oncogenic viruses or transforming genes, but dependent only upon normal gene expression. Thus, complementary DNA libraries prepared from cells not expressing *fgr* proto-oncogene mRNA were screened with a DNA segment representing the tyrosine kinase coding sequence of v-*fgr*.[27] Several cDNA clones, ranging in size from 1.1 to 2.5 kbp, were isolated and compared with each other. By restriction enzyme mapping studies it was demonstrated that all of the cDNAs were overlapping and represented the same transcript. When human cellular DNAs were hybridized with v-*fgr*, v-*yes* or v-*src* probes, bands readily distinguishable from those detected with our cDNA probe were observed. These findings demonstrated that this cDNA, designated *slk*, was a new human gene distinct from closely related *fgr*, *yes* or *src* proto-oncogenes.

The nucleotide sequence of the *slk* cDNA clone was determined by the method of Sanger et al.[47] Analysis of this sequence revealed that the *slk* cDNA clone was 2435 bp in length and contained a long open reading frame of 1611 nucleotides. An ATG codon at position 371–373 conforming to Kozak's rules for translation initiation and preceded by a TAG termination signal just two codons upstream was identified as the translation start site.[48] The amino acid sequence predicted from the long open reading frame following this codon was 537 residues in length, terminating with a TAA codon at nucleotide position 1982–1984. A computer homology search revealed that the carboxy terminal 191 amino acids of the *slk* translational product were highly related to analogous regions of proteins specified by v-*yes*, v-*fgr* and v-*scr* at levels of 85%, 75% and 74% identity, respectively (Table 16.3). A lesser degree of homology was observed with other tyrosine kinases, including v-*erbB* and v-*fms* which represent known growth factor receptors.

Of all the tyrosine kinases described to date, the putative *slk* product was most closely related to the chicken c-*src*-encoded protein, $p60^{c-src}$. A single site for tyrosine phosphorylation first identified within $p60^{v-src}$ and present in $p60^{c-src}$ at position 416 is homologous to the tyrosine residue at amino acid position 420 of the *slk*-coded protein.[49] Regions of $p60^{c-src}$ thought to be responsible for ATP binding at positions 274–279 and 295 are also present in the *slk* translational product at positions 278–283 and 299.[50,51] Moreover,

**TABLE 16.3** Amino Acid Sequence Homology Between Putative *slk* Proteins and v-*onc* Gene Products

| Product of Retroviral Onc Gene | Percent Amino Acid Identity* |
|---|---|
| v-*yes* | 85 |
| v-*fgr* | 75 |
| v-*src* | 74 |
| v-*abl* | 38 |
| v-*fes* | 38 |
| v-*erb*B | 24 |
| v-*fms* | 24 |

*Positions 346 to the carboxy terminus of the putative *slk* translational was compared with analogous regions of each *onc* gene translational product.

these two proteins are almost identical in size and share significant homology over a region of 455 amino acids. Despite its high degree of relatedness to p60$^{c\text{-}src}$, the amino terminal region of the predicted *slk* gene product, 82 amino acids in length, showed no significant homology, with p60$^{c\text{-}src}$ or any other previously described protein. Thus, this region, which corresponds to that encoded by the first two exons of c-*src*,[52] may be involved in determining unique interactions of these related proteins with specific cellular targets. The single feature in this amino terminal domain shared with p60$^{c\text{-}scr}$ or p60$^{v\text{-}scr}$ was a glycine residue at amino acid position 2, followed by lysine residues at positions 7 and 9. This region has been shown to be important for the addition of a myristic acid residue to the amino terminus of p60$^{v\text{-}src}$. This post-translational modification appears to mediate attachment of p60$^{v\text{-}src}$ to the inner face of cell membranes and to play a critical role in v-*src*-induced transformation.[53,54]

## Human slk Gene Possesses Transforming Potential

Structural relatedness between *slk* and members of the v-*src* transforming gene family suggested that the *slk*-coded protein might possess oncogenic potential. To test this possibility, we constructed a chimeric molecule utilizing a biologically active Gardner-Rasheed feline sarcoma virus (GR-FeSV) plasmid DNA as a vector. Our strategy was based upon the presence of a common ApaI restriction enzyme site at position 1028 in *slk* cDNA and at position 1066 in the GR-FeSV *onc* gene v-*fgr* (Fig. 16.8). The resulting construct, designated pv-*fgr*/*slk*, contained the GR-FeSV 5' LTR, p15, and γ-actin coding sequences, as well as 219 nucleotides of v-*fgr*.[26] The contribution of *slk* consisted of 945 bp of coding sequence as well as a portion of its 3' untranslated stretch. As shown in Fig. 8, the pv-*fgr*/*slk* plasmid induced foci of transformation upon transfection of NIH/3T3 cells with a specific focus-forming activity which was within four-fold of that displayed by pv-*fgr*. In contrast, the vector plasmid alone, pv-*fgr* Δ3', was unable to induce morphologic transformation in these same assay cells. We conclude from these findings that pv-*fgr*/*slk* has oncogenic properties and that *slk* can be activated as a transforming gene.

In an effort to detect the protein specified by the chimeric transforming DNA, cells transformed with pv-*fgr*/*slk* were metabolically labeled with $^{35}$S-methionine and examined by immunoprecipitation utilizing anti-feline leukemia virus p15 serum that recognizes the major GR-FeSV translational product P70$^{gag\text{-}actin\text{-}fgr}$.[25] Cells transformed by the chimeric molecule expressed at 71,000 dalton protein, designated P71, that could be clearly distinguished from P70$^{gag\text{-}actin\text{-}fgr}$. This size difference was consistent with the fact that P71 was predicted to possess seven additional residues at its carboxy

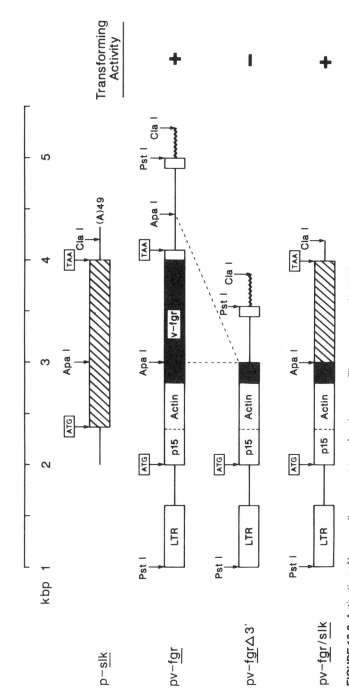

**FIGURE 16.8** Activation of human *slk* gene as a transforming gene. The structures of individual molecules as well as their ability to morphologically transform NIH/3T3 cells upon transfection are indicated.

terminus as compared to the GR-FeSV translational product. In other experiments, the P71 hybrid protein was tested in an immune complex assay for protein kinase activity. Our findings demonstrated that P71 was a tyrosine-specific protein kinase. All of these findings, combined with the observed structural relatedness of the *slk* translational product to known kinases, strongly suggested that the *slk* gene encoded a tyrosine-specific protein kinase.

## THE HUMAN SLK GENE IS STRUCTURALLY DISTINCT FROM KNOWN POLYPEPTIDE GROWTH FACTOR RECEPTORS

Within the larger tyrosine kinase family are the genes encoding receptors for epidermal growth factor (EGF),[20,21] CSF-1,[22] insulin,[55,56] and possibly other growth promoting polypeptides.[57] Recently, two tyrosine-kinase encoding retrovirus *onc* genes have been defined as altered versions of EGF and CSF-1 receptor genes.[20-22] These findings have suggested that tyrosine kinases specified by other retrovirus transforming genes might also represent growth factor receptors. Of the proto-oncogene products identified to date, p60$^{c-src}$ is the only tyrosine kinase, other than those identified as growth factor receptors, whose entire amino acid sequence is known. Our comparisons have revealed that p60$^{c-src}$ and the putative c-*slk* translational product, p60$^{c-slk}$, are almost identical in size and are highly related in amino acid sequence over a stretch which accounts for 85% of their extent. In contrast, even within their conserved tyrosine kinase domains, only distant relationships exist between either protein and known growth factor receptors. Moreover, p60$^{c-src}$ and p60$^{c-slk}$ do not possess hydrophobic domains capable of spanning cellular membranes. Such domains are hallmarks of the known polypeptide growth factor receptors described to date. Thus, p60$^{c-slk}$ would appear to represent a second tyrosine-specific protein kinase whose structure is not consistent with that of known polypeptide growth factor receptors.

## IMPLICATIONS

Investigations such as those discussed in the present report have identified roughly two dozen normal cellular genes which are capable of acquiring oncogenic properties. Although it is likely that additional oncogenes will be found, several lines of evidence indicate that the number of such genes may be limited. First, there are a number of instances where two or more distinct retrovirus *onc* genes have arisen from a single proto-oncogene. For example, the *fes* proto-oncogene of the cat gave rise to *onc* genes of two different feline sarcoma virus strains.[58] This same proto-oncogene present in the chicken genome was the progenitor of *fps*, the Fujinami sarcoma virus *onc* gene.[59] Secondly, identification of the dominant human tumor-derived oncogene, T24, revealed that this gene was a form of the *ras* proto-oncogene earlier described as the cellular cognate of the Harvey- or BALB-murine sarcoma virus *onc* genes. In addition, other distinct genes, implicated in the carcinogenic process by virtue of their amplification in certain tumor cells, have been identified because of their genetic relatedness to known oncogenes. Examined from another perspective, normal cellular functions that have been linked to proto-oncogenes have thus far implicated only growth factors and their receptors in the neoplastic process. These findings suggest an even more limited number of pathways that might lead to the malignant state.

The discovery of oncogenes was dependent upon their ability to act in a dominant fashion to induce malignant disease in experimental animals or morphologic transformation of cells in culture. In attempting to reconcile this fact with knowledge that carcinogenesis is likely a multistep process, it becomes clear that our understanding is not yet adequate to explain the etiology of cancer. However, the study of proto-oncogenes, as well as alterations capable of activating them as oncogenes, has provided important insights into molecular events that can lead to malignancy. Thus, continued efforts to understand the action of such genes can only help to unravel the carcinogenic process.

## SUMMARY

Investigations to uncover the molecular events responsible for conversion of normal cells to cancer cells have led to the identification of genetic elements, or oncogenes, that alone are capable of inducing malignant transformation of cells in tissue culture. Typically, oncogenes represent altered versions of normal cellular genes, termed proto-oncogenes. Since proto-oncogenes are highly conserved in an evolutionary sense, they must be required for normal cellular processes such as growth and development. Genetic alterations affecting proto-oncogenes have been shown to activate their oncogenic potential in model systems and in certain human tumors as well, suggesting their etiologic role in tumorigenesis. Recent discoveries revealing functions for a few of the two dozen normal proto-oncogenes thus far identified have implicated polypeptide growth factors and their cellular stimulatory pathways in the malignant process. Insights gained from these discoveries promise to provide molecular approaches of value in diagnosis and possibly prevention of human cancer.

# REFERENCES

1. Aaronson SA: Biologic characterization of mammalian cells transformed by a primate sarcoma virus. Virology 1973;52:562–567.
2. Robbins KC, Devare SG, Aaronson SA: Molecular cloning of integrated simian sarcoma virus: Genome organization of infectious DNA clones. Proc Natl Acad Sci 1981; 78:2918–2922.
3. Devare SG, Reddy EP. Law JD, et al: Nucleotide sequence of the simian sarcoma virus genome: Demonstration that its acquired cellular sequences encode the transforming gene product, p28$^{sis}$. Proc Natl Acad Sci 1983;80:731–735.
4. Robbins KC, Devare SG, Reddy EP, Aaronson SA: In vivo identification of the transforming gene product of simian sarcoma virus. Science 1982;218:1131–1133.
5. Antoniades HN, Hunkapiller MW: Human platelet-derived growth factor (PDGF): Amino terminal amino acid sequence. Science 1983;220:963–965.
6. Doolittle RF, Hunkapiller MW, Hood LE, et al: Simian sarcoma virus *onc* gene, v-*sis*, is derived from the gene (or genes) encoding a platelet-derived growth factor. Science 1983;221:275–277.
7. Waterfield MD, Scrace GT, Whittle N, et al: Platelet-derived growth factor is structurally related to the putative transforming protein p28$^{sis}$ of simian sarcoma virus. Nature 1983;304:35–39.
8. Robbins KC, Antoniades HN, Devare SG, et al: Structural and immunological similarities between simian sarcoma virus gene product(s) and huma platelet-derived growth factor. Nature 1983;305:605–608.
9. Robbins KC, Leal F, Pierce JH, Aaronson SA: The v-*sis*/PDGF-2 transforming gene product localizes to cell membranes but is not a secretory protein. EMBO J 1985;4:1783–1792.
10. Leal F, William LT, Robbins KC, Aaronson SA: Evidence that the v-*sis* gene product transforms by interaction with the receptor for platelet-derived growth factor. Science 1985;230:327–330.
11. Chiu I-M, Reddy EP, Givol D, et al: Nucleotide sequence analysis identifies the human c-*sis* proto-oncogene as structural gene for platelet-derived growth factor. Cell 1984;37:123–129.
12. Joseph SF, Guo C, Ratner L, Wong-Staal F: Human proto-oncogene nucleotide sequence corresponding to the transforming region of simian sarcoma virus. Science 1984; 223:487–491.
13. Johnsson A, Heldin C-H, Wasteson A, et al: The c-*sis* gene encodes a precursor of the B chain of platelet-derived growth factor. EMBO J 1984;3:921–928.
14. Gazit A, Igarashi H, Chiu I-M, et al: Expression of the normal human *sis*/PDGF-2 coding sequence induces cellular transformation. Cell 1984;39:89–97.
15. Eva A, Robbins KC, Anderson PR, et al: Cellular genes analogous to retroviral *onc* genes are transcribed in human tumor cells. Natural 1982;295:116–119.
16. Collins T, Ginsburg D, Boss JM, et al: Cultured human endothelial cells express platelet-derived growth factor B chain: cDNA cloning and structural analysis. Nature 1985;316:748–750.
17. Rao CD, Igarashi H, Chiu I-M, et al: Structure and sequence of the human c-*sis*/PDGF-2 transcriptional unit. Proc Natl Acad Sci (in press).
18. Wolfe LG, Smith RK, Dienhardt F: Simian sarcoma virus type 1 (Lagothrix): Focus assay and demonstration of nontransforming associated virus. J Natl Cancer Inst 1972;48:1905–1907.

19. Wolfe LG, Deinhardt F, Theilen GJ, et al: Induction of tumors in marmoset monkeys by simian sarcoma virus, Type 1 (Lagothrix): A preliminary report. J Natl Cancer Inst 1971;47:1115–1120.

20. Downward J, Yarden Y, Mayes E, et al: Close similarity of epidermal growth factor receptor and v-erbB oncogene protein sequences. Nature (London) 1984;307:521–527.

21. Ullrich A, Coussens L, Hayflick JS, et al: Human epidermal growth factor receptor cDNA sequence and aberrant expression of the amplified gene in A431 epidermoid carcinoma cells. Nature 1984;309:418–425.

22. Sherr CJ, Rettenmier CW, Sacca R, et al: The c-*fms* proto-oncogene product is related to the receptor for the mononuclear phagocyte growth factor, CSF-1. Cell 1985;41:665–676.

23. Bishop JM: Cellular oncogenes and retroviruses. Annu Rev Biochem 1983;52:301–354.

24. Rasheed S, Barbacid M, Aaronson SA, Gardner MB: Origin and biological properties of a new feline sarcoma virus. Virology 1982;117:238–244.

25. Naharro G, Dunn CY, Robbins KC: Analysis of the primary translational product and integrated DNA of a new feline sarcoma virus, GR-FeSV. Virology 1983;125:502–507.

26. Naharro G, Robbins KC, Reddy EP: Gene product of v-*fgr onc*: hybrid protein containing a portion of actin and a tyrosine-specific protein kinase. Science 1984;223:63–66.

27. Tronick SR, Popescu NC, Cheah MSC, et al: Isolation and chromosomal localization of the human *fgr* proto-oncogene, a distinct member of the tyrosine kinase gene family. Proc Natl Acad Sci USA 1985;82:6595–6599.

28. Mitelman F, Levan G: Clustering of aberrations to specific chromosomes in human neoplasms. Hereditas 1981;95:79–139.

29. Gilbert F, Balaban G, Moorhead P, et al: Abnormalties of chromosome 1p in human neuroblastoma tumors and cell lines. Cancer Genet Cytogenet 1982;7:33–42.

30. Brito-Babapulle V, Atkin NB: Breakpoints in chromosome #1 abnormalities of 218 human neoplasms. Cancer Genet Cytogenet 1981;4:215–225.

31. Haag MM, Soukup SW, Neely JE: Chromosome analysis of a human neuroblastoma. Cancer Res 1981;41:2995–2999.

32. Brodeur GM, Green AA, Hayes FA, et al: Cytogenetic features of human neuoblastomas and cell lines. Cancer Res 1983;41:4678–4686.

33. Gilbert F: Chromosomes, genes, and cancer: a classification of chromosome abnormalities in cancer. JNCI 1983;71:1107–1114.

34. Yunis JJ, Soreng AL: Constitutue fragile sites and cancer. Science 1984;226:1199–1204.

35. Morton CC, Taub R, Diamond A, et al: Mapping of the human Blym-1 transforming gene activated in Burkitt lymphomas to chromosome 1. Science 1984;223:173–175.

36. McBride OW, Swan DC, Tronick SR, et al: Regional chromosomal localization of N-*ras*, K-*ras*-1, *K-ras*-2 and *myb* oncogenes in human cells. Nucleic Acids Res 1983; 11:8221–8236.

37. Rabin M, Watson M, Barker PE, et al: N-*ras* transforming gene maps to region p11-p13 on chromosome 1 by in situ hybridization. Cytogenet Cell Genet 1984;38:70–72.

38. Popescue NC, Amsbaugh SC, DiPaolo JA, et al: Chromosomal localization of three human *ras* genes by in situ molecular hybridization. Somatic Cell and Mol Genet 1985; 11:149–155.

39. Davis M, Malcolm S, Hall A, Marshall CJ: Localization of the human N-*ras* oncogene to chromosome 1cen-p21 by in situ hybridization EMBO J 1983;2:2281–2283.

40. Franke U, de Martinville B, Coussens L, Ullrich A: The human gene for the beta subunit of nerve growth factor is located on the proximal short arm of chromosome 1. Science 1983;222:1248–1251.

41. Cheah MSC, Ley TJ, Tronick SR, Robbins KC: *fgr* proto-oncogene mRNA induced in B-lymphocytes by Epstein-Barr virus infection. Nature 1983;319:238–240.

42. Klein G, Klein E: Evolution of tumours and the impact of molecular oncology. Nature 1985;315:190–195.
43. Geser A, deThe G, Lenoir G, et al: Final cast reporting from the Ugandan prospective study of the relationship between EBV and Burkitt's lymphoma. Internatl J Cancer 1982;29:397–400.
44. Taub R, Kirsch I, Morton C, et al: Translocation of the c-*myc* gene into the immunoglobulin heavy chain locus in human Burkitt's lymphoma and murine plasmacytoma cells. Proc Natl Acad Sci USA 1982;79:7837–7841.
45. Dalla-Favera R, Bregni M, Erikson J, et al: Human c-*myc onc* gene is located on the region of chromosome 8 that is translocated in Burkitt's lymphoma cells. Proc Natl Acad Sci USA 1982;79:7824–7827.
46. Kitamura N, Kitamura A, Toyoshima K, et al: Avian sarcoma virus Y73 genome sequence and structural similarity of its transforming gene product to that of Rous sarcoma virus. Nature 1982;297:205–208.
47. Sanger F, Nicklen S, Coulson AR: DNA sequencing with chain terminating inhibitors. Proc Natl Acad Sci USA 1977;74:5463–5467.
48. Kozak M: Compilation and analysis of sequences upstream from the translational start site in eukaryotic mRNAs. Nucleic Acids Res 1984;12:857–872.
49. Smart JE, Oppermann H, Czernilofsky AP, et al: Characterization of sites for tyrosine phosphorylation in the transforming protein of Rous sarcoma virus (pp60$^{v-src}$) and its normal cellular homologue (pp60$^{c-src}$). Proc Natl Acad Sci USA 1981;78:6013–6017.
50. Barker WC, Dayhoff MO: Viral *src* gene products are related to the catalytic chain of mammalian cAMP-dependent protein kinase. Proc Natl Acad Sci USA 1982;79:2836–2839.
51. Privalsky ML, Ralston R, Bishop JM: The membrane glycoprotein encoded by the retroviral oncogene v-*erb*-B is structurally related to tyrosine-specific protein kinases. Proc Natl Acad Sci USA 1984;81:704–707.

# CHAPTER 17

# Chemoprevention in Head and Neck Cancer

*Isaiah W. Dimery, MD and*
*Waun Ki Hong, MD*

## INTRODUCTION

The concept of chemoprevention implies that a carcinogen-induced preneo-plastic transformation of a tissue is a reversible process. Such tissues, then, must be susceptible to an antineoplastic or differentiating agent that has the capability to halt the neoplastic process in those cells that are not irreversibly differentiated, and to eliminate those cells that are. Evaluation and effective treatment would require the identification of patient populations at highest risk either for development of tumor, or for development of recurrence or second primaries. Such populations are found in patients with premalignant oral lesions together with those having a history of head and neck malignancies. There is a clear relationship between the development of head and neck cancer, the presence of premalignant oral lesions, and such environmental risk factors as alcohol and tobacco use. The natural or synthetic vitamin A analogues, the retinoids, may provide an option in the prevention and treatment of cancer in these populations. This chapter discusses current studies and future directions in the use of retinoids in this regard.

## HEAD AND NECK CANCER
### Etiology and Epidemiology

Carcinoma of the upper aerodigestive tract accounts for 5% of all human tumors, with 95% of cases of squamous cell histology. These tumors typically occur in patients between the ages of 40 and 70 years. It is estimated that in 1986 there will be approximately 40,000 new cases of, and 13,000 deaths from this disease.[1]

Major risk factors for the development of these tumors include the use of tobacco products (cigarette or smokeless) and alcohol, which have a synergistic carcinogenic interaction. The primary constituent responsible for oral cancers is thought to be $N'$-nitrosonornicotine, which has tumor-promoting properties in animals and is present in cigarette smoke condensate, chewing tobacco, and snuff. The combined risk for smokers and heavy drinkers to develop oral carcinoma is sixfold higher than for a control population.[2] These risk factors have a maximum effect in the oral cavity and oropharynx in the horseshoe-shaped area extending from the anterior floor of the mouth to the tonsillar pillar-retromolar trigone where saliva pools.[3] Although this is only 20% of the surface area of the oral cavity, 75% of oral cancers originate here.

A small percentage of patients neither smoke nor drink; the risk factors in this group are as yet unknown. Evidence indicates that certain types of human viruses, such a papillomaviruses, may be involved in the development of either benign or malignant neoplasms occurring in the skin and aerodigestive tract.[4] In a study of various benign and malignant lesions of the head and neck, an immunocytochemical method searching for genus-specific structural antigens of human papillomavirus was used to evaluate patients with abnormal oral pathology.[5] Specimens positive for the antigen were from patients with laryngeal papilloma, oral papillomas, or glossal leukoplakia. Recently, in verrucous carcinoma of the larynx, Brandsma et al. found evidence of papillomavirus DNA sequences.[6] Herpes simplex virus (HSV) has also been implicated in the development of labial and oral carcinoma, with viral particles demonstrated in representative tissue samples.[7]

By various methods of analysis, the sera from patients with oral carcinoma were evaluated by Shillitoe et al. for antibody to HSV.[8-10] Elevated levels of these antibodies correlated directly with the stage of the tumor. Antibody titers in control individuals who smoked but were otherwise normal approached levels obtained in the oral cancer patients. Cigarette smoke and latent HSV infection, therefore, seem to predispose the mucosal surface to the development of oral carcinoma.

## Patterns of Failure

Marked improvements in the treatment of head and neck cancer have been made in the 1980s in comparison with therapies offered in the 1950s and 1960s. Currently, there are new surgical techniques and radiotherapeutic approaches, and chemotherapy is used earlier in the patient's management.

Nonetheless, because of neglect of symptoms and/or rapid tumor growth, patients continue to present at an advanced stage of disease that is not curable even under the most favorable of circumstances; consequently, their prognosis is poor. Notwithstanding these modern approaches and treatment techniques, patients must have radical and disfiguring surgical procedures in an attempt to render them disease-free and save their lives.

The rate of recurrence in the loco-regional area or at distant sites is 60% or more within 2 years of treatment for those individuals with advanced disease of T3, T4, N2b, or N3 stage.[11]

Hong et al. evaluated the patterns of relapse in patients who achieved complete remission after receiving combined-modality therapy including induction chemotherapy for locally advanced stage III and IV previously untreated squamous cell carcinoma.[12] Forty-two percent developed recurrent disease (18% at the primary site; 12% with distant metastases to the lung, bone, and liver; and 12% with primary recurrence plus distant metastases) within the first 3 years, with 8% developing second primary lesions.

Only patients with early-stage carcinomas can be effectively treated and cured with the surgical and radiotherapeutic techniques currently available. In the majority of patients with more advanced disease, treatment only yields a 0 to 40% 5-year survival. In the surviving patients, the incidence of development of second primary tumors is 6% per year and may closely depend on the continued use of tobacco and alcohol.[13–15] The sites of occurrence for second primary tumors are the upper aerodigestive tract, varying from 10% in the larynx to 40% in the oropharynx, with the remainder in esophagus, lung, and bladder. These second tumors usually prove to be the cause of death.

## Pathogenesis of Second Primary Tumors

Second or third primary lesions are explained by the concept of a diffuse mucosal membrane atypia known as "field cancerization."[16] Even with optimal local treatment, the mucosal surface retains this abnormality. The subclinical membrane abnormalities become clinically evident as the precancerous lesions termed leukoplakia or erythroplasia. Leukoplakia of the oral cavity is defined by the World Heath Organization as a "white patch" that does not disappear on rubbing and that cannot be ascribed clinically or histopathologically to any other disease process. Erythroplasia, by the same system of definition, is a lesion that presents as a bright red, velvety plaque that cannot be characterized clinically or pathologically as being due to any other condition. In these premalignant lesions, initiation and early promotion of the normal mucosa to atypia and metaplasia have already occurred. Further abnormal differentiation results in the development of carcinoma in situ prior to the development of invasive carcinoma.[17] These premalignant lesions commonly occur in individuals over the age of 40, but can also occur at a much younger age. The use of smokeless tobacco products (snuff and chewing tobacco) and cigarettes are usually the causative factors, although a small percentage of affected individuals have never used tobacco products. The rate of malignant transformation appears to be lowest in pure leukoplakia, intermediate in erythroleukoplakia, and highest in pure erythroplasia ranging among the three from 0.5 to 51%.[18,19]

Silverman et al. followed 275 patients with oral leukoplakia for an average of seven years; 17.5% subsequently developed squamous cell carcinoma, a result that confirms leukoplakia as a precancerous lesion that warrants aggressive management.[20] In a study of tongue carcinoma, a high incidence (116 times greater than expected) of multiple carcinomas of the oral cavity and pharynx was encountered; the incidence of multiple oral carcinomas was five times greater in those patients with leukoplakia than in those without leukoplakia.[21] Furthermore, in another series, the incidence of oral carcinoma could not be diminished by surgical removal of the leukoplakia, suggesting that all normal-appearing mucosa of patients with leukoplakia has a higher expected incidence of carcinoma.[18]

It appears that a rational approach to pursue in an effort to reduce the incidence of head and neck cancer is chemoprevention. The solution to the problem of cancer will be nearer when the basic control mechanisms that drive a cell from the proliferative to the nonproliferative and differentiated state are understood, and when the chain of events leading to the transformation of a normally functioning cell to one that is neoplastic can be altered.

## RETINOIDS AS CHEMOPREVENTIVE AGENTS
### Activity and Mechanism of Action

Normal epithelial tissues depend on certain substances to maintain their integrity and for cellular renewal. Vitamin A and its natural analogues, retinoids, are necessary for the normal development and differentiation of all epithelial tissues.[22] Animals fed a diet deficient in retinoids develop squamous metaplasia and tumors in a variety of epithelial tissues. When retinoid-deficient animals are exposed to carcinogens, a greater incidence of premalignant and malignant lesions occur.[23] The exogenous administration of retinoids can inhibit such tumor induction.[24] Retinoids thus represent a physiological approach to the problem of chemoprevention and chemotherapy in preneoplastic and neoplastic lesions.

The retinoids are a class of compounds with remarkable prophylactic and therapeutic activity in oncology, having shown activity as chemopre-

They have demonstrated antiproliferative activity against both animal and human tumors.[26-30] The history of their descriptions of basic research involving these compounds in various models, and their potential usefulness have been previously reviewed.

The exact mechanism of activity of these compounds is not known; it is believed however, that their antiproliferative activity is accomplished by their ability to induce cellular differentiation.

By the prevention or reversal of epithelial metaplasia, the development of carcinomas can be eliminated or delayed. In hamsters, high doses of vitamin A were found to inhibit tracheal and bronchial formation of squamous metaplasia induced by the intra-tracheal instillation of benzo-a-pyrene, a tobacco-related polycyclic hydrocarbon.[32] Other culture systems have demonstrated the effectiveness of retinoids in the suppression of chemical carcinogenesis in epithelial tissues.[33-36] The human tumor-cloning assay has been employed to evaluate a variety of retinoid analogues for potential antineoplastic activity in reducing tumor colony-forming units (T-CFU).[37] All-*trans*-retinoic acid, all-*trans*-retinol, and 13-*cis*-retinoic acid were equal in their ability to decrease T-CFU.[37] Lotan et al. found that retinoic acid produced differential effects on the growth of two human head and neck squamous carcinoma cell lines of well-differentiated or poorly differentiated histology.[38] The ability to inhibit the formation of colonies in soft agar was exhibited in both cell lines, whereas the anchorage-dependent growth was either inhibited or stimulated depending upon the stage of differentiation of the tumor.[38]

Since vitamin A and retinoids can reverse the abnormal differentiation in vitamin A-deficient animals or in organ culture, attempts have been made to reverse the effects of carcinogens with retinoids. A decrease in the formation of new tumors was prevented in retinoid-treated rats exposed to carcinogens.[39] It is thought that retinoids decrease the progression of preneoplastic lesions to carcinoma by suppression of the promotion stage of carcinogenesis, possibly through inhibition of the proliferation of preneoplastic cells or by redirecting the aberrant differentiation of the preneoplastic cells to normal differentiation pathways.[39] Retinoids also modulate the growth and differentiation in neoplastic cells of various histopathologic types in culture.[27,40]

A differential marker of normal and abnormal cell growth is the accumulation of products of polyamine metabolism. Ornithine decarboxylase (ODC), the rate-limiting enzyme, is markedly elevated in a variety of tumor systems and its activity is induced by chemical carcinogens.[41] Identification of increased enzyme activity may indicate that tumor promotion has been initiated.

The skin tumor promoter 12-O-tetradecanoylpho     ~~~~~~~~~
(TPA) induces the activity of the enzyme ODC in the mouse n
acid inhibited this enzyme activity and resulted in a reduction ~~~~~~~~~gen-
esis.[41] A positive correlation between this biochemical phenomenon and
skin tumor promotion has been established.[42,43] The mechanism or chemical
reaction by which retinoids inhibit TPA-induced ODC activity is, however,
not known.

Currently, we are investigating the levels of ODC activity in the oral
mucosa of patients without oral cancer who smoke and consume alcohol,
and in those who have premalignant mucosal lesions or oral cancer, to
determine if it is an early indicator of neoplastic change.

Various mechanisms have been postulated by which retinoids regulate
cell growth and differentiation, thereby exerting an anticarcinogenic and an
antitumor effect. Cellular proteins have been described that may mediate the
effects of retinoids on normal epithelial tissue, on diffusely abnormal tissues
in the area of "field cancerization," and on neoplastic tissue. Cellular retinol-binding protein (CRBP) and cellular retinoic acid binding protein
(CRABP) have been identified in varying amounts in normal mucosa and
carcinoma of the oral cavity and oropharynx.[44-46] Investigation into the
significance of these proteins continues, with consideration given to a possible steroid hormone–like activity, with CRBP and CRABP acting as receptors resulting in biochemical alterations of cell membrane protein.[47-49] Retinoids may modulate a variety of immune functions, culminating in
enhancement of the host response, and thus diminish the potential for metastases by subsequent growth inhibition.[50-53]

## Retinoid Trials on Premalignant Lesions

With a direct relationship established between the presence of leukoplakia
and the development of oral carcinoma, retinoid trials were developed to
assess the usefulness and toxicity of various compounds used either topically
or systemically to reverse this premalignant process. In early uncontrolled
trials, oral treatment with retinoic acid led to the regression of leukoplakia in
the mouth, tongue, and larynx; however, carcinomas did not respond to
such treatment.[54] In a broad phase II study to assess the antitumor effects of
the analogue isotretinoin, there were objective responses in patients with a
variety of preneoplastic lesions. In this same study, patients with squamous
cell carcinoma of the head and neck had objective regression of lesions in the
skin and subcutaneous metastases, as well as in several preneoplastic lesions.[55] Koch reported his study of 75 patients with oral leukoplakia who
were treated with a variety of retinoic acid analogues.[56] Major initial response rates of 87% were seen, with 44 to 50% of patients continuing in

remission after 2 to 4 years of follow-up. In another early study conducted by Koch, 48 patients received all-*trans*-retinoic acid, either as a 75-mg oral dose or as a 50-mg oral dose combined with 0.1% aromatic retinoid paste applied locally for 6 weeks.[57] Response rates of 71% and 83%, respectively, were achieved; however, relapses were observed within 2 months of terminating treatment. Toxic effects were mild, consisting of dry oral mucosa and cutaneous desquamation. Shah et al. utilized 13-*cis*-retinoic acid in the form of a 3- to 10-mg lozenge in the treatment of 11 evaluable patients; the response rate was 81%.[58] Again, relapses occurred after cessation of treatment. The treatment was well tolerated, with mucositis and dry lips being the major objective findings of toxicity.

In a double-blind randomized trial of 13-*cis*-retinoic acid (13-CRA) versus placebo in the treatment of oral leukoplakia, results in 26 evaluable patients were analyzed. After 3 months of therapy and 6 months of follow-up, major objective response occured in 71% of CRA treated patients versus 9% of placebo-treated patients (p = 0.004).[59] Histological reversal of mucosal dysplasia was observed in the 13-CRA-treated patients. Toxic effects consisted primarily of reversible cutaneous reactions and conjunctivitis. The 13-CRA was therefore felt to be an effective treatment for oral leukoplakia; however, maintenance treatment appears to be required.

### Retinoids as Adjuvant Therapy for Squamous Cell Carcinoma

To facilitate our understanding of retinoids as differentiating and cytostatic agents, their use as adjuvant treatment is currently being studied. A high rate of local recurrence and distant metastases occurs in advanced T and N-stage disease despite initial control with surgery, radiotherapy, and cytotoxic induction chemotherapy.[60] Adjuvant cytotoxic chemotherapy has made no impact on survival and is difficult for these patients to tolerate.[61] Therefore, we recently initiated a program to evaluate the efficacy of 13-*cis*-retinoic acid versus placebo in a double-blind randomized trial for the prevention of local recurrence, distant metastases, and seocnd primary lesions. The selected population includes patients who had stage II, III, or IV (N2a or less) disease and who are clinically free of disease after surgery, radiotherapy, or both; these patients are randomized to 13-*cis*-retinoic acid or placebo taken for 1 year. We estimate that it will be five years before any meaningful conclusions can be made.

### CONCLUSION

There appears to be a role for retinoid compounds in chemoprevention trials for head and neck cancer. These trials would exploit the various postulated mechanisms of action by which retinoids function and would focus on the ability of these substances to reverse or differentiate histologically proven malignancy to a normal-appearing histological pattern. This differentiating activity would also apply to subclinical mucosal derangement, so that retinoids could be useful in (1) preventing the development of cancer in an identifiable high-risk population whose premalignancy is not clinically evident; (2) treating minimal·residual disease or micrometastases in an adjuvant setting in those patients who have had definitive treatment with either surgery, radiotherapy, or both; and (3) preventing the occurrence of second primary malignancies in patients who have been presumably cured of their primary neoplasm.

These are studies that require a prolonged treatment period; therefore, a truly nontoxic regimen is desirable. Our present armamentarium is not devoid of side effects, and newer analogues are actively being sought. Perhaps with dosage modification (if lower doses are active), or structural changes through research into analogues, toxicity can be minimized. Furthermore, while the population of patients who qualify for adjuvant therapy or therapy of a premalignant lesion is easily identified, it is an entirely different situation to accurately identify those patients who will develop cancer for the first time. Epidemiological studies have revealed an association of low serum retinol levels and a general risk for cancer, but results have been inconclusive.[62-64] Evaluation of oral biopsies for the presence of elevated levels of ODC to identify those individuals most likely to benefit from retinoid treatment is a conceivably useful approach. Perhaps an assay of the serum retinol level in patients with a strong history of alcohol and cigarette use would identify a subpopulation who would benefit from interventional replacement therapy. Currently, trials with beta-carotene are being conducted since this compound can be taken for an extended period of time without any major toxic effects. This and other less toxic compounds would open new opportunities for use in conjunction with chemotherapy. We are fully aware that induction or adjuvant trials of chemotherapy alone are not accomplishing their intended goal of increasing the disease-free suvival. A potential alternative program for consideration is induction chemotherapy followed by maintenance therapy with retinoids after surgery, radiotherapy, or both.

It is clear that the types of studies we have discussed need to be initiated, and that other alternative therapies should be actively sought.

## REFERENCES

1. National Cancer Institute: Surveillance, epidemiology and end results program, 1986.
2. Winn DM, Blot WJ, Shy CM, et al: Snuff dipping and oral cancer among women in the southern United States. N Engl J Med 1981;304:745–749.

3. Moore C, Catlin D: Anatomic origins and locations of oral cancer. Am J Surg 1967;114:510–513.
4. Jensen AB, Kurman RJ, Lancaster WD: Human papillomavirus, in Belshe R (ed): Textbook of human viruses Edition I. Littleton: PSG, Inc, 1984, pp 951–968.
5. Strauss M, Jenson AB: Human papillomavirus in various lesions of the head and neck. Otolaryngol Head Neck Surg 1985;93(3):342–346.
6. Brandsma JL, Steinberg BM, Abramson AL, et al: Presence of human papillovirus type 16-related sequences in verrucous carcinoma of the larynx. Cancer Res 1986; 46:2185–2188.
7. Caron GA: Carcinoma at the site of herpes simplex infection (letter). J Amer Med Assoc 1980;243:2396.
8. Shillitoe EJ, Greenspan D, Greenspan JS, et al: Immunoglobulin class of antibody to herpes simplex virus in patients with oral cancer. Cancer 1983;51:65–71.
9. Shillitoe EJ, Greenspan D, Greenspan JS, et al: Antibody to early and late antigens of herpes simplex virus type 1 in patients with oral cancer. Cancer 1984;54:266–273.
10. Shillitoe EJ, Greenspan D, Greenspan JS, et al: Neutralizing antibody to herpes simplex virus type 1 in patients with oral cancer. Cancer 1982;49:2315–2320.
11. Goepfert H: Are we making any progress? Arch Otolaryngol 1984;110:562–563.
12. Hong WK, Bromer RH, Amato DA, et al: Patterns of relapse in locally advanced head and neck cancer patients who achieved complete remission after combined modality therapy. Cancer 1985;56:1242–1245.
13. Vikram B, Strong EW, Shah JP, et al: Second malignant neoplasms in patients successfully treated with multimodality treatment for advanced head and neck cancer. Head Neck Surg 1984;6:734–737.
14. Jesse RH, Sugarbaker EV: Squamous cell carcinoma of the oropharynx: Why we fail. Am J Surg 1976;132:435–438.
15. Moore C: Cigarette smoking in cancer of the mouth, pharynx, and larynx: a continuing study. J Amer Med Assoc 1971;218:553–558.
16. Slaughter DP, Southwick HW, Smejkal W: Field cancerization in oral stratified squamous epithelium: clinical implications of multicentric origin. Cancer 1953;5:963–968.
17. Vaughan CW, Homburgher F, Shapshay S, et al: Carcinogenesis in the upper aerodigestive tract. Otolaryngol Clin North Am 1980;13:403–412.
18. Einhorn J, Wersall J: Incidence of oral carcinoma in patients with leukoplakia of the oral mucosa. Cancer 1967;20:2189–2193.
19. Shafer WG, Waldron CA: Erythroplakia of the oral cavity. Cancer 1975;36:1021–1028.
20. Silverman S Jr, Gorsky M, Lozada F: Oral leukoplakia and malignant transformation. A follow-up study of 257 patients. Cancer 1984;53:563–568.
21. Shibuya H, Amagasa T, Seto K, et al: Leukoplakia-associated multiple carcinomas in patients with tongue carcinoma. Cancer 1986;57:843–846.
22. Moore T: Effect of vitamin A deficiency in animals: pharmacology and toxicology of vitamin A, in Sebrell SH, Harris RS (eds): The vitamins, 2nd ed, New York: Academic Press, 1967, pp 245–266, 280–294.
23. Sporn MB, Dunlop NM, Newton DL, et al: Prevention of chemical carcinogenesis by Vitamin A and its synthetic analogs (retinoids). Fed Proc 1976;35:1332–1338.
24. Bollag W: Prophylaxis of chemically induced benign and malignant epithelial tumors by Vitamin A acid (retinoic acid). Eur J Cancer 1972;8:689–693.
25. Sporn MB, Dunlop NM, Newton DL, et al: Relationships between structure and activity of retinoids. Nature 1976;263:110–113.
26. Haddox MK, Russell DH: Cell cycle-specific locus of vitamin A inhibition of growth. Cancer Res 1979;39:2476–2480.

27. Lotan R: Effects of vitamin A and its analogs (retinoids) on normal and neoplastic cells. Biochim Biophys Acta 1980;605:33–91.
28. Lotan R, Nicolson GL: Heterogeneity in growth inhibition by beta-trans-retinoic acid of metastatic B16 melanoma clones and in vivo-selected cell variant lines. Cancer Res 1979;39:4767–4771.
29. Lotan R, Lotan D: Stimulation of melanogenesis in a human melanoma cell line by retinoids. Cancer Res 1980;40:3345–3350.
30. Meyskens FL Jr, Fuller BB: Characterization of the effects of different retinoids on the growth and differentiation of a human melanoma cell lines and selected subclones. Cancer Res 1980;40:2194–2196.
31. Bollag W, Matter A: From vitamin A to retinoids in experimental and clinical oncology: achievements, failures and outlook. Ann NY Acad Sci 1981;359:9–23.
32. Saffiotti U, Montesano R, Sellakumar AR, et al: Experimental cancer of the lung: inhibition by vitamin A of the induction of tracheobronchial squamous metaplasia and squamous cell tumors. Cancer 1967;20:857–864.
33. Lasnitski I: The influence of a hypervitaminosis on the effect of 20-methylcholanthrene on mouse prostate glands grown in vitro. Brit J Cancer 1955;9:434–441.
34. Bollag W, Hartman HR: Prevention and therapy of cancer with retinoids in animals and man, in Sporn MB (ed): Advances and Prospects in Clinical Epidemiology and Laboratory Oncology Cancer Surgery, Vol 2. Oxford: Oxford University Press, 1983, pp 293–314.
35. Sporn MB, Roberts AB: Role of retinoids in differentiation and carcinogenesis. Cancer Res 1983;43:3034–3040.
36. Moon RC, Itri LM: Retinoids and cancer, in Sporn MB, Roberts AB, Goodman DS (eds): The Retinoids, New York: Academic Press, 1984, pp 327–371.
37. Cowan JD, Von Hoff DD, Dinesman A, et al: Use of a human tumor cloning system to screen retinoids for antineoplastic activity. Cancer 1983;51:92–96.
38. Lotan D, Sacks P, Lotan R, et al: Differential effects of retinoic acid on the growth of two human head and neck squamous cell carcinoma (HHSCC) lines. Amer Assn Cancer Res (Abstr) 1986;27:410.
39. McCormick DL, Sowell ZL, Thompson CA, et al: Inhibition by retinoid and ovariectomy of additional primary malignancies in rats following surgical removal of the first mammary cancer. Cancer 1983;51:594–599.
40. Roberts AB, Sporn MB: Cellular biology and biochemistry of the retinoids, in Sporn MB, Roberts AB, Goodman DS (eds): The Retinoids, Vol 2, New York: Academic Press, 1984, pp 209–286.
41. Verma AK, Boutwell RK: Vitamin A acid (retinoic acid), a potent inhibitor of 12-O-tetradecanoylphorbol-13-acetate-induced ornithine decarboxylase activity in mouse epidermis. Cancer Res 1977;37:2196–2201.
42. Verma AK, Rice HM, Shapas BG, et al: Inhibition of 12-0-tetradecanoylphorbol-13-acetate-induced ornithine decarboxylase activity in mouse epidermis by vitamin A analogs (retinoids). Cancer Res 1978;38:793–801.
43. Verma AK, Shapas BG, Rice HM, et al: Correlation of the inhibition by retinoids of tumor promoter-induced mouse epidermal ornithine decarboxylase activity and of skin tumor promotion. Cancer Res 1979;39:419–425.
44. Ong DE, Goodwin WJ, Jesse RH, et al: Presence of cellular retinol and retinoic acid-binding proteins in epidermoid carcinoma of the oral cavity and oropharynx. Cancer 1982;49:1409–1412.
45. Bichler E, Daxenbichler G: Retinoic acid-binding protein in human squamous cell carcinomas of the ORL region. Cancer 1982;49:619–622.

46. Gates RE, Rees RS: Altered vitamin A-binding proteins in carcinoma of the head and neck. Cancer 1985;56:2598–2604.

47. Niles RM, Logue MP: Retinoic acid increases cyclic AMP-dependent protein kinase activity in B16-F1 mouse melanoma cells. (Abstr) Proc Am Assoc Cancer Res 1979;20:166.

48. Chytil F, Ong DE: Cellular retinol-binding proteins, in Sporn MB, Roberts AB, Goodman DS (eds): The Retinoids, Vol 2, New York: Academic Press, 1984, pp 89–123.

49. Lotan R, Neumann G, Deutsch V: Identification and characterization of specific changes induced by retinoic acid in cell surface glycoconjugates of S91 murine melanoma cells. Cancer Res 1983;43:303–312.

50. Eccles SA, Alexander P: Immunologically mediated restraint of latent tumor metastases. Nature 1975;257:52–53.

51. Davey GC, Currie GA, Alexander P: Immunity as the predominant factor determining metastasis by murine lymphomas. Brit J Cancer 1979;40:590–596.

52. Alexander P, Eccles SA: Host factors in metastases: immunostimulatory actions of retinoids. Transplant Proc 1984;16:486–488.

53. Bollag W: Prophylaxis of chemically induced epithelial tumors with an aromatic retinoic acid analog (RO 10–9359) Eur J Cancer 1975;11:721–724.

54. Ryssel HJ, Brunner KW, Bollag W: Die peroral anwendung von vitamin-A-saure bei leukoplakien, hyperkeratosen und plattenepithelkarzinomen: ergebnisse und vertralichkeit. Schweiz Med Wochenschr 1971;101:1027–1030.

55. Meyskens FL Jr, Gilmartin E, Alberts DS, et al: Activity of isotretinoin against squamous cell cancers and preneoplastic lesions. Cancer Treat Rep 1982;66:1315–1319.

56. Koch H: Biochemical treatment of precancerous oral lesions: the effectiveness of various analogs of retinoic acid. J Maxillofac Surg 1978;6:59–63.

57. Koch HF: Effect of retinoids on precancerous lesions of oral mucosa, in Orfanos CE (ed): Retinoids, Berlin: Springer-Verlag, 1981, pp 307–312.

58. Shah JP, Strong EW, DeCosse JJ, et al: Effect of retinoids on oral leukoplakia. Am J Surg 1983;146:466–470.

59. Hong WK, Itri L, Endicott J, et al: 13-cis-retinoic acid in the treatment of oral leukoplakia. N Engl J Med 1986;315:1501–1505.

60. Hong WK, Bromer R: Chemotherapy in head and neck cancer. N Engl J Med 1983;308:75–79.

61. Kun LE, Toohill RJ, Holoye PY, et al: A randomized study of adjuvant chemotherapy for cancer of the upper aerodigestive tract. Int J Radiat Oncol Biol Phys 1986;12:173–178.

62. Wald N, Idle M, Boreham J, et al: Low serum vitamin A and subsequent risk of cancer: preliminary results of a prospective study. Lancet 1980;2:812–815.

63. Kark JD, Smith AH, Switzer BR: Serum vitamin A (retinol) and cancer incidence in Evans County, Georgia. JNCI 1981;66:7–16.

64. Willett WC, Polk BF, Underwood BA, et al: Relation of serum vitamin A and E and carotenoids to the risk of cancer. N Engl J Med 1984;310:430–434.

# CHAPTER 18

# The Radiobiology of Head and Neck Cancer

*Stephen A. Sapareto, PhD*

Many of the currently accepted standards in the radiotherapy of head and neck malignancies, like those for most other tumor sites, have developed from the empirical study of clinical results during the last 50 years. It has only been in the last few decades that biological techniques have developed to the point where basic research studies have contributed to our understanding of the radiobiological factors involved in the successful treatment of these malignancies. Major advances in biological techniques, such as the in vitro growth and clonogenic assay of cells and the ability to study cells as a synchronous cohort throughout the cell cycle,[1,2] have led to a number of ideas for the improvement of radiation therapy.

While our current knowledge of radiobiology has not definitively identified any single cause for radiotherapy failure, it has identified a number of important factors that are most likely to affect the success or failure of radiation treatment of solid tumors. These have come to be known as the 4 R's of radiobiology.[3] They represent the four major factors after a radiation treatment which are most likely to determine the effectiveness of subsequent treatments. They are: *repopulation* by division and regrowth of cells, *redistribution* of cells throughout the cell cycle, *repair* of sublethal and potentially lethal radiation damage, and *reoxygenation* of cells.

The identification of these factors has led to the development of several strategies currently under investigation to improve radiation therapy. These strategies include: (1) increased oxygenation of tumors (e.g., using hyperbaric oxygen and blood transfusions); (2) high LET radiations (e.g., using neutrons, pions, or heavy ions); (3) hyperfractionation of radiation treatment; (4) radiosensitizers and protectors; and (5) radiation combined with hyperthermia (see other chapters in this book and reference no. 4 for reviews of these strategies). By far, the most common factor that is targeted by these strategies is the oxygenation of tumor cells. This is the single factor that is most likely to be consistently different between normal tissues and those tumor cells believed to cause local failure of radiotherapy.[5]

## TUMOR OXYGENATION

The importance of oxygen concentration in radiation sensitivity was first noted in the early part of this century by several investigators using plant and parasite biological systems.[6,7] These and many subsequent studies have shown that the lack of oxygen (hypoxia) causes a significant increase in cellular resistance to radiation-induced damage. This change in radiosensitivity caused by hypoxia occurs at extremely low partial pressures of oxygen —from 0 to 30 mm Hg.[8] This phenomenon is quantitatively expressed by the oxygen enhancement ratio (OER), that is, the ratio of the doses in the absence and presence of oxygen required to achieve a given level of survival. OER values range from 1.0 (no effect) for densely ionizing or high linear energy transfer (LET) radiation to over 2.5 for sparsely ionizing or low LET radiation; intermediate LET radiations, such as energetic neutrons, show intermediate values of OER (Fig. 18.1).

In 1955, Thomlinson and Gray postulated from histologic evidence that, due to inadequate vascularization, solid tumors were likely to contain poorly oxygenated or hypoxic cells that would be resistant to radiation exposure.[10] Subsequently, in 1963, Powers and Tolmach first demonstrated the presence of hypoxic cells which were resistant to radiation treatment in a murine solid tumor (Fig. 18.2).[11] Based upon this original work, tumors have been thought to consist of three cellular compartments (Fig. 18.3): cells with adequate nutrient and oxygen supply (adjacent to blood vessels), cells that are dead because they have suffered long periods of inadequate oxygen and nutrient levels, and cells that are viable but are radiobiologically hypoxic — either because of intervening cells that utilize most of the available oxygen or because of vascular occlusion from various causes. This hypoxic compartment of a tumor is a transient state, since continuous exposure to radiobiologically hypoxic levels of oxygen eventually leads to cell death. The ability of cells to survive under prolonged periods of hypoxia have been reported to range from several hours to several days (Fig. 18.4).

Numerous attempts have been made to determine the proportion of radiobiologically hypoxic cells in a number of different tumors (Table 18.1). The results demonstrate a considerable amount of variability even within similar tumor types. With the exception of determinations on the human tumors noted in the table, three basic techniques have been used to estimate

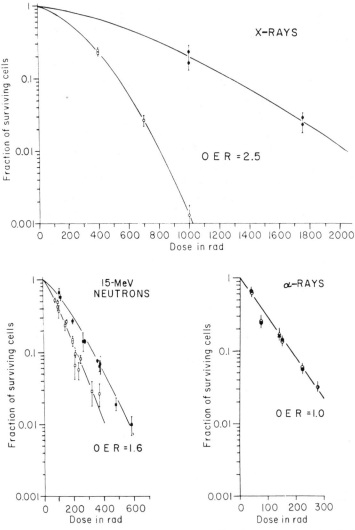

**FIGURE 18.1** Survival curves illustrating the oxygen effect for three types of radiation with different LET's. (Reproduced with permission from reference 9; see 9 for original references).

hypoxia in tumors. These are the paired survival curve assay, the clamped tumor control dose (TCD$_{50}$) assay, and the clamped tumor growth delay assay. Moulder and Rockwell have recently published a comprehensive review providing a description of these techniques and a critical evaluation of the utility and problems of each.[15] In compiling the published data on tumor hypoxia determinations, they have identified a number of inconsistencies. For example, comparable determinations of hypoxic fractions using different techniques for several rodent tumors from their review are shown in Table 18.2. Despite the fact that these are comparisons performed within the same laboratory or, in some cases, in different laboratories but with tumors for which there was no evidence of significant alteration in any other tumor characteristic, in general, the data yield imcompatable results. For example, while clamped $TCD_{50}$ values are generally lower than paired sur-

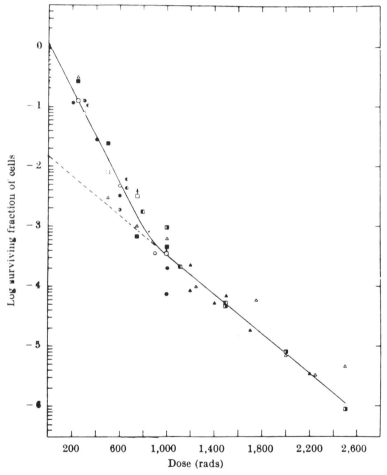

**FIGURE 18.2** Survival as a function of radiation dose for cells irradiated in vivo in the 6C3HED murine lymphosarcoma demonstrating the presence of approximately 1.5% hypoxic cells. (Reproduced with permission from reference 11).

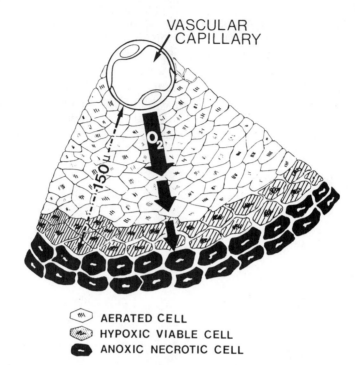

**FIGURE 18.3** Illustration of three radiobiologically important cellular compartments of tumors. (Reproduced with permission from reference 12).

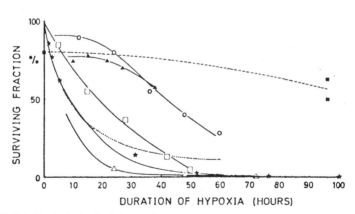

**FIGURE 18.4** Survival of cells during prolonged hypoxia as reported by several investigators. (Reproduced with permission from reference 13; see 13 for original references.)

**TABLE 18.1** Proportion of Hypoxic Cells in Tumours

| Tumors in Rats and Mice (%) | | | |
|---|---|---|---|
| CBA Sarcoma F | >50 | Adenocarcinoma MTG-B | 21 |
| Gardner lymphosa | 1 | Sq. Carcinoma D | 18 |
| C3H Sarcoma KHT | 14 | C3H mammary Ca | 7 |
| Rhabdomyosa BA 1112 | 15 | Carcinoma KHJJ | 19 |
| Osteosarcoma C22LR | 14 | C3H mammary (females) | 1 |
| | | CA          (males) | 17 |
| Fibrosarcoma RIB5 | 17 | Squamous Ca. G (intraderm.) | <1 |
| Fibrosarcoma KHT | 12 | (subcut.) | >46 |
| Sarcoma EMT6 | 35 | Carcinoma DC | 10–30 |
| CBA sarcoma F (in situ) | <10 | C3H mammary Ca (small) | 0.2 |
| (excised) | 50 | (large) | >20 |
| Sarcoma S | <0.01 | WHT anaplastic (in situ) | >80 |
| Sarcoma S (fast) | 1–30 | MT          (excised) | 5 |
| Sarcoma FA | 30–70 | Sarcoma RH | 2–25 |
| Sarcoma BS 2b | 5–25 | Carcinoma NT | 7–18 |
| Human: tumor nodules[a] | 12–20 | | |
| Human: tumor nodules[a] | 1–80 | | |

[a]Determined from misonidazole studies, see reference 14.
Reproduced with permission from reference 5.

vival curve values for the BA1112 rat tumor, the opposite is seen for the MT mouse tumor. Although Moulder and Rockwell discuss a number of possible explanations for these and other discrepancies, both between techniques and within a given technique, no satisfactory explanation could be found and their conclusion is that some of the assumptions of the various techniques may not be valid under certain conditions. Another possible explanation for these inconsistencies is that individual tumor variability prevents any such comparison. Certainly, in light of the wide confidence limit values shown in Table 18.2, the validity of pooling measurements for any tumor system and comparing averages is highly questionable. In order to investigate this hypothesis, methods must be found which will allow comparative studies in individual tumors.

Other methods with the potential to measure hypoxic fraction in individual tumors have been reported. The use of a radioactive labelled nitroheterocyclic compound ($^3$H or $^{14}$C-misonidazole) to identify hypoxic cells has been demonstrated by Chapman, et al.[16] Using relatively low, nontoxic levels of $^{14}$C-misonidazole, they have been able to visualize and quantitatively estimate the hypoxic areas of EMT6 tumor sections by autoradiography (Figure 18.5). In a somewhat analogous manner, Olive has demonstrated the use of fluorescent nitroheterocyclic compounds to identify

**TABLE 18.2** A Summary of Published Values for the Hypoxic Fraction of Rodent Tumors Assayed by Different Methods.[a]

| Tumor System | Hypoxic Fraction by Assay[b,c] | | | |
|---|---|---|---|---|
| | PS (%) | TC (%) | GD[d] (%) | GD[e] (%) |
| RIB5C (rat) | 13 (7.4–24)% | — | 0.13 (0.02–1.0)% | 0.05 (0–0.24)% |
| EMT6 (mouse) | 5.4 (3.6–7.9)% | — | 69 (51–81)% | 23 (11–42)% |
| BA1112 (rat) | 21 (15–29)% | 1.1 (0.37–2.7)% | 1.6 (0.4–7.4)% | 9.9 (5.5–19)% |
| | 17 (9.3–30)% | 2.1 (0.41–11)% | | |
| | 40 (21–76)% | 11 (4.1–45)% | | |
| | | 0.38 (0.05–2.6)% | | |
| | | 6.1 (1.1–43)% | | |
| MT (mouse) | 6.5 (4.1–10)% | >51 | | |

[a]See reference 15 for individual references.
[b]PS: paired survival assay, TC: clamped $TCD_{50}$ assay, GD: clamped tumor growth delay assay.
[c]Values in each column represent different measurements for the same tumors.
[d]Calculated hypoxic fraction from growth delay in a manner similar to paired survival curves assay.
[e]Calculated hypoxic fraction from growth delay in a manner similar to $TCD_{50}$ assay.

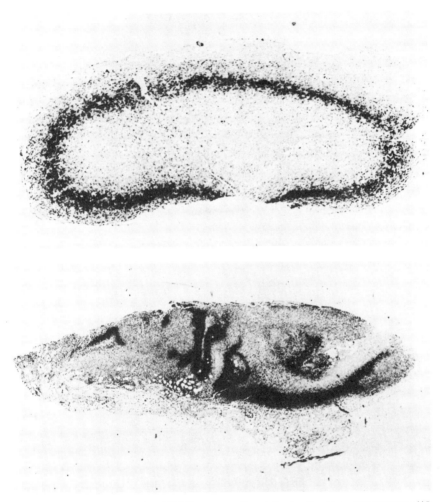

**FIGURE 18.5** Autoradiographs of EMT6 tumor sections following three hour exposures to $^{14}$C labelled misonidazole (50 $\mu$M). Two different size tumors are shown: 1.5 $\times$ 0.5 mm (top) and 5.0 $\times$ 2.0 mm (bottom). (Reproduced with permission from reference 16)

hypoxic cells by spectrofluorometry or flow cytometry.[17] Both of these techniques are applicable to the determination of hypoxic fraction in individual tumors and can be used in human studies,[18] however, since they require tissue biopsy, they are subject to nonrepresentative sampling problems as well as to limited repeatability preventing their use to monitor dynamic changes.

Understanding the dynamic changes in hypoxic fraction of individual tumors is essential to determine the importance of reoxygenation of tumors on the success or failure of radiotherapy. Hypoxic cells are believed to become important in clinical failure when they are reoxygenated by the death of intervening well-oxygenated cells (making more oxygen available) following radiotherapy. In addition, other mechanisms such as reversal of transient vascular occlusion might lead to the reoxygenation of cells that were radioresistant at the time of radiation due to hypoxia and thus were able to survive an initial treatment. To date, studies have demonstrated marked variability of tumor reoxygenation both between and within histological categories of model animal tumor systems (Fig. 18.6). This variability has been attributed to a number of factors, including the rates of cell growth and loss and the architecture and perfusion characteristics of the tumor.[13,15,19] Although not shown in Figure 18.6, there are large confidence limits associated with data points for these measurements.[14,20] Clearly, the distribution of cells between oxygenated and hypoxic states is a dynamic balance of a number of cellular and physiological factors that appear to vary tremendously between individual tumors.

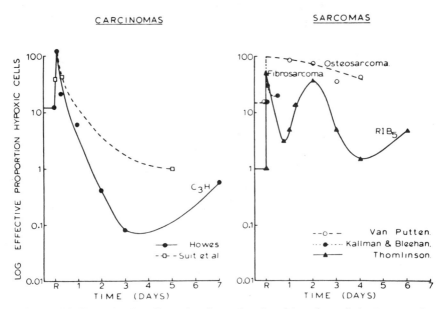

**FIGURE 18.6** The proportion of hypoxic cells as a function of time after radiation treatment for published studies of animal model tumors categorized as carcinomas or sarcomas. (Reproduced with permission from reference 5; see reference 5 for original references)

## DETERMINATION OF TUMOR PHYSIOLOGY

Early investigators[10,21] categorized the histology of tumors into three generally defined types: those that are peripherally vascularized with penetrating vessels, those peripherally vascularized with few penetrating vessels, and those with central or more evenly distributed vascularization (Fig. 18.7). While these initial categorizations of a number of model tumor systems have provided much of our current understanding of the importance of tumor environment in radiotherapy, the extrapolation of this knowledge from in vivo animal model systems to new clinical protocols, to date, has not been as successful as hoped.[5,22] This failure, in part, may be due to the possibility that individual tumor variability of the factors important to successful radiotherapy completely overshadows any possibility of simple categorization. This possibility emphasizes the importance of the conclusion by Fowler that methods to identify patients having tumors with poor reoxygenation characteristics will be essential to fairly judge new therapeutic strategies.[22] Clearly, the ability to determine the distribution of cells within various environments in individual tumors and the dynamic changes that alter this composition with time are essential to address this question.

The presence of poorly oxygenated cells in tumors is dependent on several physiological factors that include: blood flow to the tumor, oxygen and nutrient content in the blood, perfusion of oxygen and nutrients throughout the tumor, and metabolic rates of cells within the tumor. Each of these factors is interdependent upon the others. In order to better understand the tumor environment and the dynamic changes that occur, it is essential to study each of these physiological factors.

Surface coil NMR (SC-NMR) is a recently developed technique that provides a nondestructive, noninvasive in vivo measure of several of these important physiological characteristics.[23] Chemical shift spectra of $^{31}$P provide a quantitative measure of phosphorus-containing metabolites that are intimately involved in energy metabolism (e.g., phosphocreatine [PCr], nucleoside triphosphates [NTP] and inorganic phosphate [$P_i$]) and pH ($pH_{NMR}$). Pioneering work in the application of SC-NMR spectroscopy in oncology has focused on observation of the $^{31}$P nuclide. The results of $^{31}$P SC-NMR studies of rodent and human tumors suggest that $^{31}$P SC-NMR provides a sensitive monitor of tumor metabolism and therapeutic response.[16]

To illustrate the usefulness of $^{31}$P SC-NMR, the effects of hyperglycemia on the $pH_{NMR}$ of subcutaneous murine RIF-1 tumors is shown in Figure 18.8. Following intraperitoneal injection of an aqueous glucose solution (~7.5 g/kg dose), the $pH_{NMR}$ decreased from an initial pH value of about 7.0 to about 6.6. In addition, the PCr concentration decreased by ~50% and the

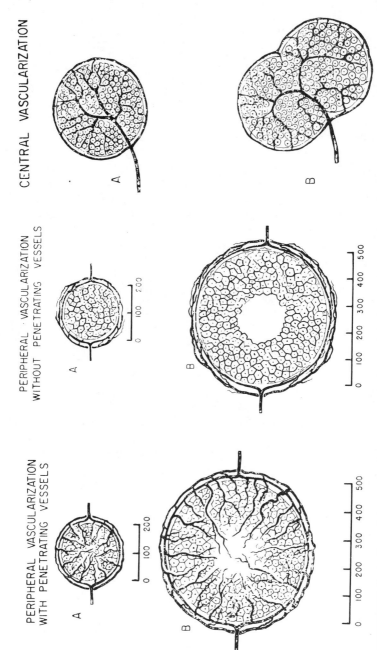

**FIGURE 18.7** Illustrations of three general categories of tumor vascularization based on histological studies. (Reproduced with permission from reference 21.)

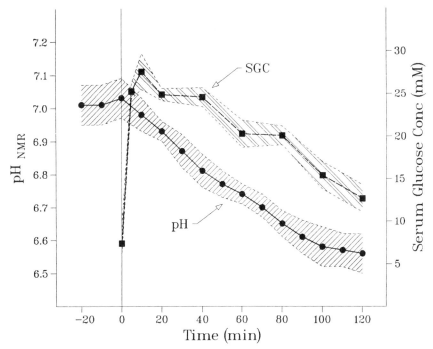

**FIGURE 18.8** Average tumor pH (n = 9) and average serum glucose concentration (n = 2-4), of RIF-1 tumor transplanted in C3H/Anf mice, after bolus i.p. injection of 7.5 g glucose/Kg body weight at time 0 min. Circles correspond to average $pH_{NMR}$, squares correspond to average SGC (m*M*). The shaded regions represent ± SE. The SGC curve was determined using mice not employed for other experiments. (Reproduced with permission from reference 26)

NTP concentration remained relatively constant. No significant changes were observed in normal murine leg muscle following similar glucose injection. These results are consistent with previously reported studies using pH microelectrodes.[23] While the exact mechanism for this tumor selective effect has not been proven, it is likely that two important factors in this phenomenon are glucose-induced alteration of tumor blood flow and cellular metabolism.

An important observation from these studies of the RIF-1 tumor is that there is a great deal of variability in the relative levels of PCr, NTP and inorganic phosphate ($P_i$) as well as $pH_{NMR}$ even when the tumors are roughly the same size and age (Figure 18.9). While these studies have shown that the $pH_{NMR}$ and the $P_i$ : NTP ratio are inversely correlated, indicating the acidification of ischemic tissue, no correlation between tumor size and any of the NMR observations is seen (Fig. 18.10).

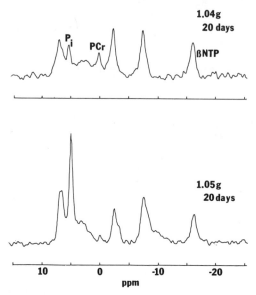

**FIGURE 18.9** 81 MHz NMR spectrum of two in vivo RIF-1 tumors transplanted in C3H/Anf mice. The size and age of tumors are indicated to the right. Both tumors began from $5 \times 10^5$ cell subcutaneous inocula from the same tumor on the same day. $pH_{NMR}$ is 7.16 and 6.91 for the top and bottom tumor, respectively. (Redrawn from reference 27)

The relationship of these measurements to other tumor physiological characteristics provides strong support for their validity and further emphasis for individual tumor variability. This is well illustrated in combined studies of $^{31}P$ NMR spectra and perfusion measurements taken on the same RIF-1 tumors.[27] These studies have utilized a unique method to measure tumor perfusion noninvasively by high energy photon activation of oxygen in situ followed by the detecton of $^{15}O$ washout from positron emission.[28] In addition to measuring the volume-averaged perfusion rate of tumors, this is the only blood flow measurement technique with the ability to quantify the well-perfused fraction of the tumor (Fig. 18.11).

The results of these studies indicate that the well-perfused fraction of the tumor correlates well with the $pH_{NMR}$ and with the PCr : NTP ratio (Fig. 18.12), and correlates inversely with the $P_i$ : NTP ratio. Neither the perfusion rate in the well-perfused fraction nor the volume-averaged perfusion rate correlate with any of the $^{31}P$ NMR observables. As might be expected, these correlations suggest a greater population of cells in an ischemic environment (as indicated by low $pH_{NMR}$ and high $P_i$ : NTP ratio) for tumors which have a greater portion of their volume poorly-perfused.

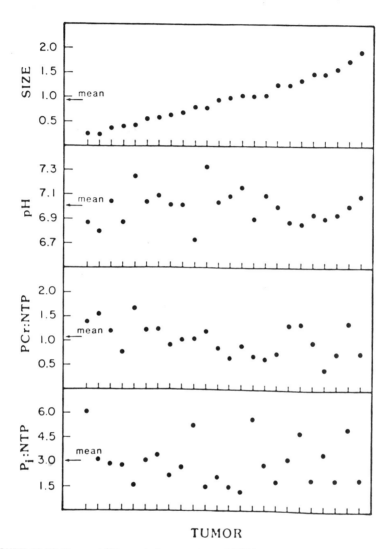

**FIGURE 18.10** Size and $^{31}$P spectral parameters of RIF-1 tumors transplanted in C3H/Anf mice. Size in cm$^3$; pH$_{NMR}$; PCr : NTP peak height ratio; P$_i$ : NTP peak height ratio. Average values are indicated by arrows on the ordinate of each plot. Tumors have been ordered as a function of increasing size.

## DETERMINATION OF TISSUE AND CELLULAR COMPARTMENTS

Although intuitively one would expect the poorly-perfused fraction of a tumor as determined by $^{15}O$ washout and the $^{31}P$ NMR indicators of ischemia to correlate with the hypoxic fraction, these relationships have not yet been established. The values of the $P_i : NTP$ ratio and the $pH_{NMR}$ are dependent on the concentration and relaxation time of $P_i$, and the pH in various environments or compartments within the tissue. These factors are, in turn, dependent on the relative volumes of intracellular, interstitial, and vascular spaces and the volume distribution of tumor cell environments (i.e., normoxic, hypoxic, and necrotic).

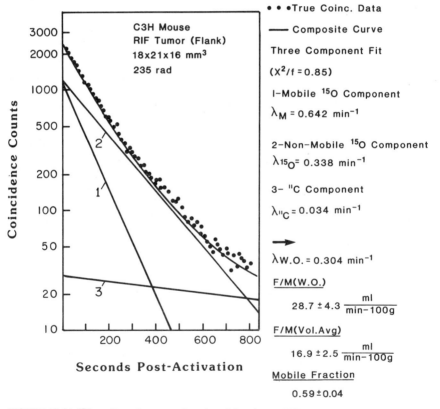

**FIGURE 18.11** $^{15}O$ positron decay as a function of time from a RIF-1 tumor activated in situ with 30 Mev photons. The labeled lines represent the three components of the least squares fit for (1) mobile $^{15}O$, (2) non-mobile $^{15}O$, (3) and $^{11}C$. Mobile fraction = 0.59 and perfusion rate (well-perfused) = 28.7 ± 4.3 ml/min/100 g. (Reproduced with permission from reference 29)

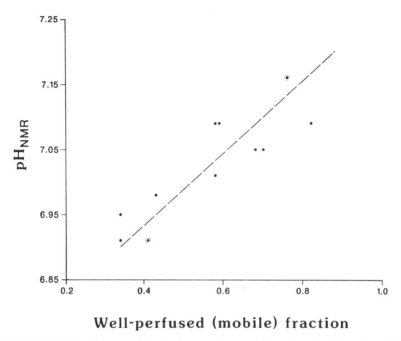

**Well-perfused (mobile) fraction**

**FIGURE 18.12** Plot of the correlation between $pH_{NMR}$ and the well-perfused fraction of RIF-1 murine tumors transplanted in C3H/Anf mice. The line indicates the results of least squares stepwise linear regression analysis of the data represented by the solid circles. The two data points that are encircled correspond to the tumors for which the $^{31}P$ NMR spectra are shown in Figure 18.8. (Reproduced with permission from reference 27)

In tumors, the distribution of intracellular, interstitial, and vascular spaces is varied and inhomogeneous due to the abnormal and inadequate vascular architecture.[10,21] The variability in vascular space of tumors has been described by Jain and is summarized in Table 18.3.[19] As can be seen, the vascular space has been reported to vary from 0.4 to 27.5%. Along with the variation in vascular space, the distribution of intracellular and interstitial space also varies between tumors (Fig. 18.13). With the exception that tumors, in general, seem to have less vascular and more interstitital space than normal liver tissue, this data is of limited usefulness in the interpretation of the physiological factors discussed above. Although not directly addressed by either Gullino or Jain, this may again be due to the possibility that individual tumor variability masks important conclusions.[19,30] Clearly, an examination of these factors in individual tumors will aid in the correct interpretation of in vivo $^{31}P$ NMR measurements.

**TABLE 18.3** Summary of Published Measurements of Vascular Space of Tumors

| Tumor | Weight Range (gm) | Vascular Space (%) |
|---|---|---|
| Walker (256) carcinoma | 3.5–13.0 | 10.6 |
| Walker (256) carcinoma | 1.0–4.0 | 4.0 |
| Mammary carcinoma | 0.1–2.4 | 16.0 |
| Mammary carcinoma | 0.1–2.4 | 15.0–18.0 |
| Fibrosarcoma 4956 | 5.6–14.8 | 1.0 |
| Hepatoma 5123 | 1.0–12.9 | 4.5 |
| Hepatoma 3683 | 1.4–10.5 | 5.0 |
| Novikoff hepatoma | 1.8–6.9 | 4.5 |
| Hepatoma LC | 7.0–32.1 | 8.0 |
| Hepatoma HC | 5.0–9.4 | 12.4 |
| Hepatoma A | 2.7–4.1 | 5.8 |
| Hepatoma S | 2.3–4.9 | 8.1 |
| Rat Liver | 7.8–8.5 | 18.5 |
| Canine lymphosarcoma | — | 14–27.5 |
| DS carcinosarcoma | 3.0–11.0 | 0.4–4.0 |

LC = low catalase; HC = high catalase; A = ascites form; S = solid subcutaneous form.
See reference 19 for individual references.

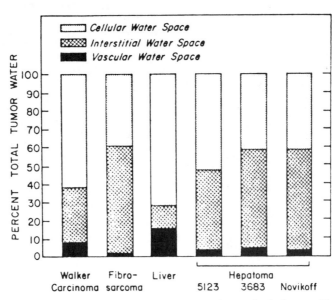

**FIGURE 18.13** The relative proportions of water spaces in neoplastic tissues. (Reproduced with permission from reference 30)

## SUMMARY

Of the radiobiological factors that are most likely to affect the success or failure of radiation treatment of solid tumors, the oxygen availability both before and during radiotherapy is one of the most likely to affect success or failure of radiotherapy and, thus, is the most common factor targeted by new therapeutic strategies. The radioresistant hypoxic fraction of a tumor is a population of cells in which dynamic changes occur due to a number of cellular and physiological factors including growth rate, blood flow and metabolism. Past efforts to understand these factors have been hampered by the tremendous variability of individual tumors and the use of destructive techniques that prevent correlation of the measurement of these factors on individual tumors. The development of new techniques that allow the non-invasive monitoring of physiological processes so that dynamic temporal changes may be studied on individual tumors will pave the way for a more fundamental understanding of the role of these important radiobiological factors in successful clinical radiotherapy.

## REFERENCES

1. Puck TT, Marcus PI: Action of x-rays on mammalian cells. J Exp Med 1956;103:653–666.
2. Terasima R, Tolmach LJ: X-ray sensitivity and DNA synthesis in synchronous populations of HeLa cells. Science 1963;140:490–492.
3. Withers HR: The 4 R's of Radiotherapy, in Lett J, Adler H (eds): Advances in Radiation Biology, New York: Academic Press, 1975;5:341–371.
4. Steel GG, Adams GE, Peckham MJ, (eds): The Biological Basis of Radiotherapy. New York: Elsevier, 1983.
5. Denekamp J: Does physiological hypoxia matter in cancer therapy?, in Steel GG, Adams GE, Peckham MJ (eds): The Biological Basis of Radiotherapy. New York: Elsevier, 1983, pp 139–155.
6. Holthusen H: Beitrage sur biologie der strahlenwirkung, Pfluger's Archiv fur die Gesamte Physiologie. 1921;187:1–24.
7. Petri E: Zur Keuntnis der Bedingungen der biologischen Wirkung der Roentgenstralen. Biochem. Zeitschr. 1923;135:353.
8. Koch CJ: Oxygen effects in radiobiology, in Bicher HI, Bruley DF (eds): Hyperthermia. Advances in Experimental Medicine and Biology. New York: Plenum Press, 1982;157:123–144.
9. Hall E: Radiobiology for the Radiologist, 2nd ed. Hagerstown: Harper and Row: 1978, p 83.
10. Thomlinson RH, Gray LH: The histological structure of some human lung cancers and the possible implications for radiotherapy. Brit J Cancer 1955;9:539–549.
11. Powers WE, Tolmach LJ: A multicomponent x ray survival curve for mouse lymphosarcoma cells irradiated in vivo. Nature 1963;197:710–711.
12. Hall E: Radiobiology for the Radiologist, 2nd ed. Hagerstown: Harper and Row p 90.

13. Born R, Hug O, Trott KR: The effect of prolonged hypoxia on growth and viability of Chinese hamster cells. Int J Radiat Oncol Biol Phys 1976;1:687–697.
14. Denekamp J, Fowler JF, Dische S: The proportion of hypoxic cells in a human tumor. Int J Radiat Oncol Biol Phys 1977;2:1227–1228.
15. Moulder JE, Rockwell S: Hypoxic fractions of solid tumors: Experimental techniques, methods of analysis, and a survey of existing data. Int J Radiat Oncol Biol Phys 1984;10:695–712.
16. Chapman JD, Franko AJ, Sharplin J: A marker for hypoxic cells in tumors with potential clinical applicability. Brit J Cancer 1981;43:546–550.
17. Olive PL, Durand RE: Fluorescent nitroheterocycles for identifying hypoxic cells. Cancer Res 1983;43:3276–3280.
18. Urtasun R, Chapman JD, Franko AJ, Koch CJ: Binding of tritiated (3-H) misonidazole to solid tumors as a measure of tumor hypoxia. Int J Radiat Oncol Biol Phys (in press), 1986.
19. Jain RK: Mass transport in tumors, in Advances in Transport Processes 1983;3:205–239.
20. Dorie MJ, Kallman RF: Reoxygenation in the RIF-1 tumor. Int J Radiat Oncol Biol Phys (in press), 1986.
21. Rubin P, Cassaret G: Microcirculation of tumors. Part I: anatomy, function and necrosis. Clin Radiol 1966;17:220–229.
22. Fowler JF: Rationales for high linear energy transfer radiotherapy, in Steel GG, Adams GE, Peckham MJ (eds): The Biological Basis of Radiotherapy. New York: Elsevier, 1983, pp 261–268.
23. Jahde E, Rajewsky MF: Tumor selective modification of cellular microenvironment in vivo. Cancer Res 1982;42:1498–1512.
24. Ackerman JJH, Grove TH, Wong GG, et al: Mapping of metabolites in whole animals by $^{31}$P NMR using surface coils. Nature 1980;283:167–170.
25. Ng TC, Evanochko WT, Hiramoto RN, et al: $^{31}$P NMR spectroscopy of in vivo tumors. J Magn Reson 1982;49:271–286.
26. Evelhoch JL, Sapareto SA, Jick DEL, Ackerman JJH: In vivo metabolic effects of hyperglycemia in murine radiation-induced fibrosarcoma: A $^{31}$P NMR investigation. Proc Natl Acad Sci USA 1984;81:6496–6500.
27. Evelhoch JL, Sapareto SA, Nussbaum GH, Ackerman JJH: Correlations between $^{31}$P NMR spectroscopy and $^{15}$O perfusion measurements in RIF-1 murine tumor in vivo. Radiat Res 1986;106:122–131.
28. Ten Haken RK, Nussbaum GH, Emami B, Hughes WL: Photon-activation $^{15}$O decay studies of tumor blood flow. Med Phys 1981;8:324–336.
29. Nussbaum GH, Purdy JA, Granda CO, et al: Use of the Clinac-35 for tissue activation in noninvasive measurement of capillary blood flow. Med Phys 1983;10:487–490.
30. Gullino PM: Extracellular compartments of solid tumors, in: Becker F, (ed): Cancer: A Comprehensive Treatise. New York: Plenum Press, 1975, pp 327–350.

# CHAPTER 19

# Radiosensitizers
# and Radioprotectors

*Gisele Sarosy, MD and*
*Frederick A. Valeriote, PhD*

## INTRODUCTION

Since the discovery of the usefulness of ionizing radiation in cancer therapy, attempts have been made not only to understand the mechanism of its lethal effect at both the biochemical and cellular levels, but also to find ways to modify the action in order to increase therapeutic efficacy in the tumor-bearing host. As shown in Figure 19.1, ionizing radiation not only interacts directly with biological macromolecules, with DNA certainly being the central target, but also interacts with the water molecules in the cell generating a variety of free radicals. These radicals can diffuse to the site of DNA and cause a variety of reactions to produce damage. Subsequently, the damage produced on the DNA can be repaired, either chemically or enzymatically, with the consequent survival of the cell or fixed by agents such as $O_2$ (and radiation sensitizers) with the consequent death of the cell.

One could modify the effect of radiation at either the level of radical formation or DNA damage; for example, modifying the concentration of the radicals by interposing agents that react with them, or modifying the DNA damage itself. Radiosensitizers and radioprotectors can affect both of the sites. Sensitizers could decrease the level of thiol ($-SH$) groups in the cell, inhibit repair (enzymes) of DNA, or interact with the damaged DNA so that the damage becomes irreversible (fixed). Protectors could increase the level of thiols which then interact with either the radicals and ions formed or the damaged DNA site, or decrease the level of agents such as oxygen that fix the DNA damage.

A new element that has recently been introduced into this field of study

**267**

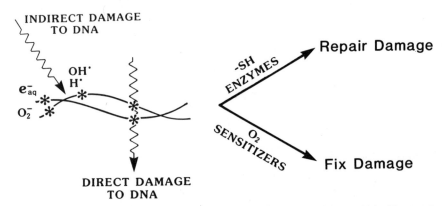

**FIGURE 19.1** Modes of interaction of radiation with DNA and the pathways which either repair or fix the damage.

is the interactions noted by both of these classes of compounds with chemotherapeutic agents, and in particular, with the alkylating agents. Because of the importance of alkylating agents such as cisplatin in the treatment of head and neck cancer, this area of study will also be discussed here.

## RADIOSENSITIZERS

There are many physical and chemical factors that can increase the sensitivity of a cell population to radiation and hence be termed radiation sensitizers.[1] Such sensitizers include hyperbaric oxygen (or even low concentrations in the case of hypoxic cells), oxygen-carrying emulsified perfluorochemicals, halogenated pyrimidines such as 5-fluorouracil, inhibitors of potentially lethal damage such as the DNA repair inhibitor caffeine, hyperthermia, hypoxic cell sensitizers, and glutathione depletors such as buthionine sulfoximine. In this review, however, we will consider only hyperbaric oxygen and the 2-nitroimidazole hypoxic cell sensitizers.

### The Oxygen Effect

One major difference between tumor and normal cell populations is in their sensitivity to radiation; this is a reflection of their different growth kinetics and vascularity such that the architecture of the tumor results in the development of radiation resistant, hypoxic cells. Such cells exist in even relatively small-sized tumors. These "radiobiological" hypoxic cells rarely exist in normal cell populations. One of the first observed therapeutic consequences of this difference in oxygenation status was that much larger doses of radiation were required to kill hypoxic cells than non-hypoxic cells. This is shown in Figure 19.2 for CHO cells in tissue culture where a three-fold difference in the slopes of the dose-survival curve is noted for aerated versus hypoxic cells.[2] This ratio is termed the oxygen enhancement ratio (OER).

That this is an important consideration for tumor cells in vivo was demonstrated in 1963 by Powers and Tolmach consequent to the construction of a dose-survival curve to radiation for a murine lymphosarcoma.[3] They concluded that about 1% of the tumor cells were radiobiologically hypoxic, that is, demonstrated this dramatic difference in sensitivity to radiation exposure. Over the last two decades, the existence of such hypoxic cells in animal solid tumors has been repeatedly demonstrated to comprise between 1 and 50% of the tumor cell population.[4] In humans, the effect of hemoglobin level on local control and subsequent cure rate provides evidence for the importance of hypoxia in clinical radiotherapy.[5]

Significant controversy has surrounded the question of the importance of such hypoxic cells in the effective delivery of radiation therapy. Examination of a variety of fractionation regimens, computer modelling of various schedule scenarios, and analysis of rates of reoxygenation of residual tumor cells following radiation treatment all have occupied a prominent place in the thoughts and work of radiation biologists and radiation therapists. The

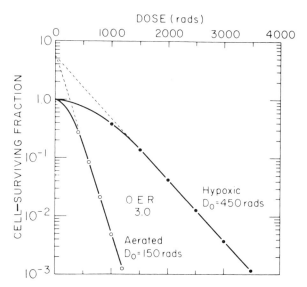

**FIGURE 19.2** Survival curve for cultured CHO cells exposed to x-rays under aerated conditions and under hypoxic conditions. (Reproduced with permission from ref. 2).

consensus remains that such hypoxic cells limit the effectiveness of therapy and local control, and consequently, many attempts have been made to destroy more effectively the hypoxic cell population. One strategy to increase their sensitivity to radiation would be to increase the oxygen tension to the hypoxic cells by increasing the oxygen pressure exposing the host.

## Hyperbaric Oxygen Trials

The first clinical trials of hyperbaric oxygen began in the mid 1950's. Limitations to its widespread use included the expense of the machines and the small size of the treatment chambers which prevented therapy of patients who were either claustrophobic or who had large tumors. In addition, due to the physical limitations imposed by the shape and size of the treatment units, technical difficulties were frequently encountered administering the dose; only in the Cardiff and Leeds trials were the same beam direction techniques used for those patients treated in hyperbaric oxygen and those treated in air.[6] Because of the difficulty in administering radiation therapy in hyperbaric oxygen, therapy was frequently administered in several large fractions rather than in a conventional fractionation scheme.

Five prospective randomized trials were undertaken in head and neck carcinoma, the largest of which were performed in England. In the first Cardiff trial (Table 19.1), sponsored by the Medical Research Council (MRC), 295 patients were randomized to receive 3500–4600 rads in ten fractions over 22 days either in hyperbaric oxygen or in air. At 5 years, the local control rate was significantly improved in those patients treated with hyperbaric oxygen (53% compared to 30%, p ≤ 0.001). However, there was no significant improvement in survival, and there was increased morbidity in those patients in whom the larynx was in the treatment field.[7]

In the second Cardiff trial (Table 19.1), 103 patients were randomized

**TABLE 19.1** MRC Hyperbaric Oxygen Trials Carcinoma of Head and Neck

|  |  | HBO | Air | Comments |
|---|---|---|---|---|
| 1st Trial (276 pts.) |  |  |  |  |
| Local control | (5 yr) | 53% | 30% | p < 0.001 |
| Survival | (5 yr) | 40% | 40% |  |
| 2nd Trial (103 pts.) |  |  |  |  |
| Local control | (5 yr) | 60% | 41% | p < 0.01 |
| Survival | (5 yr) | 55% | 31% | — |

No difference in complications.
10% lower dose to larynx fields only.
Data taken from refs. 7–11.

between a regimen identical to the first Cardiff trial in hyperbaric oxygen and a conventional daily fractionation in air. In addition, the dose of radiation was reduced by 10% for those treated in hyperbaric oxygen whose larnyx was in the treatment field.[10] Five-year follow-up showed a survival of 55% among those patients treated in hyperbaric oxygen and 31% among those treated in air; the local control rates were 60% and 41%, respectively. The greatest advantage to treatment with hyperbaric oxygen was seen in patients with tumors less than 5 cm in diameter.[8,11,12] Although an improvement was seen in this trial among those treated with hyperbaric oxygen, the difference in the fractionation regimen in these two arms makes comparisons difficult.

Three other prospective randomized trials have been undertaken in head and neck cancer, all of which show a tread towards improved local control among those treated with hyperbaric oxygen. These three trials involved small numbers of patients, and the fractionation schedule differed between those treated with hyperbaric oxygen and those treated in air.[11,12]

The results in other disease sites have been less encouraging. Although a trail showed an increase in local control in patients with carcinoma of the cervix, most marked in patients with stage III disease treated in hyperbaric oxygen, other trials have failed to confirm this finding.[8,13] Trials in other sites, such as bladder, have failed to show an improvement among those patients treated with hyperbaric oxygen.[8]

Hyperbaric oxygen trials have been abandoned in view of the generally negative results, with the possible exception of head and neck carcinoma.[6] The physiologic changes induced by hyperbaric oxygen, such as vasoconstriction, may offset the potential benefits of increased oxygen tension.

## Hypoxic Cell Sensitizers

Beginning in the early 1960's, attempts were made to either obtain or synthesize chemicals that could mimic the effect of oxygen in sensitizing hypoxic cells to radiation. The electron-affinic nitroimidazoles, metronidazole and misonidazole (Fig. 19.3), became the major candidates in the 1970's for further experimental and clinical study as well as the basis for analog development.

As shown in Figure 19.4, significant radiation sensitization can be achieved by misonidazole. These data demonstrate no change in the extrapolation number but a dose-dependent increase in the slope of the dose-survival curve. This experiment demonstrated that 2 mM misonidazole was nearly as effective as oxygen; also, no sensitization was noted for well-oxygenated cells. These, and other, in vitro studies were quickly tested in vivo models using murine tumor[4]; an example is shown in Figure 19.5 for a mammary carcinoma.[15] A significant decrease in the dose of radiation neces-

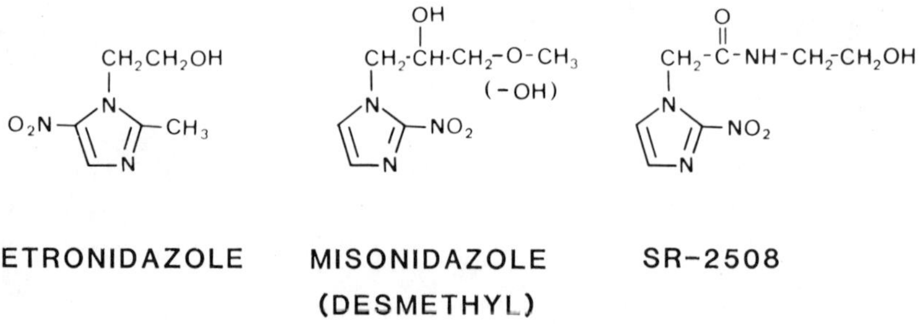

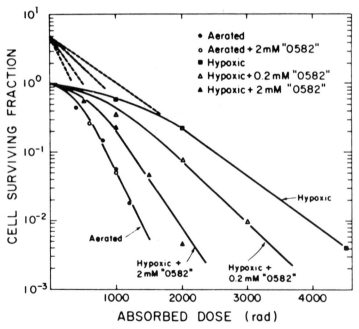

METRONIDAZOLE  MISONIDAZOLE  SR-2508
(DESMETHYL)

**FIGURE 19.3** Structures of major nitroimidazoles being studied in experimental and clinical research.

**FIGURE 19.4** Cell survival for V79 cells irradiated with $^{60}$Co gamma rays under aerated and hypoxic conditions and exposed to various concentrations of misonidazole. (Reproduced with permission from ref. 14).

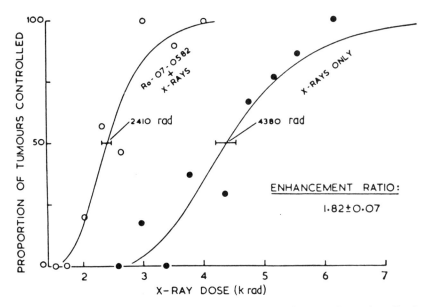

**FIGURE 19.5** Proportion of tumors controlled at 150 days as a function of x-ray dose. For the combination study, misonidazole (1 mg/g body weight, i.p.) was administered 30′ before a single dose of radiation. (Reproduced with permission from ref. 15.)

sary to control the tumors (cure the mice) is evident from the displacement of the dose-response curves. In this case, a significant enhancement ratio of 1.82 was obtained; that is, pretreatment with misonidazole increased the effectiveness of 2410 rads x-radiation to that noted by 4380 rads alone. This parameter is comparable in concept to the OER and is generally termed Sensitizer Enhancement Ratio (SER).

These results together with a host of others demonstrating in vivo effectiveness of misonidazole as a radiation sensitizer led to the initiation of a number of clinical trials of radiosensitizers.

## Clinical Trials

Extensive clinical trials of the sensitizer misonidazole in combination with radiotherapy have been carried out by RTOG in this country as well as similar groups in the U.K. and Japan. Initial clinical trials of misonidazole, which began in the late 1970's, sought to define both the maximally tolerated dose and the dose limiting toxicity of multiple dose administration. In addition, plasma and tumor levels of misonidazole were obtained in an attempt to define the SER that could be achieved together with its frequency during a course of radiation therapy.

The primary dose-limiting toxic effect of misonidazole is peripheral neuropathy, which is related to the total cumulative dose administered. The mildest neuropathies are sensory only, but at higher grades involve motor weakness as well. In the phase I trial of orally administered misonidazole conducted by the RTOG, 99 courses were evaluable for neurotoxicity. The incidence was 36% at cumulative doses below 12 $g/M^2$ and 74% above 12 $g/M^2$. However, there was a wide variation in the threshold dose at which peripheral neuropathy appeared; some patients developed neuropathy with a total cumulative dose as low as 6 $g/M^2$. The maximally tolerated single dose of misonidazole was $4-5$ $g/M^2$, and was associated with nausea, vomiting and diarrhea. Misonidazole has a long serum half life, with a $t^{1/2}_\beta$ of $13.8 \pm 5.1$ hours. Based on pharmacologic data obtained during this trial, a dose of misonidazole of 2 $g/M^2$ should produce an SER in tumor tissue of approximately 1.6.[16]

Once the MTD of misonidazole was established, a variety of clinical trials were undertaken. The aim of phase II trials was to establish the tolerance of radiation therapy combined with misonidazole in a variety of disease sites, and to determine whether there was a marked improvement in activity compared to historical controls. Phase III trials would then provide the definitive means of determining whether the addition of a radiosensitizer improved the activity of radiation therapy alone. The cumulative dose-related peripheral neuropathy greatly limited the amount of misonidazole that could be administered. In some trails, patients received several large fractions of radiotherapy, each of which was preceded by a relatively large dose of misonidazole. In such a fashion each dose of radiotherapy was administered with a maximal SER, however, by giving radiotherapy in several large doses, the advantages of reoxygenation in a conventional regimen o fractionation are lost. The opposite approach was to administer radiotherapy in a conventional fractionation regimen with a small dose of misonidazole, 400 $mg/M^2$, before each fraction. However, the SER associated with such a small dose ($<1.1-1.2$) would not likely be of significant clinical benefit (Table 19.2).

Most trials tried to compromise between these two extremes. In some trials, patients received a larger dose of radiation therapy once weekly, associated with a dose of 2$g/M^2$ misonidazole and conventional radiotherapy the remaining days of each week. In other trials, patients received two fractions of radiotherapy within 24 hours after administration of one dose of 2$g/M^2$ to take advantage of the long half life of misonidazole; radiotherapy without misonidazole was administered the remaining three days each week. Therefore, interpreting the results of many phase II/III trials is difficult because of the many different radiation therapy schemes employed.

**TABLE 19.2** Radiotherapy Doses (SER)

| Fractionation | Dose g/m² | Plateau Plasma Concentration | | Probable Levels in Hypoxic Tumor Cells | |
|---|---|---|---|---|---|
| | | ug/ml | Enhancement | $\mu$g/g | Enhancement |
| 6 | 2 | 80 | 1.65 | 40 | 1.50 |
| 10 | 1.2 | 50 | 1.55 | 25 | 1.40 |
| 20 | 0.6 | 24 | 1.40 | 12 | 1.20 |
| 24 | 0.5 | 20 | 1.35 | 10 | 1.20 |
| 30 | 0.4 | 16 | 1.25 | 8 | 1.15 |

Reproduced from ref. 17.

Two phase II trials in head and neck cancer were performed in the United States with oral misonidazole (Table 19.3).[18] In the first trial, 45 evaluable patients with advanced disease (T3 and T4) primaries received misonidazole weekly in conjunction with two doses of radiotherapy; the patients then received the remaining three doses each week in a conventional fractionation regimen without misonidazole.[19] Of the 32 patients who received the full treatment regimen of radiation therapy and sensitizer, 56% had a complete response and 34% had a partial response.[20] A second phase II trial explored the same schedule of radiation therapy used in the hyperbaric oxygen trials conducted by the MRC, but was closed prior to completion when the RTOG decided to pursue a phase III trial with the regimen used in the first trial.[20]

**TABLE 19.3** Misonidazole: Advanced Head and Neck Cancer

| Treatment | Type of Trial |
|---|---|
| 250 rad (4 hrs after Miso) q wk $\times$ 5 wks | Phase II |
| 210 rad (8 hrs after Miso) q wk $\times$ 5 wks | |
| 180 rad q day $\times$ 3 per wk $\times$ 5/wks then 180 rad q day $\times$ 5/wk $\times$ 2–3 wks | |
| Total dose = 6600–7200 rad | |
| Misonidazole 2.5 g/m² q wk $\times$ 6 = 15 g/m² modified to 2.0 g/m² q wk $\times$ 6 = 12 g/m² | |
| 400 rad $\times$ 2 $\times$ wk then 3 $\times$/wk = 4800–5600 rad | Phase II |
| Misonidazole 1.25 g/m² (reduced to 1.0 g/m²) biw-tiw $\times$ 5 wks = 12–15 g/m² | |
| 1. XRT 400 rad $\times$ 12 fx/2.5 wks = 4800 rad | Randomized |
| 2. XRT + Miso 1.5 g/m² tiw $\times$ 7 = 10.5 g/m² | Phase II |
| 1. XRT — 6600–7380 rad 33–41 fxs at 180–200 rad/fx, 5 fxs/week | Phase III |
| 2. XRT + Miso | |
|     XRT — 2 fxs q Mon, 1 fx q Tues, Thurs, Fri 6600–7380 rad/6.6–7 wks | |
|     Miso — 2.0 g/m² q wk $\times$ 6 = 12 g/m² | |

Two comparative trials were then undertaken (Table 19.3). In a randomized phase II trial, no major difference in either response or toxicity was seen in patients with advanced head and neck cancer who received 400 rads daily 5 days/week for a total of 12 treatments with or without misonidazole (1.5 g/$M^2$ three times per week for seven doses).[20] A randomized phase III trial was undertaken to determine whether misonidazole given in conjunction with two doses of radiotherapy would be significantly better than radiation alone in a conventional fractionation regimen. Although the analysis is not complete, no significant benefit has been seen among those receiving the radiosensitizer.[21]

A summary of the date from many clinical trials in head and neck cancer with misonidazole conducted outside the U.S. is presented in Table 19.4 taken from Dische et al.[22] Although in 8/12 trials there was some improvement in local control or survival at an early interim period, this was frequently lost with further follow-up. One randomized trial has recently shown a statistically significant increase in local control rate in patients with enlarged cervical nodes.[21] In a trial conducted by the Danish Head and Neck Cancer Study Group, not shown on this table, 494 patients with all stages of disease (except larynx stage 1) were randomized to treatment with one of two different split course radiation regimens with either misonidazole (11 g/$M^2$) or placebo during the initial month of therapy. A benefit to treatment with misonidazole was statistically significant in male patients with pharyngeal carcinoma at 3 years (46% vs. 26%, p < 0.02).[23]

Since the start of clinical trials, more than 5000 patients have been enrolled in more than 120 randomized controlled clinical trials. At least 750 patients have developed some degree of peripheral neuropathy secondary to administration of misonidazole.[17] To date, the overall results have been negative, with the possible exception of an occasional subgroup of patients with head and neck cancer.[24] In virtually all trials, this early improvement in response and survival has been lost with further follow-up.

## Conclusion and Future Studies

While the results to date with radiosensitizers are not very promising, it is important to understand why the exciting experimental studies have not resulted in clinical benefit. Limitations which have been recognized for many years are discussed below and future studies suggested.[4,25-27]

Limitations in the effectiveness of the misonidazole result from chemical, pharmacologic, toxicologic and other biological considerations. Each of these problems underlies one area of ongoing drug development of radiation sensitizers.[14,25] First is the problem of sensitizer dose. Because of the dose limiting toxicities, even the maximal single tolerated dose does not yield an

**TABLE 19.4** Misonidazole: Head and Neck Cancer

| Investigator/Title | Location | Case Material | Total No. | Total Dose G/M$^2$ |
|---|---|---|---|---|
| Sealy | Cape Town, South Africa | Advanced oral cancer | 97 | 12 |
| Sealy | Cape Town, South Africa | Advanced oral cancer | 64 | 12 |
| Bataini | Paris, France | Oral cavity | 84 | 14 |
| | | Oropharynx | | |
| Dahanca | Denmark | Pharynx | 153 | 11 |
| | | Larynx | | |
| Arcangeli | Rome, Italy | Secondary cancer | 25 | 12 |
| | | Neck nodes (multi. lesions) | | |
| Medical Research Council | United Kingdom | Oral | 164 | 12 |
| | | Pharyngeal | | |
| | | Laryngeal | | |
| Cattan | Rheims, France | Advanced head and neck tumor | 71 | 12 |
| Giaux | Lille, France | Bucco pharyngeal | 56 | 12 |
| Bataini | Paris, France | Larynx | 65 | 14 |
| | | Hypopharynx | | |
| Medical Research Council | United Kingdom | Oral | 93 | 12 |
| | | Pharyngeal | | |
| | | Laryngeal | | |
| Dahanca | Denmark | Pharyngeal | 143 | 11 |
| | | Larynx | | |
| Gil Govarre | Madrid, Spain | Head and neck (include some cervical cancer) | 40 | 15 |

enhancement ratio of 3; usually the value is closer to 2.[4,28] Furthermore, this effect in animal models is observed with a plasma concentration often much higher than that which can be achieved in humans (i.e., for misonidazole it is approximately 150 $\mu$g/ml). The higher concentration achievable in the mouse is due to the shorter half-life when compared to humans, although a similar C x t at maximum tolerated doses may in fact equalize the sensitizing effect between the two species. The cumulative total dose is limited in humans by neurotoxicity. Therefore, in order to achieve higher plasma levels, with a greater number of radiation therapy treatments, new sensitizers with decreased neurotoxicity are being studied.

A second problem arises due to the required scheduling of radiation. Since radiation is administered in fractionated schedules, the sensitizer must also be fractionated. However, as cumulative toxicity limits the individual dose that can be administered, and since there is a relationship between the sensitizing ratio and the dose of sensitizer, the decrease in dose for the fractionation schedule significantly compromises the degree of sensitization (Table 19.2).[29,30] As a possible solution to this problem, as with dose limitations, new agents with decreased lipophilicity and possibly decreased neurotoxicity have been synthesized. An example is SR-2508 (Fig. 19.3), which is significantly less toxic than misonidazole, yet retains molar equivalent activity in terms of sensitization.[31]

Thirdly, while the extent of hypoxia is quite variable, it is probably in the order of 10% for a given tumor. Thus, only that small, albeit critical, fraction will be affected by exposure to a radiosensitizer. Of more importance, however, is the kinetics of reoxygenation following radiation therapy. If, for a given tumor, it is rapid and complete following a few radiation treatments, then subsequent sensitizer courses would obviously be ineffective.[32] Indeed, such an effect with a concomitant compromise of sensitizer effect in only a five-fraction radiation course was demonstrated by Denekamp and Harris.[33] While the results to date seem to indicate a compromise of sensitizer effect with fractionation, the picture is far from clear, and more studies with experimental tumors and different fractionation regimens are necessary.[26] One possible approach to this problem might be to schedule therapy (with or without sensitizer as well as the dose of sensitizer) in relation to the hypoxic fraction at a given treatment. This value might be obtained through the use of a radioactive, fluorescent or NMR-sensitive tag to the hypoxic cell population.[34,35]

Finally, a better understanding of the mechanism of action of the hypoxic cell sensitizers may allow us to design better schedules or combinations. For example, recent studies implicate the 2-nitroimidazoles as depletors of glutathione.[36] As shown in Figure 19.6, 2-nitroimidazoles can be reduced to hydroxylamines that can react with macromolecules (thereby

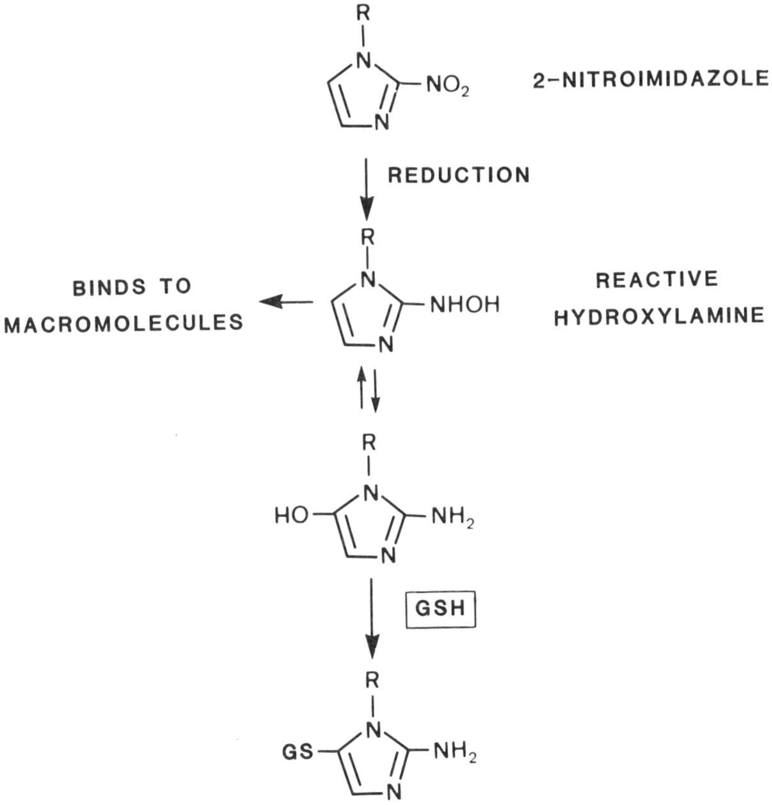

**FIGURE 19.6** Metabolic pathway of 2-nitroimidazoles.

fixing damage), or, upon rearrangement, react with glutathione (GSH) consequently decreasing the cellular content of this important reductive species.[37,38] Continued exposure of cells by these agents and the consequent glutathione depletion might explain not only the cytotoxic effect of these agents alone on cultured cells,[39] but also the "pre-incubation" effect in which prior exposure to a variety of hypoxic cell sensitizers increases hypoxic cell sensitivity to radiation.[40] Furthermore, as shown by Roizen-Towle et al,[41] there appears to be a correlation between thiol depletion by nitroimidazoles (in hypoxic cells) and sensitization to subsequent melphalan exposure.

In conclusion, many of the problems that restrict the effectiveness of radiation sensitizers are understood, and it is hoped that the clinical results from the next generation of the 2-nitroimidazoles will indicate that we are heading in the right direction. Furthermore, scheduling of the agents in an attempt to optimally deplete cellular glutathione appears promising.

## Chemosensitization

It is important to consider the limitations of hypoxic cell sensitizers in radiation therapy since a number of these limitations do not occur for chemosensitization.

Of recent interest is the observation that hypoxic cell sensitizers modulate the cytotoxicity of chemotherapeutic agents. It was noted in 1975 that misonidazole was inherently cytotoxic to hypoxic cells.[42] A recent study by Geard et al, is presented here to demonstrate this cytotoxic effect (Fig. 19.7)[39]; it was noted both that SR-2508 is more active than misonidazole and that it requires a long duration of exposure to kill aerated cell.

While this finding led to the initial experimental trials of these agents in combination with anticancer agents, it soon became obvious that non-cytotoxic levels could increase the sensitivity of hypoxic cells to alkylating agents.[77]

The first studies by Rose et al. demonstrated in vivo potentiation of the cytotoxicity of a variety of anticancer agents including melphalan and cyclophosphamide when 1 mg/g misonidazole was administered 30 minutes before the alkylating agents.[45] The potentiation was significantly greater for the

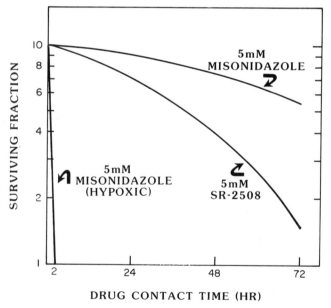

**FIGURE 19.7** Survival of aerated V-79 cells to exposure to either misonidazole or SR-2508. (Data taken from refs. 39 and 43).

tumor (Lewis lung carcinoma) than for normal tissues (bone marrow and intestinal stem cells).

Subsequently, a number of experimental studies have examined the interaction of hypoxic cell sensitizers, mainly misonidazole, and chemotherapeutic agents.[43,46,47] Alkylating agents such as cyclophosphamide, melphalan and CCNU demonstrate significant potentiation with enhancement values of 2 or more as shown in Figure 19.8 for cyclophosphamide against Lewis lung cancer. However, toxicity is also enhanced when hypoxic cell sensitizers are given before alkylating agents as shown in Figure 19.8 for cyclophosphamide against hematopoietic stem cells. Therefore, in order to derive therapeutic benefit, greater enhancement of tumor cells must occur. Fortunately, such differential enhancement is usually observed[48]; in Figure 19.8 the ratio of tumor sensitization to normal cell sensitization is 2 : 1.3. For the anticancer agent cisplatin, the experimental studies have been varied. In some studies, potentiation of cytotoxicity is noted,[50] while in others, no sensitization has been noted (Fig. 19.8).[48,49,51]

The mechanism for the sensitization is not clear, however a number of effects have been noted:

1. Unlike the situation noted for radiation, hypoxia is not a requirement for the chemosensitization since: (a) enhancement of alkylating agent cytotoxicity is noted for tumors which have only a few hypoxic cells in vivo,[52] and (b) toxicity is usually enhanced even though these normal cells are not hypoxic.
2. Misonidazole pretreatment can modify the pharmacokinetics of agents such as cyclophosphamide and melphalan.[53,54]
3. Sensitizers reduce the glutathione level in hypoxic cells thereby which may sensitize them to subsequent alkylating agents.[36,43] As a corollary, addition of thiol-containing agents reduces the extent of sensitization.[50]
4. Hypoxic cell sensitizers produce single strand breaks (sub-lethal damage) that can increase the extent of DNA cross-linking of alkylating agents.[43] Indeed, increased cross-linking has been noted for both tumors and normal cells by alkaline elution.[55]
5. Inhibition of repair of potentially lethal damage (PLD),[56] although chemosensitization has been noted in cases where there is no modification of PLD.[47]

### Clinical Trials

Based on in vivo data suggesting that misonidazole and melphalan have synergistic antitumor activity, a phase I trial was undertaken to determine the maximally tolerated dose of each of these agents when misonidazole is

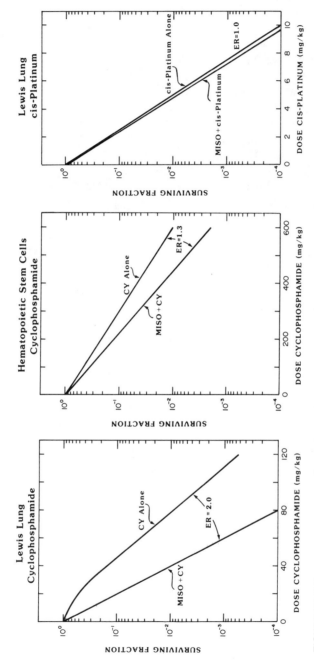

**FIGURE 19.8** Dose-response curves for cyclophosphamide, melphalan and CCNU given alone or following misonidazole pretreatment. (Redrawn from ref. 48, 49).

given orally 2 hours before intravenous melphalan. Because in vivo data suggested that misonidazole should be given simultaneously with, or slightly before the alkylating agent, a two hour interval was chosen so that orally administered misonidazole could achieve peak plasma levels. This trial established that both drugs could be given at their individual maximally tolerated doses; the hematologic toxicity of melphalan did not appear to be worsened by concomitant administration of misonidazole. Among 30 evaluable patients, 1 partial response (>50% decrease in the product of two longest perpendicular diameters) was seen in a patient with malignant melanoma.[57] NCOG then undertook a randomized phase II trial of misonidazole 4 g/$M^2$ po., followed 4 hours later by melphalan 0.6 mg/$M^2$, versus melphalan alone in patients with lung cancer (excluding small cell lung cancer). This trial recently closed; results are not yet available.

Table 19.5 summarizes the trials that have been conducted with misonidazole and cyclophosphamide. In the phase I trials by Davila et al. and Tutsch et al.,[58,59] hematologic toxicity did not appear to be worsened by concomitant administration of misonidazole, and there was no change in the pharmacokinetics of either drug. In a phase II trial in patients with non-small cell lung carcinoma conducted by Busutti et al., myelosuppression was similar to that which would be anticipated in patients treated with cyclophosphamide alone; no responses were seen.[60]

Table 19.5 also summarizes the trials that have been conducted with radiation sensitizers and nitrosoureas. Urtasun et al. treated 6 malignant glioma patients with misonidazole 2 gm/$M^2$ orally every other day for a total of 3 doses; 3 hours following the last dose of misonidazole, patients received BCNU 80 mg/$M^2$. Myelosuppression was seen, but no change was seen in the pharmacokinetics of either drug.[61] A similar study was performed by Fulton and Urtason.[62] They treated 13 malignant glioma patients with a single oral dose of misonidazole 3.5 g/$M^2$ followed 4 hours later by CCNU 120 mg/$M^2$. Toxicity and activity did not appear to differ from that induced by CCNU alone.[62] Steward et al. treated 23 patients in a broad phase II trial with metronidazole 1.5 gm/$M^2$ 1 hour and 12 hours prior to a single dose of intravenous BCNU. The dose limiting toxic effect was once again myelosuppession, and it did not appear to be enhanced by the addition of a radiosensitizer. Although there were too few patients of any histologic diagnosis to make a reliable estimate of the activity of this combination, some degree of tumor regression was seen in patients with malignant glioma, non-small cell lung cancer, and colon carcinoma.[63]

As well as exploring metronidazole and CCNU, Steward et al administered metronidazole 1.5 gm/$M^2$ 12 hours and 1 hour prior to mitomycin C 10–20 mg/$M^2$ to 40 patients.[63] Myelosuppression was dose limiting; however, four patients developed severe pulmonary toxicity following one cycle

**TABLE 19.5** Misonidazole/Metronidazole Clinical Trials: Chemosensitization

| Author | Regimen | Timing | Number of Patients |
|---|---|---|---|
| Davila | Misonidazole 1–2 gm/m² PO<br>Cyclophosphamide 0.4–1.3 g/m² IV | 4 Hr. | 42 |
| Busutti | Misonidazole 0.5–1 g/m² PO qD × 3<br>Cyclophosphamide 250–500 mg/m² IV qD × 3 | 2 Hr. or 3 Hr. | 15 |
| Tutsch | Misonidazole 0.5–5 gm/m² IV<br>Cyclophosphamide 1–1.4 g/m² IV | 2 Hr. | 34 |
| Urtason (Alberta) | Misonidazole 2 gm/m² PO qOD × 3<br>BCNU 80 mg/m² IV qOD × 3 | 3 Hr. | 6 |
| Fulton (Alberta) | Misonidazole 3.5 gm/m² PO<br>CCNU 120 mg/m² PO | 4 Hr. | 13 |
| Stewart (Ontario) | Metronidazole 1.5 gm/m² PO × 2<br>BCNU 180–240 mg/m² IV | 12 Hr. and 1 Hr. | 23 |
| Stewart (Ontario) | Metronidazole 1.5 gm/m² PO × 2<br>Mitomycin C 10–20 mg/m² | 12 Hr. and 1 Hr. | 40 |

of therapy; in two it was fatal, suggesting that metronidazole may enhance the pulmonary toxicity of mitomycin C. A recent review of this subject was done by Presant.[64]

## Conclusions and Future Studies

While the clinical studies to date do not seem as promising as the experimental data for the use of hypoxia cell sensitizers in combination with either radiotherapy or chemotherapy, our better understanding of the basis for the limited positive clinical result does provide some encouragement for further study.

First, radiotherapy trials with the more potent SR-2508 are now in progress.[65] While the single dose MTD has not been determined, the cumulative dose limiting toxicity is peripheral neuropathy noted in some patients receiving over 21 $g/M^2/3$ weeks or 30 $g/M^2/5$ weeks. However, toxicity correlates with the pharmacokinetic parameter "area under the curve" (AUC). In 23 patients, no toxicity was noted for values less than 38 mM.hr, whereas all patients whose values were greater than 34 mM.hr demonstrated toxicity. More potent sensitizers might be developed. If this occurs, we may begin to see consistant positive clinical results. Second, the SR-2508-chemotherapy trials will also begin shortly. It is possible that if sufficiently large doses can be administered before the alkylating agents, positive clinical trials may occur as a result. Thirdly, and of a more complex nature, the ability to determine the degree of tumor hypoxia during therapy will allow a more rational development of a schedule of radiation and sensitizer.

Finally, further studies to define the relation of sensitizers to glutathione levels might indicate an application of this treatment against the predominantly non-hypoxic tumor cells. This is particularly important in relation to optimal scheduling of the sensitizer such as by prolonged exposure.[66]

Because of the unique nature of chemosensitizers, clinical trials of these agents should be of different design and have different endpoints from that of a strict cytotoxic agent. A phase I trial should define the optimal dose of effect chemosensitization, which might not necessarily be the same as a maximally tolerated dose based on toxicity. Once this dose is defined, early randomized trials should be pursued, preferably in a disease with a sharp dose-response curve. An important aim of these randomized trials is to determine whether the sensitizer enhances antitumor effect more than toxicity. Another therapeutic possibility is the use of these sensitizers together with *both* radiation and chemotherapy. Indeed, laboratory studies have reported the effectiveness of such a combination (misonidazole plus radiation plus CCNU) in an in vivo tumor model (KHT sarcoma).[67]

As a final note to these experimental studies, it should be remembered that these agents have inherent cytotoxic activity against both non-hypoxic and hypoxic cells.[68] While it appears unlikely that misonidazole reaches toxic levels in clinical trials,[69] such a possibility must be kept in mind for subsequent generations of these sensitizers and for each tumor type examined.

## RADIATION PROTECTORS

Radiation protectors have been studied for many decades, as they offer the opportunity to modify the extent of radiation damage on normal tissues as well as provide insight into the basic mechanism of radiation cytotoxicity. The attractiveness of such compounds is that, if effective, they could allow higher doses of radiation to be administered to a tumor, thereby increasing the local cure rate. Or, alternatively, they could decrease the normal tissue toxicity in cases where there is already a high local control rate.

This area of research had its advent in studies carried out in the early 1950's, in which SH-containing compounds were examined as protective agents for the lethal effects of both radiation and nitrogen mustard. Patt first studied this phenomenon in animals by showing a reduction of radiation lethality to rats by cysteine pretreatment.[70,71] No potentiation occurred if cysteine was given as early as 5 minutes after the radiation. He postulated that cysteine either protected cellular components from oxidation or acted directly on the oxidating agents produced by the radiation of water.[71] He also demonstrated that other sulfhydryl compounds such as glutathione were effective.[71] A systematic study carried out by a number of investigators identified cysteamine as the best substance suitable for human use.[72-75]

The U.S. Army Anti-Radiation Drug Development Program (1959–1973) at Walter Reed Hospital produced (or contracted to laboratories such as Southern Research Institute for the phosphorothioates) and tested about 4400 potential radiation protective agents, mostly aminothiols.[76] The compound WR-2721 had the best activity of the agents (although it lacked oral activity) (Fig. 19.9).[77]

Yuhas examined the ability of a number of these agents to modify bone marrow and GI and CNS toxicity, and noted protection of the first two and sensitization of the third. WR-2721 was the most active of the compounds and demonstrated a dose-response relationship.[78-80] He examined the effect of time interval and showed maximum protection occurred when WR-2721 preceded the radiation by about 15 min. Yuhas also showed limited protection for a transplantable mammary tumor after irradiation, thus indicating the potential of WR-2721 in radiotherapy.[81]

Phillip's group has also studied WR-2721 extensively. He reasoned that

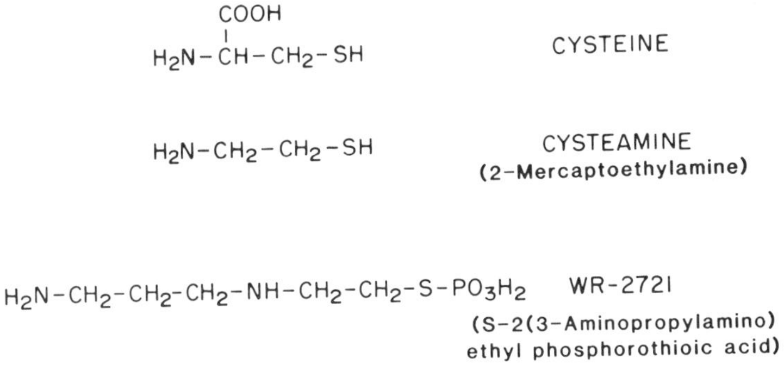

$$COOH$$
$$H_2N-\overset{|}{C}H-CH_2-SH \qquad CYSTEINE$$

$$H_2N-CH_2-CH_2-SH \qquad CYSTEAMINE$$
$$(2-Mercaptoethylamine)$$

$$H_2N-CH_2-CH_2-CH_2-NH-CH_2-CH_2-S-PO_3H_2 \qquad WR-2721$$
$$(S-2(3-Aminopropylamino)$$
$$ethyl\ phosphorothioic\ acid)$$

**FIGURE 19.9** Structure of main aminothiols used as radiation protective agents.

since protection was low for hypoxic versus non-hypoxic cells,[82,83] and since tumors have a poor blood supply, protection occurs even for fractionated therapy,[84] and tumor cure shows a steep dose-response relationship, then the protectors may have a major impact on local-regional control.[85] Phillips examined a variety of normal tissues and found protection of all, though it was demonstrated to different degrees. Unfortunately, when P388 cells and EMT-6 cells were examined, protection was also noted (as expected for non-hypoxic cells, DMF values of 2.2 for P388 and 1.3 for EMT-6 were obtained).[86]

In terms of the mechanism for any differential effect between normal and tumor cells, Yuhas demonstrated a striking difference in drug uptake between normal and tumor cells.[87] Whereas normal cells demonstrate a slow, passive uptake, tumors appear to actively absorb the compound. Even examining 1–2 mm cubes where hypoxia is not a problem, a temperature-dependent concentration mechanism is noted for normal cells but not tumor cells. This concentration of protector appears to be a facilitated diffusion, since classic inhibitors of active transport are without effect. However, others have not noted any difference in WR-2721 uptake in vitro between normal and tumor tissue, leading to the proposal that the difference in vascularity between normal and tumor tissue underlies their respective uptake differences. Furthermore, some studies have shown a strong dependence of the dose modifying factor upon tumor size, such that tumor micrometastases show significant radioprotection by WR-2721, while macroscopic tumor does not.[88]

Yuhas postulated that the splenic vasodilation noted with WR-2721 might modify oxygen tension and thus radiation sensitivity with the host tissue.[89] However, the fact that the active species WR-1065 also protects in vitro (as does cysteamine) indicates that the protection is not simply a physiologic effect.[90]

The most obvious biochemical mechanism for sulfhydryl protection is through radical scavanging or reaction with DNA radicals.[91,92] The basic hydrogen donation reaction would be:

$$PSH + R\cdot \rightarrow PS\cdot + RH$$

where P is the protector and $R\cdot$ is the radiation-produced radical species. Another possibility for mechanism of action relates to the ability of some of the aminothiols to bind to DNA, thereby preventing damage to this macromolecule.[93]

Recently, Durand proposed from studies with spheroids that WR-2721 acts as an "oxygen-depleting" agent (by thiol oxidation) that is dependent upon the dephosphorylation of WR-2721 by the specific tissue.[94] Phillips also studied the ability of normal and tumor cell homogenates to dephosphorylate WR-2721; he noted about a 15-fold difference in activity between mouse liver and duodenum, while the Ehrlich ascites cells and P388 cells fell within the range. Since uptake also appeared similar for normal and tumor cells, Phillips postulated that any differential sensitivity in the solid tumors was hypoxia-related.

Even though the thiol may protect both the normal and tumor cells to the same extent in vitro, the fact that these agents appeared to localize preferrentially in bone marrow and intestine suggests that preferrential protection may occur in vivo.[95]

At present, a large variety of both normal and tumor cell populations have been studied for the ability of WR-2721 to protect them from radiation damage, and the data support a differential effect.[96,97]

For many solid tumors the dose reduction factors noted following WR-2721 pretreatment are low (1.0 to 1.5); however, a few examples of values up to 2.8 have been observed.[98] On the other hand, protective values for normal tissue vary widely (from 1.0 to nearly 3.0), although they are usually above 1.5 for many critical tissues (skin, bone marrow, intestinal mucosa). Furthermore, protection of normal tissues shows a dependency upon radiation fraction size with increased protection at the lower (therapeutic) sizes. A dependency upon oxygen tension has also been observed, with the extent of protection diminishing with decreased oxygen tension.[99] Thus, care is required in translating this radioprotective prescription to human solid tumors *in general*, and to the specific tumor type. Normal tissue situations may or may not benefit from the introduction of a radiation protector into the therapeutic protocol.

## Clinical Studies

During the initial development of WR-2721, normal volunteers were given excalating doses of drug. Some volunteers tolerated doses as high as 5000 mg/M$^2$; toxicities were primarily gastrointestinal.[100]

Two parallel phase I trials of WR-2721 as a radioprotector have been conducted by the RTOG. The first trial sought to define the MTD of WR-2721 when given as a single bolus 15 to 20 minutes prior to radiation therapy, whereas the second sought to define the MTD of WR-2721 when given in multiple doses for several weeks. During the course of the trial, the formulation and manner of reconstitution was changed. The reconstituted solution used in the first part of the trial was acidic, which might have caused hydrolysis of 30% of the parent compound, leading to enhanced toxicity and perhaps decreased efficacy.[101] Toxicities seen during the phase I trials have included nausea, vomiting, sneezing, and most significantly, hypotension. Hypocalcemia was also noted.[102]

## Chemoprotection

Brandt and Griffin carried out experiments patterned upon those of Patt with nitrogen mustard (HN2) and cysteine, and demonstrated a six- to eight-fold decrease in the LD$_{50}$ value when cysteine preceded HN2. These investigators were interested in the reduction of host toxicity as a way to increase the dose of HN2 so as to kill more leukemia cells in vivo.

In Denmark, Therkelsen and others similarly studied cysteine analogs to discover more effective agents in preventing HN2 toxicity against host, bone marrow, and intestinal tract damage. These studies demonstrated that, in mice, cysteamine analogs could be more active than the parent compound,[104,105] that combinations of sulfhydryl compounds such as glutathione and cysteamine could be of increased effectiveness,[106] and, most importantly, that cysteamine exerted *no* protective effect on HN2 for a transplanted leukemia, while at the same time it allowed a greater dose of HN2 to be administered.[107] Yuhas later demonstrated a similar lack of protection for a solid tumor.[108]

The protective effect does not seem to act on all alkylating agents, as it was demonstrated that neither cysteine nor cysteamine were able to protect against thio-TEPA, TEM, or L-PAM, and they had minimal activity against cyclophosphamide.[109-111] One proposed mechanism for the difference may be that cysteine is metabolized rapidly in vivo, and if the alkylating agents is "slow acting," not much protection will occur.[109]

The next important development in the study of chemoprotective agents was the demonstration by Yuhas in 1979 that the phosphorothioate

WR-2721 was capable of protecting mice from HN2 toxicity (DMF = 2.2).[112] He also showed the dose-response relationship for the effect, examined the interval dependency, and demonstrated little, if any, effect on protection of a HN2-responsive solid tumor.[112] A further study with the MCa-11 mammary tumor demonstrated protection from Cis-Pt nephrotoxicity and host toxicity without compromising tumor cytoxicity.[113]

One of the most studied systems for quantification of cytotoxic effects of agents on a normal tissue is the hematopoietic stem cell. Wasserman et al. recently showed the pronounced protective effect of WR-2721 for radiation (DMF = 2.4) HN2 (4.6), cis-PT (3.2), CY (2.4), BCNU (1.5) and 5-FU (2.7).[114] In the same study, he demonstrated no protective effect with any of these drugs using a tumor growth delay assay for EMT-6 tumors. A crucial therapeutic element in all of these studies was the degree of protection of tumor cells compared to normal cells in the same host. There is no question that the compound WR-2721 can provide some degree of protection to *some* tumor cell populations exposed to radiation[115-117]; however, tumor protection is more often not observed, or is of a lower magnitude than that noted for normal tissues, and is dependent on factors such as tumor size and oxygenation.[118,119] Most important for this discussion, however, is that tumor protection by alkylating agents has not been seen in systems where pronounced protection of normal cells by WR-2721 pretreatment has been observed.[120]

A recent novel finding is the *chemosensitization* by WR-2721 and other thiols with specificity for transplanted leukemia.[121,122] Figure 19.10 demonstrates this pronounced potentiation noted for I.V. administered HN2 preceded by I.P. administered WR-2721. At the maximum tolerated dose of HN2, which is about 0.2 mg/mouse, the extent of potentiation is approximately 1000-fold.

The biochemical basis for this potentiation is not known, and is even more pronounced for other thiols such as disulfiram and diethyldithiocarbamate.[123] Given the two profound effects of chemoprotection in normal cells and chemopotentiation in tumor cells for a number of thiol-containing agents, the underlying biochemical mechanism for these effects are important to discern.

Salerno and Friedell early postulated that the effect of cysteamine was simply a direct interaction of – SH with the reactive imonium ion of HN2[124]; however, the fact that there was no decrease in the activity of HN2 in a number of tumors, along with the simultaneously decreasing host toxicity argues against this interpretation being the sole mechanism. Two other observations provide some rationale for the chemoprotection of normal tissues. First, normal cells appear to have an active uptake of WR-2721 compared to tumor cells[87]; in addition, because of the vasculature of solid

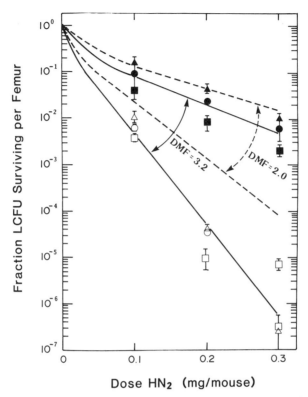

**FIGURE 19.10** Survival of AKR leukemia cells (LCFU) as a function of dose of HN2 administered I.V. (open symbols). Closed symbols are results obtained when 15 mg WR-2721/mouse was administered I.P. 15′ before the HN2. Dashed lines are for comparison with previously published results for I.P. administered HN2 together with I.P. administered WR-2721.[121]

tumors, WR-2721 has a difficulty of penetrating the tumor compared to normal tissues.[125]

Thiophosphates must be de-phosphorylated to become active. In vitro studies show that the dephosphorylated compound WR-1065 is significantly more active as a protector than WR-2721. WR-1065 is readily oxidized to the disulfide (inactive) product. WR-2721 is gradually hydrolyzed intracellularly by enzymes. It is known to enter cells by passive diffusion and is hydrolyzed by a saturable hydrolytic enzyme system.[126] Also, WR-1065 seems to be transported slowly into cells.

There is increasing evidence not only that the level of nonprotein sulfhydryls in cells is an important factor in radiation and alkylating agent sensitivity,[127] but also that thiol manipulation represents a potentially important biochemical modulator to sensitize cells to radiation or alkylating agents.[128-130]

With regard to head and neck cancers, protection of normal tissue toxicity to cisplatin has been well demonstrated, while at the same time, little or no decrease in the antitumor effect has been found.[115,131] An example is shown in Figure 19.11 where WR-2721 pretreatment allowed the larger doses of cisplatin to be administered to mice bearing the mammary

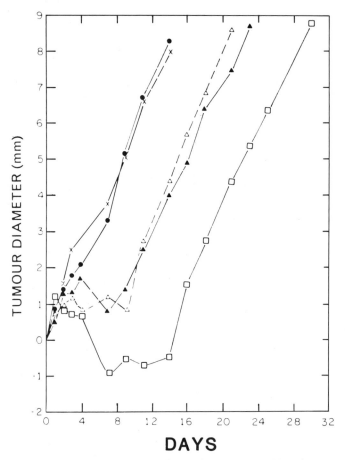

**FIGURE 19.11** Growth of MCa-11 tumor in Balb/c mice given no treatment (x), 5 daily doses of 1 mg/kg of cis-Pt (●), 5 daily doses of 2 mg/kg of cis-Pt (▲), 5 daily doses of 2 mg/kg, each pretreated 30 min earlier with an injection of 100 mg/kg of WR-2721 (△), and 5 daily doses of 3 mg/kg of cis-Pt each pretreated 30 min earlier by an injection of 100 mg/kg of WR-2721 (□). (Reproduced with permission from ref. 132).

tumor, while no detrimental effect on the significant tumor response to cisplatin resulted.

This area of research involving radiation protectors and alkylating agents is of increasing importance and potential clinical significance.[133,134] The finding of protection of alkylating agents added a further dimension to the importance of these compounds.

## Clinical Studies

The first clinical application was done in 1951 by Weisberger et al,[135] who administered L-cysteine (10–30 g) either I.V. or orally to patients 1 hour prior to HN2 therapy, and noted hematological protection and the ability to administer nearly four-fold higher doses of HN2.

Concomitant with the phase I trials of WR-2721 and radiation, chemo-protection trials have been carried out with escalating doses of cyclophosphamide, HN2, and cisplatin.[136]

Table 19.6 summarizes clinical trials that have been performed using WR-2721 and either cisplatin or cyclophosphamide.

The first of these combination trials was initiated prior to the completion of the phase I trial of WR-2721 as a single agent. In this trial, patients received WR-2721 450–740 mg/m$^2$ prior to the chemotherapeutic agent. WR-2721 was administered in an unbuffered solution over 20 to 50 minutes. Patients who received cisplatin in this trial were hydrated but did not receive mannitol. There were no controls among those patients treated with cisplatin; among ten patients treated with cyclophosphamide and WR-2721, five received cyclophosphamide alone during a subsequent course. Among patients treated with cisplatin, drug-induced toxicity occurred, suggesting that WR-2721 did not afford clinically significant protection in this situation. The only suggestion of benefit in this trial was that myelosuppression appeared less severe in patients treated with both cyclophosphamide and WR-2721 than with cyclophosphamide alone.[136] Several other trials suggest that WR-2721 may protect against cyclophosphamide-induced marrow toxicity,[137,141,143] however, one trial conducted by Wooley et al. failed to confirm this finding.[142] Trials with WR-2721 and cisplatin suggest that WR-2721 may protect against cisplatin-induced nephrotoxicity and neurotoxicity,[139,140] however, this has not been shown in a controlled, randomized trial.

Although it remains unclear whether WR-2721 protects against the toxicity induced by cytotoxic agents, antitumor activity has been seen thus far. In 16 patients with advanced head and neck cancer treated with WR-2721 450–910 mg/m$^2$, nine had objective partial responses.[144] Among 19 patients with malignant melanoma receiving WR-2721, 740 mg/m$^2$, and

**TABLE 19.6** Clinical Trials: WR-2721 as a Chemoprotector

| Institution | # PTS./(#Courses) | Regimen | Reference |
|---|---|---|---|
| U. of Penna. | 12/(22) | WR-2721 450–740 mg/m$^2$<br>Cisplatin 50–120 mg/m$^2$ (no mannitol) | 137 |
| U. of Penna. | 16/(—) | WR-2721 740 mg/m$^2$<br>Cisplatin 120–150 mg/m$^2$ | 138 |
| U. of Penna. | 19/(—) | WR-2721 450–910 mg/m$^2$<br>Cisplatin 50–120 mg/m$^2$ (no mannitol) | 139,140 |
| | 40/(125) | WR-2721 740–910 mg/m$^2$<br>Cisplatin 80–150 mg/m$^2$ (mannitol) | |
| U. of Penna. | 21 | 1st Cycle: Cyclophosphamide 1500 mg/m$^2$<br>2nd Cycle: Cyclophosphamide 1500 mg/m$^2$<br>WR-2721 740 mg/m$^2$ | 141 |
| Georgetown | (13) | 1st Cycle: Cyclophosphamide 1000 mg/m$^2$<br>2nd Cycle: Cyclophosphamide 1000 mg/m$^2$<br>WR-2721 250–1000 mg/m$^2$ | 142 |
| U. of Penna. | 15 | 1st Cycle: Cyclophosphamide 1200–1800 mg/m$^2$<br>WR-2721 450–1100 mg/m$^2$<br>2nd Cycle: Cyclophosphamide<br>versus | 143 |
| | 25 | 1st Cycle: Cyclophosphamide 1200–1800 mg/m$^2$<br>2nd Cycle: Cyclophosphamide<br>WR-2721 450–1100 mg/m$^2$ | |
| U. of Penna. | 5 | Cyclophosphamide 1200–1800 mg/m$^2$<br>WR-2721 450 mg/m$^2$ | 137 |
| | 5 | 1st Cycle: Cyclophosphamide 1200–1800 mg/m$^2$<br>WR-2721 450 mg/m$^2$<br>2nd Cycle: Cyclophosphamide | |

cisplatin, 80–150 mg/m², 11 partial responses were seen. This might indicate that although WR-2721 may protect against chemotherapy-induced toxicity, it does not prevent antitumor activity.

Despite some encouraging preclinical data, WR-2721 has not yet demonstrated clinical benefit as a chemoprotector in a controlled, randomized, clinical trial. In addition, it is possible that higher doses of WR-2721, if clinically tolerated, will be more likely to provide protection.

## DISCUSSION

While progress in the use of radiosensitizers and radioprotectors has seemed incredibly slow over the past decade or more in terms of clinical utility, the potential for clinical impact remains bright. A number of the limitations of previous sensitizers for radiotherapy trials may be overcome with the present generation of hypoxic cell sensitizers; the concern about appropriate scheduling would be put on a firmer footing if some measure of tumor hypoxia were available during the course of therapy.

The use of hypoxic sensitizers for chemosensitization is only beginning, and the trials with SR-2508 will likely be critical to the development of this field of study. The use of radiation protectors together with either radiation or chemotherapy remains in an experimental endeavor, and new agents seem required before positive clinical results are forthcoming.

### ACKNOWLEDGMENTS

This work was supported by Public Health Service Grant CA-34144 from the National Cancer Institute and by the Wayne State University Ben Kasle Trust for Cancer Research.

## REFERENCES

1. Brown JM, Biaglow JE, Hall EJ, et al: Sensitizers and protectors to radiation and chemotherapeutic drugs. Cancer Treatment Symposium 1984;1:85–101.
2. Hall EJ: Radiobiology for the Radiologist, 2nd Ed, Hagerstown: Harper & Row, 1982.
3. Powers WE, Tolmach LJ: Multicomponent x-ray survival curves for mouse lymphosarcoma cells irradiated in vivo. Nature 1963;197:710–711.
4. Fowler JF, Denekamp J: A review of hypoxic cell radiosensitization in experimental tumors. Pharmacol Ther 1979;7:413–444.
5. Bush RS, Jenkin RDT, Allt WEC, et al: Definitive evidence for hypoxic cells influencing cure in cancer therapy. Brit J Cancer 37, Supp III 1978;302–306.

6. Henk JM: Does hyperbaric oxygen have a future in radiation therapy? Int J Radiat Oncol Biol Phys 1981;17:1125–1128.

7. Henk JM, Kunkler PB, Smith CW: Radiotherapy and hyperbaric oxygen in head and neck cancer. Lancet 1977;ii:101–103.

8. Henk JM, Smith CW: Radiotherapy and hyperbaric oxygen in head and neck cancer. Interum report of 2nd clinical trial. Lancet 1977;ii:104–105.

9. Fowler JH: in Meyn RE, Withers HR (eds): Radiation Biology in Cancer Research, New York: Raven Press, 1980, pp 533–546.

10. Dische S: Hyperbaric oxygen: The medical research council trials and their clinical significance. Med J Radiol 1979;51:888–894.

11. Henk JM: Long-term result of hyperbaric oxygen and radiotherapy in head and neck cancer. Proceedings of the Conference on Chemical Modifiers of Cancer Treatment, (Abstr 4–22), October 20–24, 1985.

12. Chang CH, Conley JJ, Herbert C: Radiotherapy of advanced carcinoma of the oropharyngeal region under hyperbaric oxygenation. Amer J Roentgenol 1973;117:509–516.

13. Watson ER, Halnam KE, Dische S, et al: Hyperbaric oxygen and radiotherapy: A Medical Research Council trial in carcinoma of the cervix. Brit J Radiology 1978;51:879–887.

14. Hall EJ, Roizin-Towle L: Hypoxic sensitizers: Radiobiological studies at the cellular level. Radiology 1975;117:453–457.

15. Sheldon PW, Foster JL, Fowler JF: Radiosensitization of C3H mouse mammary tumours by a 2-nitroimidazole drug. Brit J Cancer 1974;30:560–565.

16. Phillips TL, Wasserman TH, Johnson RJ, et al: Final report on the United States phase I clinical trials of the hypoxic cell radiosensitizer, misonidazole (RO-07-0582 NSC #261037). Cancer 1981;48:1697–1704.

17. Dische S: Clinical trials of hypoxic cell sensitizers—the European experience. in Liss A (ed): 13th International Cancer Conference, Part D—Research and Treatment, New York: Alan R. Liss, 1983, pp. 293–303.

18. Wasserman TH, Phillips TL, Ross G, Kane LJ: Differential protection against cytotoxic chemotherapeutic effects on bone marrow CFUs by WR-2721. Cancer Clin Trials 1981;4:3–6.

19. Fazekas JT: The value of adjuvant misonidazole in the definitive irradiation of advanced head and neck squamous cancer. An RTOG pilot study (Abstr). Int J Radiat Oncol Biol Phys (Suppl 2) 1979;5:186.

20. Phillips TL, Wasserman TH, Atetz J: Clinical trials of hypoxic cell sensitizers. Int J Radiat Oncol Biol Phys 1982;8:327–334.

21. Coleman CN: Hypoxic cell radiosensitizers: Expectations and progress in drug developments. Int J Radiat Oncol Biol Phys 1985;11:323–329.

22. Dische S: Chemical sensitizers for hypoxic cells: A decade of experience in clinical radiotherapy. Radiother Oncol 1985;3:97–115.

23. Overgaard J: Misonidazole combined with split-course radiotherapy in the treatment of invasive carcinoma of the larynx and pharynx. cf. ref. 11. (Abstr 1–23).

24. Urtasun RC, Coleman CN, Wasserman TH, Phillips TL: Clinical trials with hypoxic cell sensitizers: Time to retrench or time to push forward? Int J Rad Oncol Biol Phys 1984;10:1691–1699.

25. Fowler JF: Chemical modifiers of radiosensitivity—theory and reality: A review. Int J Radiat Oncol Biol Phys 1985;11:665–674.

26. Hill RP: Sensitizers and radiation dose fractionation: Results and interpretation. Int J Rad Oncol Biol Phys (in press).

27. Brown JM: Clinical trials of radiosensitizers: What should we expect? Int J Rad Oncol Biol Phys 1984;10:425–429.

28. Denekamp J, Hirst DG, Stewart FA, Terry NHA: Is tumour radiosensitization by misonidazole a general phenomenon? Brit J Cancer 1980;41:1–9.

29. Sheldon PW, Hill SA, Foster JL, Fowler JF: Radiosensitization of $C_3H$ mouse mammary tumours using fractionated doses of x-rays with the drug RO-07-0582. Brit J Radiol 1976;49:76–80.

30. Denekamp J, McNally NJ, Fowler JF, Joiner MC: Are many small fractions best? Brit J Radiol 1980;53:981–990.

31. Brown JM, Workman P: Partition coefficient as a guide to the development of radiosensitizers which are less toxic than misonidazole. Radiat Res 1986;82:171–190.

32. Urtasun RC, Coleman CN, Wasserman TH, Phillips TL: Clinical trials with hypoxic cell sensitizers: Time to retrench or time to push forward. Int J Radiat Oncol Biol Phys 1984;10:1691–1696.

33. Denekamp J, Harris SR: The response of a transplantable tumor to fractionated radiation. 1. X-Rays and the hypoxic cell radiosensitizer RO-07-0582. Radiat Res 1976;66:66–75.

34. Chapman JD, Franko AJ, Sharplin J: A marker for hypoxic cells in tumours with potential clinical applicability. Brit J Cancer 1981;43:546–550.

35. Hirst DG, Hazelhurst JL, Brown JM: Changes in misonidazole binding with hypoxic function in mouse tumors. Int J Rad Oncol Biol Phys 1985;11:1349–1355.

36. Bump EA, Taylor YC, Brown JM: Role of glutathione in the hypoxic cell cytotoxicity of misonidazole. Cancer Res 1983;43:997–1002.

37. Varghese AJ: Glutathione conjugates of misonidazole. Biochem Biophys Res Comm 1983;112:1013–1020.

38. Varghese AJ, Whitmore GF: Misonidazole-glutathione conjugates of CHO cells. Int J Rad Oncol Biol Phys 1984;10:1341–1345.

39. Geard CR, Spunberg JJ, Rutledge-Freeman M, Harding T. Genotoxic and cytotoxic effects of three electronic-affinic sensitizers on hypoxic and aerated mammalian cells. Int J Rad Oncol Biol Phys 1982;8:713–717.

40. Hall E, Astor M, Biaglow J, Parkam JC: The enhanced sensitivity of mammalian cells to killing by x-rays after prolonged exposure to several nitroimidazoles. Int J Radiat Oncol Biol Phys 1982;8:447–451.

41. Roizen-Towle L, Hall EJ, Flynn M, et al: Enhanced cytotoxicity of melphalan by prolonged exposure to nitroimidazole: The role of endogenous thiols. Int J Radiat Oncol Biol Phys 1982;8:759–760.

42. Hall EJ, Roizen-Towle L, Hypoxic Sensitizers: Radiobiological studies at the cellular level. Radiology 1975;117:453–457.

43. Brown JM: The mechanisms of cytotoxicity and chemosensitization by misonidazole and other nitroimidazoles. Int J Radio Oncol Biol Phys 1982;8:675–682.

44. Siemann DW: Modification of chemotherapy by nitroimidazoles. Int J Radiat Oncol Biol Phys 1984;10:1585–1594.

45. Rose CM, Millar JL, Peacock JH, et al: Differential enhancement of melphalan cytotoxicity in tumor and normal tissue by misonidazole, in Brady LW (ed): Radiation Sensitizers, Their Use in the Clinical Management of Cancer, New York: Masson Publishing 1980, pp 250–257.

46. McNally NJ. Enhancement of chemotherapy agents. Int J Radiol Oncol Biol Phys 1982;8:593–598.

47. Siemann, DW: Modification of chemotherapy by nitroimidazoles. Int J Radiol Oncol Biol Phys 1984; 10:1584–1594.

48. Clement JJ, Gorman MS, Wodinsky I, et al: Enhancement of antitumor activity of alkylating agents by the radiation sensitizer misonidazole. Cancer Res 1980;40:4165–4172.

49. Stephens TC, Courtenay VD, Mills J, et al: Enhanced cell killing in Lewis lung carcinoma and a human pancreatic-carcinoma xenograft by the combination of cytotoxic drugs and misonidazole. Brit J Cancer 1981;43:451–457.

50. Roizin Towle LA,, Hall EJ: Enhanced cytotoxicity of antineoplastic agents following prolonged exposure to misonidazole. Brit J Cancer 1981;44:201–207.

51. Stratford IJ, Williamson C, Adams GE: Combination studies with misonidazole and a cis-platinum complex: Cytotoxicity and radiosensitization in vitro. Brit J Cancer 1980;41:517–522.

52. Brown JM, Hirst DG: Effect of clinical levels of misonidazole on the response of tumour and normal tissues in the mouse to alkylating agents. Brit J Cancer 1982;45:700–708.

53. Tannock, IF: In vivo interaction of anti-cancer drugs with misonidazole or metronidazole: Cyclophosphamide and BCNU. Brit J Cancer 1980;42:871–880.

54. Horsman MR, Evans JW, Brown JM: Enhancement of melphalan-induced tumour cell killing by misonidazole: An interaction of competing mechanisms. Brit J Cancer 1984;50:305–316.

55. Murray D, Meyn RE: Enhancement of the DNA cross-linking activity of melphalan by misonidazole in vivo. Brit J Cancer 1983;47:195–203.

56. Law MP, Hirst DG, Brown JM: Enhancing effect of misonidazole on the response of the RIF-1 tumour to cyclophosphamide. Brit J Cancer 1981;44:208–218.

57. Coleman CN, Griedman MK, Jacobs C, et al: Phase I trial of intravenous L-phenylalanine mustard plus the sensitizer misonidazole. Cancer Res 1983;43:5022–5025.

58. Davila E, Klein L, Vogel CT, et al: Phase I trial of misonidazole plus cyclophosphamide in solid tumors. J Clin Oncol 1985;3:121–127.

59. Jutsch K, Koeller JM, Earhart RN, et al: Phase I trial and pharmacokinetics of concurrent I.V. Misonidazole and cyclophosphamide. Proc Amer Assoc Clin Oncol 1983;2:29.

60. Bussetti L, Breccia A, Atagn G, et al: Clinical trials with cyclophosphamide and misonidazole combination for maintaining treatment after radiation therapy of lung carcinoma. Int J Rad Oncol Biol Phys 1984;10:1739–1743.

61. Urtason RC, Janasichuk H, Fulton D, et al: Pharmacokinetic interaction of BCNU and misonidazole in humans. Int J Radiat Oncol Biol Phys 1982;8:381–386.

62. Fulton DS, Urtason RC: Misonidazole and CCNU chemotherapy for recurrent primary malignant brain tumor. Proc Amer Soc Clin Oncol 1984;3:266.

63. Stewart DJ, Maroun JA, Young V, et al: Feasibility of combining metronidazole with chemotherapy. J Clin Oncol 1983;1:17–23.

64. Presant CA: Modulation of alkylating agents by radiation sensitizers – clinical aspects, in Valeriote R, Johnson R, Baker L (ed): Biochemical Modulators: Experimental and Clinical Approaches. New York: Martinus Nijhoff, 1986.

65. Coleman CN, Urtasun RC, Wasserman TH, et al: Initial report of the phase I trial of the hypoxic cell radiosensitizer SR-2508. Int J Rad Oncol Biol Phys 1984;10:1749–1753.

66. Hirst DG, Brown JM: The therapeutic potential of misonidazole enhancement of alkylating agent cytotoxicity. Int J Radiol Oncol Biol Phys 1982;8:639–642.

67. Siemann DW, Hill SA: Increased therapeutic benefit through the addition of misonidazole to a nitrosourea-radiation combination. Cancer Res 1986;46:629–632.

68. Brown JM: Cytotoxic effects of the hypoxic cell radiosensitizer RO 7-0582 to tumor cells in vivo. Radiat Res 1977;72:469–486.

69. Brown JM, Yu NY: Cytotoxicity of misonidazole in vivo under conditions of prolonged contact of drug with the tumour cells. Brit J Radiol 1979;52:893–896.

70. Patt HM, Tyree EB, Straube RL, Smith DE: Cysteine protection against x-irradiation. Science 1949;110:213–214.

71. Patt HM, Smith DE, Tyree EB, Straube RL: Further studies on modification of sensitivity to x-rays by cysteine. Proc Soc Exp Biol Med 1950;73:18–21.

72. Bacq ZM, Dechamps G, Fischer P, et al: Protection against x-rays and therapy of radiation sickness with B-mercapto-ethylamine. Science 1985;117:633–636.

73. Alexander P, Bacq ZM, Cousens SF et al: Mode of action of some substances which protect against the lethal effects of x-rays. Radiat Res 1955;2:392–413.

74. Doherty DG, Burnett WT Jr: Protective effect of S,B-Amino-ethylisothiuronium.Br.HBr and related compounds against x-radiation death in mice. Proc Soc Exp Biol Med 1955;89:312–314.

75. Doherty DG, Burnett WT Jr, Shapiro R: Chemical protection against ionizing radiation II. Mercaptoalkylamines and related compounds with protective activity. Radiat Res 1957;7:13–21.

76. Piper JR, Stringfellow CR Jr, Elliott R, Johnston TP: S-2-(W-amino-alkylamino) ethyl dihydrogen phosphorothioates and related compounds as potential antiradiation agents. J Med Chem 1969;12:236–243.

77. Davidson DE, Grenan MM, Sweeney TR: Biological characteristics of some improved radioprotectors. cf. ref. 45, pp. 309–320.

78. Yuhas JM, Storer JB: Chemoprotection against three modes of radiation death in the mouse. Int J Radiat Biol 1969;15:233–237.

79. Yuhas JM, Spellman JM, Culo F: The role of WR-2721 in radiotherapy and chemotherapy. Clin Cancer Trials 1980;3:211–216.

80. Yuhas JM: Biological factors affecting the radioprotective efficiency of S-2-[3-aminopropylamino]-ethylphosphorothioic acid (WR-2721). $LD_{50}(30)$ doses. Radiat Res 1970;44:621–628.

81. Yuhas JM, Storer JB: Differential chemoprotection of normal and malignant tissues. J Natl Cancer Inst 1969;42:331–335.

82. Harris JW, Phillips TL: Radiobiological and biochemical studies of thiophosphate radioprotective compounds related to cysteamine. Radiat Res 1971;46:362–379.

83. Utley JF, Phillips TL, Kane LJ, et al: Differential radioprotection of euoxic and hypoxic mouse mammary tumors by a thiophosphate compound. Radiology 1974;110:213–216.

84. Utley JF, Phillips TL, Kane LJ: Protection of normal tissues by WR-2721 during fractionated irradiation. Int J Radiat Oncol Biol Phys 1976;1:679–703.

85. Phillips T: Rationale for initial clinical trials and future development of radioprotectors. Cancer Clin Trials 1980;3:165–173.

86. Phillips TL, Kane L, Utley JF: Radioprotection of tumor and normal tissues by thiophosphate compounds. Cancer 1973;32:528–535.

87. Yuhas JM: Active versus passive absorption kinetics as the basis for selective protection of normal tissues by S-2-(3-aminopropylamino)-ethylphosphorothioic acid. Cancer Res 1980;40:1519–1524.

88. Milas L, Hunter N, Ito H, et al: Factors influencing radioprotection of tumors by WR-2721, in Nygaard OF, Simic MG (eds): Radioprotectors and Anticarcinogens, Academic Press, 1983, pp. 695–718.

89. Yuhas JM, Proctor JO, Smith LH: Some pharmacologic effects of WR-2721: Their role in toxicity and radioprotection. Radiat Res 1979;54:222–233.

90. Purdie JW: A comparative study of the radioprotective effects of cysteamine, WR-2721 and WR-1065 in cultured human cells. Radiat Res 1979;77:303–311.

91. Laffeur MVM, Woldhuis J, Loman H: Effects of sulfhydryl compounds on the radiation damage in biologically active DNA. Int J Radiat Biol 1980;37:493–498.

92. Livesey JC, Reed DJ, Adamson LF (eds). Radiation-Protective Drugs and Their Reaction Mechanisms, New Jersey: Noyes Publications, 1985.
93. Brown PE: Mechanism of action of aminothiol radioprotectors. Nature 1967;213:363–364.
94. Durand RE: Radioprotection by WR-2721 in vitro at low oxygen tensions: Implications for the mechanisms of action. Brit J Cancer 1983;47:387–392.
95. Shapiro B, Schwartz EE, Kollmann G: The distribution and the chemical forms of the radiation-protective agent AET in mammary tumor-bearing mice. Cancer Res 1963;23:223–228.
96. Yuhas JM, Phillips TL: Pharmacokinetics and mechanism of action of WR-2721 and other protective agents. cf. ref. 88, pp. 639–653.
97. Ito H, Meistrich ML, Barkley T, et al: Protection of acute and late radiation damage of the gastrointestinal tract by WR-2721. Int J Radiat Oncol Biol Phys 1986;12:211–219.
98. Denekamp J, Rojas A, Stewart FA: Is radioprotection by WR-2721 restricted to normal tissues. cf. ref. 88, pp. 655–679.
99. Denekamp J, Michael BD, Rojas A, Stewart FA: Radioprotection of mouse skin by WR-2721: The critical influence of oxygen tension. Int J Radiat Oncol Biol Phys 1982;8:531–534.
100. Phillips TL: Rationale for initial clinical trials and future development of radioprotectors. Cancer Clin Trials 1980;3:165–173.
101. Blumberg AL, Nelson DF, Gramkowski M, et al: Clinical trials of WR-2721 with radiation therapy. Int J Rad Biol Phys 1982;8:561–563.
102. Klingerman MM, Blumberg AL, Glick JW: Phase I trials of WR-2721 in combination with radiation therapy and the alkylating agents cyclophosphamide and cis-platinum. Cancer Clin Trials 1981;4:469–474.
103. Brandt EL, Griffin AC: Reduction of toxicity of nitrogen mustards by cysteine. Cancer 1951;4:1030–1035.
104. Therkelsen AJ: Protective effect of cysteamine on mice injected with nitrogen mustard, in, Mitchell JS, Holmes BE, Smith CL (eds): Progress in Radiobiology, London: Oliver and Boyd, 1956, pp. 260–266.
105. Therkelsen AJ: Studies on the protective action of cysteamine and related compounds against nitrogen mustard (HN2) injected into mice. Acta Radiol 1958;49:49–65.
106. Peczenik O: Influence of cysteineamine, methylamine and cortisone on the toxicity and activity of nitrogen mustard. Nature 1953;172:454–455.
107. Therkelsen AJ: Studies on the mechanism of the protective action of sulphydryl compounds and amines against nitrogen mustard (HN2) and roentgen irradiation in mice. Biochem Pharmacol 1958;1:258–266.
108. Therkelsen AJ: Combined treatment of a transplantable mouse tumor with cysteamine (B-mercaptoethylamine) and nitrogen mustard (HN2). Biochem Pharmacol 1958;1:245–257.
109. Goldenthal EI, Nadkarni MV, Smith PK: A study of comparative protection against lethality of triethylenemelamine, nitrogen mustard and x-irradiation in mice. Radiat Res 1959;5:571–583.
110. Conners TA, Elson LA: Reduction of the toxicity of "radiomimetic" alkylating agents in rats by thiol pretreatment. Biochem Pharmacol 1962;11:1221–1232.
111. Rutman RJ, Lewis FS, Price CC: Experimental chemotherapy studies. IV. The protective action of mercaptoalkylamines against alkylating agents. Cancer Res 1964;24:626–633.
112. Yuhas JM: Differential protection of normal and malignant tissues against the cytotoxic effects of mechlorethamine. Cancer Treat Rep 1979;63:971–976.

113. Yuhas JM, Spellman JM, Jordan SW, et al: Treatment of tumours with the combination of WR-2721 and cis-dichloro-diammineplatinum (11) or cyclophosphamide. Brit J Cancer 1980;42:574–585.

114. Wasserman TH, Phillips TL, Ross G, Kane LJ: Differential protection against cytotoxic chemotherapeutic effects on bone marrow CFUs by WR-2721. Cancer Clin Trials 1981;4:3–6.

115. Phillips TL, Yuhas JM, Wasserman TH: Differential protection against alkylating agent injury in tumors and normal tissues. cf. ref. 88, pp. 735–748.

116. Clement JJ, Johnson RK: Influence of WR-2721 on the efficacy of radiotherapy and chemotherapy of murine tumors. Int J Radiat Oncol Biol Phys 1982;8:539–542.

117. Denekamp J, Stewart FA, Rojas A: Is the outlook grey for WR-2721 as a clinical radioprotector? Int J Rad Oncol Biol Phys 1983;9:1247–1249.

118. Milas L, Hunter N, Ito H, Peters LJ: Effect of tumor type, size and endpoint on tumor radioprotection by WR-2721. Int J Rad Oncol Biol Phys 1984;10:41–48.

119. Stewart FA, Rojas A, Denekamp J: Radioprotection of two mouse tumors by WR-2721 in single and fractionated treatments. Int J Radiat Oncol Biol Phys 1983;9:507–513.

120. Brown JM, Biaglow JE, Hall EJ, et al: Sensitizers and protectors to radiation and chemotherapeutic drugs. Cancer Treat Symp 1984;1:85–101.

121. Valeriote F, Tolen S: Protection and potentiation of nitrogen mustard cytotoxicity by WR-2721. Cancer Res 1982;42:4330–4331.

122. Valeriote F, Grates H: Dose and interval relationship for the interaction of WR-2721 and nitrogen mustard with normal and malignant cells. Int J Radiat Oncol Biol Phys 1984;10:1561–1564

123. Valeriote F, Grates H: Potentiation of nitrogen mustard cytotoxicity to leukemia cells by sulfur-containing compounds administered in vivo. Int J Radiat Oncol Biol Phys (in press).

124. Salerno P, Friedell HL: Studies on the nature of the protective actions of B-mercaptoethylamine and cysteine against x-rays and a nitrogen mustard. Western Reserve Univ., Atomic Energy Medical Research Project, Cleveland, U.S. Atomic Energy Comm. Nuclear Sci. Contract W31-109-eng-78, 1955.

125. Millar JE, McElwain TJ, Clutterbuck RD, Wist EA: The modification of melphalan toxicity in tumour bearing mice by S-2-(3-aminopropylamino)-ethylphosphorothioic acid (WR-2721). Amer J Clin Oncol 1982;5:321–328.

126. Purdie JW: Dephosphorylation of WR-2721 to WR-1065 in vitro and effect of WR-1065 and misonidazole in combination in irradiated cells. cf. ref. 45, pp. 330–333.

127. Deschavanne PJ, Malaise EP, Revesz L: Radiation survival of glutathione-deficient human fibroblasts in culture. Brit J Radiol 1981;54:361–362.

128. Dethmers JK, Meister A: Glutatione export by human lymphoid cells: Depletion of glutathione by inhibition of its synthesis decreases export and increases sensitivity to radiation. Proc Natl Acad Sci 1981;78:7492–7496.

129. Bump EA, Yu NY, Brown JM: Radiosensitization of hypoxic cells by depletion of intracellular glutathione. Science 1982;217:544–545.

130. Murray D, Meyn RE: Enhancement of the DNA cross-linking activity of nitrogen mustard by misonidazole and diethyl maleate in a mouse fibrosarcoma tumor in vivo. Cancer Res 1984;44:91–96.

131. Yuhas JM: A more general role for WR-2721 in cancer therapy. Brit J Cancer 1980;41:832–834.

132. Yuhas JM, Spellman JM, Jordan SW, et al: Treatment of tumours with the combination of WR-2721 and cis-dichlordiamnine platinum (11) or cyclophosphamide. Brit J Cancer 1980;42:574–585.

133. Conference on Chemical Modification: Radiation and Cytotoxic Drugs (Key Biscayne). Int J Radiat Oncol Biol Phys 1982;8:323–815.
134. Chemical Modifiers of Cancer Treatment (Banff). Int J Radiat Oncol Biol Phys 1984;10:1161–1828.
135. Weisberger AS, Heinte RW, Levine B: The effect of L-cysteine on nitrogen mustard therapy. Amer J Med Sci 1951;224:201–211.
136. Glick JH, Glover DJ, Turris A, et al: Clinical trials of WR-2721 with chemotherapy. cf. ref. 88, pp. 719–734.
137. Glick JH, Glover DJ, Weller C, et al: Phase I clinical trials of WR-2721 with alkylating agent chemotherapy. Int J Radiat Oncol Biol Phys 1982;8:575–580.
138. Weisman RA, Glover DJ, Schwartz DM: Limitation of cis-platinum ototoxicity by a protector agent, WR-2721. cf. ref. 11, (Abstr 7–29).
139. Glover D, Glick JH, Weller C, et al: Phase I/II trials of WR-2721 and cis-platinum. cf. ref. 11, (Abstr 7–25).
140. Glover D, Glick JH, Weller C, et al: Phase I trials of WR-2721 and cis platinum. Int J Radiat Oncol Biol Phys 1984;10:1781–1784.
141. Glover D, Glick J, Weller C, Klegerman M: WR-2721 protects against the hematologic toxicity of cyclophosphamide: A controlled Phase II trial. cf. ref. 11 (Abstr 7–28).
142. Woolley PV, Ayoob MJ, Smith J, Dritschelo A: Clinical trial of the effect of S-2-(3-amino-propylamino)-ethyl-phosphorothioic acid (WR-2721) (NSC 296961) on the toxicity of cyclophosphamide. J Clin Oncol 1983;3:198–203.
143. Glick JH, Glover D, Weller C, et al: Phase I controlled trials of WR-2721 and cyclophosphamide. Int J Radiat Oncol Biol Phys 1984;10:1777–1780.
144. Glover D, Weller C, Glick J: Phase II trial of WR-2721 and cis-platinum in metastatic carcinoma of the head and neck. cf. ref. 11, (Abstr 7–26).

# CHAPTER 20

# Principles and Clinical Results of Neutron Therapy of the Head and Neck

*Frank R. Hendrickson, MD*
*K.R. Saroja, MD, and*
*JoAnne Mansell, RN, PA*

## INTRODUCTION

The effective interaction of major cancer treatment disciplines has been clearly demonstrated for the cancers of the upper airway and food passages. In no other major cancer site has the effectiveness of each discipline and the complementary interactions of all of the disciplines been so thoroughly established. In order to develop effective strategies of management to integrate the complementary effects of each of the disciplines, it is imperative that the principles underlying the tumor response to radiation therapy and chemotherapy be thoroughly understood. These principles have been addressed in another chapter in this book; several are of sufficient importance to warrant re-emphasis, particularly with relation to high linear energy transfer (LET) radiations.

A cardinal principle of both radiation therapy and chemotherapy is the exponential response of cells as a function of linear increases in dose. This means that larger tumors require larger doses than small tumors and that sub-clinical disease can be controlled with a lesser dose than needed for overt disease. A second major principle relates to the impact of oxygen on ionizing radiation effects. Cells deficient in oxygen require approximately three times as much dose for the same degree of injury. Cells sufficiently far from the capillary network to be deficient in oxygen almost certainly receive lower concentrations of chemotherapeutic agents as well. This may account for some of the variation in the response of some tumors to chemotherapy. In addition, hypoxia may also impede the effectiveness of specific chemotherapeutic agents.

The use of neutron radiation for the treatment of certain tumors is dependent upon some of the biologic differences in the interaction of photons or other low LET radiations and neutrons. At the molecular level, the distribution of energy from X-rays and electrons is sparse, with many molecules between each of the discreet molecular ionizations. With heavier particles (neutrons are 2000 times the size of electrons), the focal depositions or energy are much closer together, giving a densely ionizing tract. This translates into more effective injury to the principal target of ionizing radiation for cell division, i.e., the DNA molecule.

The relative biologic effectiveness of neutron radiation varies somewhere between 2.5 and perhaps 5 or 6, depending on the tissue evaluated and upon the fraction size of the photon radiation. This greater effectiveness of the densely ionizing tract also reduces the effect of hypoxia from roughly a factor of three to a factor of about 1.5. This means that cells that are protected from low LET radiation because of their oxygen deficiency are much less protected from neutron radiation. An additional difference relates to the cell cycle or cell age at the time of radiation. Cells in $G_1$ phase are generally more resistant to standard forms of radiation therapy than cells in $G_2$ or mitosis. This difference can be several-fold in magnitude. The variation in response to neutrons throughout the cell cycle is significantly decreased and may account for part of the improved effect of neutrons on slowly growing tumors that often have a large proportion of their cells in a prolonged $G_1$ phase.[1] When neutrons are used, the reduction in the magnitude of the shoulder on the surviving fraction curve translates into several important clinical factors. Because of the small or absent shoulder, the summation of neutron doses is essentially linear, meaning that the number of fractions into which the total dose is divided is relatively less important. For photon radiation, the size of the fraction or the total number of fractions is highly important in describing the ultimate biologic effect. The fact that neutrons have a small or absent shoulder means that there is little or no repair of the less than lethal damage and therefore, the timing or interval between fractions is less important than for low LET radiation.

All of these factors interplay in the development of a rationale or strategy for selecting appropriate tumors for neutron radiation. The first factor predictive of a more favorable neutron response would be slow tumor growth. Slow growing tumors respond slowly over a prolonged period of time, since the manifestation of response is a function of when the tumor cells die. Because tumor cells basically die at their next attempt at cell division, tumors that are making an infrequent effort at cell division i.e., with a long cell cycle, will not shrink quickly. Therefore, these tumors will not reoxygenate well and will leave significant hypoxic cells behind that will fail to respond to subsequent fractions. More rapidly proliferating tumors manifest their cell death promptly and show clinical shrinkage, facilitating reoxygenation of the remaining cells. In addition, slow growing tumors tend to have long $G_1$ phases in their cell cycle, leading to a larger proportion of their cells in this relatively X-ray insensitive portion of the cycle. Neutrons, having less cycle dependence, would have a greater effectiveness on $G_1$ cells.

A second factor predictive of a more favorable neutron response would be large tumor size, particularly among those tumors with significant areas of necrosis. The necrotic cells are obviously not a clinical problem, but immediately contiguous to the necrosis are areas of anoxia or hypoxia that are preferentially protected from low LET radiation injury. This type of large tumor may therefore benefit from neutron radiation therapy. Neutrons would be expected to be of less clinical advantage for tumors that have good re-oxygenation or where the tumor has a rapid repopulation. If the tumor repopulation rate approaches or exceeds the repopulation rate of the normal cell renewal system in the region, neutrons and photons would be equally effective.

Several physical characteristics of the neutron beam must be understood from the point of view of normal tissue injury, particularly in the upper airway and food passages. Firstly, neutrons (in comparison to x-rays) are absorbed less in the bone than they are in other tissues. Since the primary interaction of neutrons is with hydrogen atoms, there is preferential protection of bone. In contrast, there is greater absorption in fat, since fat has a high hydrogen content. This puts the subcutaneous fatty tissues and the spinal cord and brain at somewhat greater risk of injury.

Clinical experience with the use of neutrons in the treatment of upper airway and food passage cancers goes back to the early 1940's when Dr. Stone treated a number of patients at a facility in San Francisco.[2,3] The relative biologic effectiveness of neutrons was not well understood at that time and patients were given as much as 50% more dose than was planned. This led to excellent tumor control, but it also led to devastating normal tissue complications. Subsequent clinical trials were delayed until further biologic knowledge was secured. The next major studies came from Dr. Catterall in England in the 1960's.[4-9] These preliminary, but randomized, studies had indicated a superior response by neutrons both in producing complete clinical regression as well as permanent local control. These early studies were so dramatic, both for epidermoid cancers and for various salivary gland histologic types, that is was suspected that the results might look good because the control patients were treated poorly. Subsequent studies done through the Radiation Therapy Oncology Group and other individual observations have tended to confirm a minimal or modest superiority for neutrons for stage IV epidermoid cancers and a highly significant superiority for treatment of salivary tumor types, both in the major salivary gland sites as well as minor salivary gland locations throughout the mouth and throat.[10,11]

## MATERIALS AND METHODS

Groups of 118 patients with salivary gland tumors and 81 patients with epidermoid carcinoma were treated with fast neutrons at Fermi National Accelerator Laboratory, Neutron Therapy Facility, between September 1976 and December 1984. Table 20.1 shows distribution of patients with salivary gland tumors according to location.

Sixty-three patients (53.4%) had major salivary gland tumors. Fifty-one pe⁻ients (80.9%) had parotid gland tumors and 12 patients (19%) had submaxillary gland involvement. Fifty-five patients (47%) had minor salivary gland tumors; major locations were in the oropharynx, maxillary sinus (29% each) and oral cavity (18.2%). There were five patients (9.1%) with the trachea as the primary location of the disease.

Tables 20.2 and 20.3 show the distribution of patients with epidermoid carcinoma in head and neck according to site and stage.

The oral cavity and oropharynx were the primary sites in 49 patients (60.5%); 64 patients (89%) had stage III and IV cancers. There were 72 patients with primary lesions and nine with recurrent lesions.

A total of 113 patients with salivary gland tumors and 81 patients with

**TABLE 20.1** Distribution of Salivary Gland Tumors: Head and Neck

| Site | Number of Patients |
|---|---|
| Major (63) | |
| Parotid | 51 (81%) |
| Submaxillary | 12 (19%) |
| Minor (55) | |
| Oropharynx | 16 (29%) |
| Oral cavity | 10 (18.2%) |
| Maxillary sinus | 16 (29%) |
| Nasal cavity | 3 (5.5%) |
| Nasopharynx | 3 (5.5%) |
| Trachea | 5 (9.1%) |
| Larynx | 1 (1.8%) |
| Neck (unknown primary) | 1 (1.8%) |
| TOTAL | 118 |

**TABLE 20.2** Epidermoid Carcinoma: Head and Neck by Site

| Site | Number of Patients |
|------|--------------------|
| Oral cavity | 23 (28%) |
| Oropharynx | 26 (32%) |
| Larynx | 12 (15%) |
| Hypopharynx | 13 (16%) |
| Neck nodes | 6 (4%) |
| Sinuses | 1 (1.2%) |
| TOTAL | 81 |

epidermoid carcinoma who completed the treatments were analyzed for local control, sites of failure, survival, and treatment-related morbidity.

## TECHNIQUE

66 MeV protons are bombarded on a thin, beryllium target to produce neutrons. The physical beam characteristics, depth dose distribution, and skin sparing effects, are similar to 6 MeV X-rays.[12] The relative biological effectiveness of this beam for soft tissue is three, and for the central nervous system, it is estimated to be four.[13] Because of the fixed horizontal beam, the patients are treated in a seated position in an isocentrically mounted chair with capabilities of front to back, side to side, and rotational movements. The patients are immobilized with Lightcast II tape. Treatment plans are individualized for each patient. The target volume included at least a 1 cm margin around the tumor. An attempt was always made to spare the contralateral mouth and neck, especially in patients with salivary gland tumors. In planning, efforts were made to keep the spinal cord dose limited to 12.5 Gy.

Typical isodose distributions for patients with tumors of the parotid gland and other locations in the head and neck area are shown in Figures 20.1 and 20.2.

**TABLE 20.3** Epidermoid Carcinoma: Head and Neck by Stage

| Stage | Number of Patients |
|-------|--------------------|
| Stage I | 0 (0%) |
| Stage II | 8 (11.1%) |
| Stage III | 13 (18.1%) |
| Stage IV | 51 (71%) |
| Recurrent | 9 |
| TOTAL | 81 |

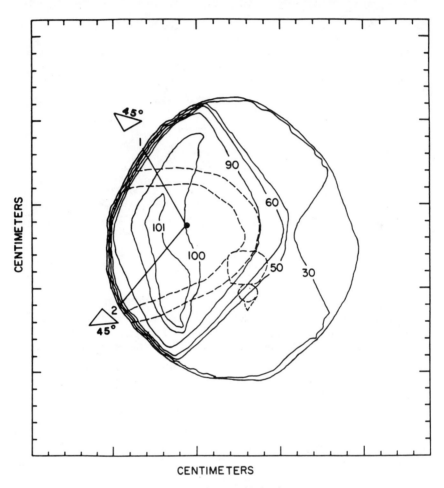

**FIGURE 20.1** Typical isodose distribution for parotid gland tumor.

## FOLLOW-UP

Most of the patients had regular follow-up examinations at the Neutron Therapy Facility. A few of the out-of-state patients were followed by radiation oncologists who also are familiar with our facility, and evaluations were sent to us. The follow-up evaluation included a complete physical examination, with special attention to neutron treatment related side effects. Periodic CT scans and chest X-rays were obtained as indicated. All suspected recurrent disease was confirmed by biopsy.

## RESULTS

The results of local control for salivary gland tumors are shown in Table 20.4 and Table 20.5. Forty-one (67.2%) of 61 patients in the group of major salivary gland tumors had local tumor control. Fourteen patients (23%) had persistent disease and only six (9.8%) had local recurrence. Out of 41 patients with local control, 10 patients (24.4%) developed distant metastatic disease and five patients (12.2%) developed regional disease. Of fourteen patients with persistent disease, six (43%) had regional failures, and two (14.3%)

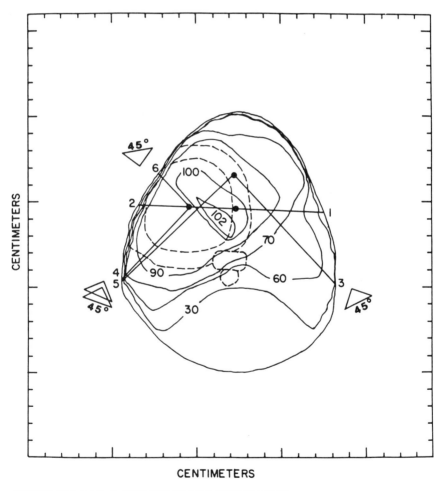

**FIGURE 20.2** Isodose distribution for head and neck tumors.

**TABLE 20.4** Major Salivary Gland Tumors: Local Control and Sites of Failure (%)

| Dose Range (Gy.) | Number of Patients | Local Cont. % | Local Rec. % | Persis. Disease % | Dist. Mets Only % | Reg. Rec. Only % | Reg. Rec. + Dist. Mets % | Persis. Dis. + Reg. Rec. % | Persis. Dis. + Dist. Mets % |
|---|---|---|---|---|---|---|---|---|---|
| 20.00 or less | 14 | 9 (64.3%) | 0 | 5 | 3 | 0 | 2 | 2 | 0 |
| 20.01–22.00 | 31 | 20 (65%) | 5△○ | 6 | 5 | 3 | 1 | 3 | 1 |
| 22.01–24.00 | 10 | 6 (60%) | 1△ | 3 | 1 | 1◊ | 0 | 1 | 1 |
| >24.00 | 6 | 6 (100%) | 0 | 0 | 1 | 1 | 0 | 0 | 0 |
| TOTAL | 61 | 41 (67.2%) | 6 (9.8%) | 14 (23%) | 10 (16.4%) | 5 (8.2%) | 3 (5%) | 6 (9.8%) | 2 (3.3%) |

△One patient in each group had regional recurrence.
○One patient had distant metastases.
◊One patient was salvaged by photon radiation.

**TABLE 20.5** Minor Salivary Gland Tumors: Local Control and Sites of Failure (%)

| Dose Range (Gy.) | Number of Patients | Local Cont. % | Local Rec. % | Persis. Disease % | Dist. Mets Only % | Reg. Rec. Only % | Reg. Rec. + Dist. Mets % | Persis. Dis. + Reg. Rec. % | Persis. Dis. + Dist. Mets % |
|---|---|---|---|---|---|---|---|---|---|
| 20.00 or less | 9 | 4 (44.4) | 2△○ | 3 | 2 | 0 | 0 | 2 | 1 |
| 20.01–22.00 | 21* | 14 (66.6) | 4+Φ○ | 2 | 3 | 2 | 0 | 0 | 1 |
| 22.01–24.00 | 13 | 9 (69.2) | 1○ | 3 | 3 | 1 | 0 | 0 | 1 |
| >24.00 | 9 | 3 (33.3%) | 4●†θ | 2 | 0 | 1 | 0 | 1 | 1 |
| TOTAL | 52 | 30 (57.7%) | 11 (21.2%) | 10 (19.2%) | 8 (15.4%) | 4 (7.7%) | 0 | 3 (5.8%) | 4 (7.7%) |

*Local disease status remains unknown.
△One patient had both regional recurrence and distant metastases.
○One patient in each group had distant metastases.
ΦTwo patients in the group had regional recurrence.
●One patient had regional recurrence.
†Two patients had distant metastases.
θDistant metastases status remains unknown.
+One patient was salvaged by surgery and remains locally NED.

progressed to develop distant failures. Two patients with local recurrence also had regional disease, and one had distant disease as well. One patient with regional failure was successfully treated with photons.

Thirty patients (58%) of 52 with minor salivary gland tumors had local control. Ten patients (19%) had persistent disease, and 11 (21.2%) had local recurrence. Of these 11 patients, four failed regionally and six failed distantly. One patient with local recurrence was successfully treated with radical surgery and remained NED. Of 30 patients with local control, eight developed distant metastatic disease and four developed regional disease. Of ten patients with persistent disease, three failed regionally and four progressed to develop distant metastatic disease.

In patients with minor salivary gland tumors, local control was analyzed according to the site (Table 20.6). Though the patient number in each group was small, interestingly, 13 of 14 patients with oropharynx lesions had local control (93%). Six of ten patients (60%) with oral cavity lesions had control of their disease. Four of six patients and three of five patients with nasal cavity, nasopharynx, and tracheal disease, respectively, had local control. However, only four patients of 15 with maxillary sinus disease had local control.

Local control was also analyzed according to the categories of patients based on treatment and the results are shown in Table 20.7.

No significant differences in rate of local control were noted when neutrons were used either for recurrence after primary surgical therapy (67%), or as postoperative adjuvant therapy for gross residual disease (64%). However there was significantly better local control when primarily neutrons were used after biopsy than when they were used only for boost after photons (62.1% versus 50%). An important observation was that 70% (7/10) had control of their disease when neutrons were used for patients who had recurrent disease after surgery and conventional radiation.

**TABLE 20.6** Minor Salivary Gland Tumors (Subgroups) Neutrons — Local Control

| Sites | Number of Patients | Local Control % |
|---|---|---|
| Oropharynx | 14* | 13 (93%) |
| Oral cavity | 10 | 6 (60%) |
| Maxillary sinus | 15** | 4 (27%) |
| Nasal cavity and nasopharynx | 6 | 4 (67%) |
| Trachea | 5 | 3 (60%) |
| Larynx | 1 | 0 |
| Neck | 1 | 0 |
| TOTAL | 52 | 30 (58%) |

*Status of local control in one patient is unknown.
**Local recurrence salvaged by surgery in one patient.

**TABLE 20.7** Salivary Gland Tumors Categories of Patients Based on Treatment

| Patient Groups | Number of Patients | Local Control % |
|---|---|---|
| Neutrons as primary treatment | 29 | 18 (62.1%) |
| Neutrons for boost after photons | 14** | 7 (50%) |
| Neutrons for post-op. residual disease | 36 | 23 (64%) |
| Neutrons after recurrent disease after primary surgical treatment | 24 | 16 (67%) |
| Neutrons for recurrent disease after surgery and conv. rad | 10* | 7 (70%) |
| TOTAL | 113 | 71 (63%) |

*Status of local disease in one patient is unknown.

**One patient received 7000 rads of electrons ten years prior to current 4000 rads of photons and neutron boost.

Seventy-four percent of patients (62/84) had local control when their measurable disease was less than 5 cm., and only 31% of the patients (9/29) had local control of their disease with larger lesions (Table 20.8). Nine of these 29 patients had lesions measuring larger than 8 cm, with the largest measuring 15 × 14 cm.

Table 20.9 shows local control results in patients with epidermoid cancer in the head and neck region treated with neutrons only. Six out of 8 patients (75%) with stage II disease had local control. The local control rate of stage III and IV patients together was 52% (33/64), which was lower than that for salivary gland tumors. Distant metastatic disease in epidermoid cancer occurred in 14 patients (17.3%); six of these had metastatic disease as the only site, whereas eight had distant metastatic disease in combination with regional and/or local persistant disease. Twenty percent of the patients (16/81) had regional failure. Four of these 16 patients experienced regional failure only, and ten patients had regional failure in combination with other sites. Twenty-seven patients (33.3%) had persistent disease. Thirteen patients had local recurrent disease, and eight had only local failure, whereas five patients had failures in other sites as well.

**TABLE 20.8** Salivary Gland Tumors Size of Lesion — Local Control

| Size of Lesion | Number of Patients | Local Control % |
|---|---|---|
| 5 cm or less | 84 | 62 (74%) |
| >5 cm | 29 | 9 (31%) |
| TOTAL | 113 | 71 (63%) |

**TABLE 20.9** Epidermoid Carcinoma: Head and Neck Local Control—Neutrons Only

| Stage | Number of Patients | Local Control % |
|---|---|---|
| Stage II | 8 | 6 (75%) |
| Stage III | 13 | 8 (61.5%) |
| Stage IV | 51 | 25 (49%) |
| Recurrent | 9 | 3 (33.3%) |
| TOTAL | 81 | 42 (52%) |

Table 20.10 summarizes the major treatment morbidity including both epidermoid and salivary gland tumors. Patients who received prior low LET radiation were excluded from mobidity analysis. The RTOG/EORTC late radiation morbidity scoring system was used. Persistent tumor at the primary site causing ulceration was not scored as treatment morbidity. Persistent ulceration, symptomatic severe fibrosis, and xerostomia that needed medical or surgical intervention was scored as major morbidity. Out of 168 evaluable patients, a total of 32 patients had moderate morbidity. Bone necrosis was precipitated by tooth extraction in two patients. The patient who developed severe xerostomia had smoked heavily and consumed large amounts of alcohol. In the patient who developed a loss of vision, the original extension of the tumor had necessitated inclusion of the ipsilateral eye in the high dose target volume. Necrosis of the larynx and trachea ended fatally in

**TABLE 20.10** Head and Neck Cancer—Major Morbidity Neutrons Only

| Morbidity | Number of Patients | Comments |
|---|---|---|
| Subcutaneous fibrosis | 7 | One patient required tracheostomy |
| Soft tissue necrosis | 7 | All healed with conservative management |
| Cartilage necrosis | 7 | Fatal in four patients |
| Osteoradionecrosis | 7 | Precipitated by tooth extraction in 2/7 |
| | | All but one patient functioning well with conservative management and/or partial mandibulectomy |
| Brain | 2 | Craniotomy |
| Blindness | 1 | Eye in the target volume |
| Severe xerostomia | 1 | Required gastrostomy |
| | | Patient continued heavy smoking and alcohol consumption |
| TOTAL | 32 | |

four patients. One of these patients had undergone multiple resections prior to neutron therapy; another patient developed necrosis following repeated biopsies post-therapy (no tumor was found at autopsy). Six of the seven patients with osteoradionecrosis are functioning well with minimal morbidity following either conservative management or partial resection of the mandible.

## CNS AND PERIPHERAL NERVE INJURIES

None of the patients in this series have developed overt myelopathy. Results of evaluation of patients followed for one to five years after neutron radiation has been previously published.[13] RBE for the human spinal cord for neutrons compared to conventional radiation apparently does not exceed four.

Table 20.11 shows major morbidity versus neutron dose delivered in head and neck cancer. A definite correlation was found between total dose delivered and major morbidity.

### Survival

Figures 20.3 and 20.4 show the survival curves for 81 patients with epidermoid carcinoma and 113 patients with salivary gland tumors. The observed median survival for salivary gland tumors is 38.4 months. Adjusted observed median survival, adjusted for intercurrent disease, is 47 months. Median duration of survival when this disease is locally controlled is 86.3 months. The longest follow-up period is 106 months, and the minimum follow-up period is 18 months. For epidermoid carcinomas, observed median survival is 11.5 months and adjusted observed median survival is 15.8 months. Median duration of survival when this disease is locally controlled is 23.9 months. The longest survival time in this group is 53.4 months. As it has

**TABLE 20.11** Head and Neck Cancer Dose vs. Major Morbidity Neutrons Only

| Dose Range (Gy.) | Number of Patients | Complications No./(%) |
|---|---|---|
| 16–18 | 0 | 0 (0%) |
| 18–20 | 3 | 0 |
| 20–22 | 30 | 3 (16%) |
| 22–24 | 88 | 16 |
| 24–26 | 24 | 8 (28%) |
| 26–28 | 23 | 5 |
| TOTAL | 168 | 32 (19%) |

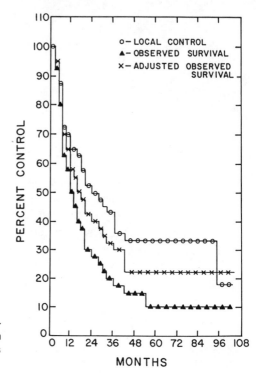

**FIGURE 20.3** Survival curves in patients with epidermoid carcinoma in the head and neck region—neutrons only.

been previously reported,[11] the patients with salivary gland tumors survive longer than patients with epidermoid carcinomas.

## DISCUSSION

Optimal management of patients with locally advanced head and neck cancers is a perpetual challenge for oncologists. Combined modalities, surgery, radiation, and chemotherapy are all used in various combinations. Fast neutron radiation therapy for treating patients with locally advanced head and neck cancer has been in vogue for at least four decades. Catterall et al. reported a local control rate with neutrons of 90% in salivary gland tumors and 76% in locally advanced head and neck cancers.[7,9] In our series, the overall control rate of 52% in stage III and stage IV disease for epidermoid carcinoma patients, although fairly comparable to reports by M.D. Anderson Hospital in Houston, Texas,[14-16] is low when compared to reports of randomized trials from Hammersmith.[7] At Hammersmith, the target volume encompassed only gross tumor and uninvolved areas were not in-

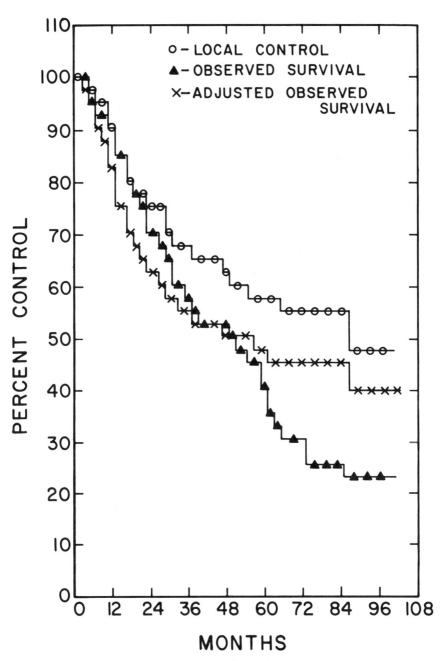

**FIGURE 20.4** Survival curves in patients with salivary gland tumors.

cluded. This probably explains the higher tumor control with greater sparing of normal tissues in their series. Superiority of neutrons in treatment of non-epidermoid tumors, especially the salivary gland type, is well established.[9,17] Results with conventional radiation therapy in controlling gross residual disease was reported between 10–40%.[18-20] Henry et al.,[21] in their series of 30 patients, reported 100% local control (4/4) with neutron treatments of lesions sized 3–6 cm and only 33% local control (2/6) with photon treatments. In the above series, the number of patients was small in each group and the period of follow-up was short. Our results in patients with lesions smaller than 5 cm is 74%, which is slightly lower when compared to the above report.

An interesting observation in the subgroup of minor salivary glands in our series is that 93% (13/14) patients with oropharyngeal lesions had local control. This needs to be confirmed in a larger group of patients. In this series, seven of ten patients with salivary gland tumors who were re-irradiated achieved local control. This finding is comparable to a recent report from Hammersmith.[22] Results in a larger group of patients who were similarly re-irradiated at our facility will be reported soon. Recently there have been reports about combining concurrent or sequential chemotherapy and conventional radiation therapy for patients with locally advanced head and neck cancers. The efficacy of this approach is suggestive but not yet firmly established.[23,24] The possible benefit of combining chemotherapy and neutron radiation has not yet been investigated. In general, the strategy for managing inoperable patients would suggest that neutrons alone may be somewhat superior to photons and electrons alone. Whether simultaneous or prior chemotherapy would be of advantage, needs yet to be investigated.

## CONCLUSIONS

Neutron therapy differs from standard photon or electron radiation therapy because of the biologic differences in the mechanisms of absorption of energy; this translates into a greater radiobiologic effectiveness and a lesser dependence on oxygen status, cell cycle status, and type of fractionation. In the mouth and throat area, this biologic advantage could lead to better management of the non-epidermoid cancers. There may also be a small, but definite advantage for epidermoid cancers, particularly among localized stage IV patients. The risks of normal tissue injury with neutrons compared to photon radiation are somewhat less for bone injury, but somewhat greater for subcutaneous fibrosis and potential spinal cord or brain injury.

Current policies for managing patients who have had all gross tumor resected suggest that postoperative low LET radiations with X-rays or electrons have a high probability of reducing local recurrence rates and that neutrons would not appear to be appropriate. The best management of patients who have had a good response to preliminary chemotherapy is still in question. Radical surgery, which may lead to disfigurement and dysfunction, seems hard to justify in the absence of demonstrable disease. Perhaps patients achieving a CR to chemotherapy should have aggressive standard irradiation to consolidate the therapeutic effect; surgery might be reserved as a salvage procedure. For patients having less than a total response to chemotherapy, neutrons might be considered an alternative to the surgical resection.

## ACKNOWLEDGMENTS

The authors would like to thank Mrs. Laurie Hanabarger for typing the manuscript and the neutron therapy staff for making this a success.

# REFERENCES

1. Battermann JJ, Breur K, Hart GAM: Observations on pulmonary metastases in patients after single doses and multiple fractions of fast neutrons and Cobalt-60 gamma rays. Eur J Cancer 1981;17:539–548.
2. Stone RS, Larkin JC Jr: The treatment of cancer with fast neutrons. Radiology 1942;39:608–620.
3. Stone RS, Lawrence JH, Aebersold PC: A preliminary report on the use of fast neutrons in the treatment of malignant disease. Radiology 1940;35:322–327.
4. Catterall, M: The treatment of patients with fast neutrons from the Medical Research Council's Cyclotron at Hammersmith Hospital, London. Proc Conf Particle Accelerators Rad Ther Los Alamos Scientific Laboratory report LA-5180-C. (U.S. Atomic Energy Commission Technical Information Center, Oak Ridge, Tenn.).
5. Catterall M: The treatment of advanced cancer by fast neutrons from Medical Research Council's Cyclotron at Hammersmith Hospital, London. Eur J Cancer 1974;10:343–347.
6. Catterall M, Vonberg DD: Treatment of advanced tumors of head and neck with fast neutrons. Brit Med J 1974;3:137–143.
7. Catterall M, Beweley DK: Second report on results of a randomized clinical trial of fast neutrons compared with X or gamma rays in treatment of advanced tumors of head and neck. Brit Med J 1977;1:1642.
8. Catterall M: Factors influencing the results of treatment with fast neutrons from the Medical Research Council's Cyclotron at Hammersmith Hospital, London, Surg. Radiother. Chemother. Cancer 1975;5:149–153.
9. Catterall M, Bewley D: Malignant Tumors of Salivary Glands. Fast Neutrons in the Treatment of Cancer, New York: Grune and Stratton, 1979, pp. 219–234.
10. Griffin TW, Davis R, Laramore G, et al: Fast neutron irradiation of metastatic cervical adenopathy: The results of a randomized RTOG study. Int J Radiat Oncol Biol Phys 1983;9:1267–1270.
11. Kurup PD, Mansell J, Ten Haken, et al: Response of epidermoid and non-epidermoid cancers of the head and neck to fast neutron irradiation: The Fermilab Experience. Int J Radiation Oncol Biol Phys, 1984;10:473–479.

12. Cohen L, Awschalom M: The cancer therapy facility at the Fermi National Accelerator Laboratory: A preliminary report. Appl Radiol 1976;5(6):51–60.
13. Cohen L, Ten Haken, Randall K: Tolerance of the human spinal cord to high energy p(66)Be(49) neutrons. Int J Radiation Oncol Biol Phys 1985;11:743–749.
14. Maor MH, Hussey DH, Barkley T Jr, Jesse RH: Further follow-up on M.D. Anderson trial on fast neutron therapy for head and neck cancer. Int J Radiat Oncol Biol Phys 1981;7:1212–1213.
15. Maor MH, Hussey DH, Fletcher GM, Jesse RH: Fast neutron therapy for locally advanced head and neck tumors. Int J Radiat Oncol Biol Phys 1981;7:155–163.
16. Batterman JJ, Breuer K: Results of the fast neutron teletherapy for locally advanced head and neck tumors. Int J Radiat Oncol Biol Phys 1981;7:1045–1050.
17. Kaul R, Hendrickson F, Cohen L, et al: Fast neutrons in the treatment of salivary gland tumors. Int J Radiat Oncol Biol Phys 1981;7:1667–1671.
18. Elkon D, Colman M, Hendrickson FR: Radiation therapy in the treatment of malignant salivary gland tumors. Cancer 1978;41:502–506.
19. Chung CT, Sagerman RH, Ryoo MC, et al: The changing role of external-beam irradiation in the management of malignant tumors of the major salivary glands. Radiology 1982;145:175–177.
20. Shidnia H, Hornback NB, Hamaker R, Lindeman R: Carcinoma of major salivary glands. Cancer 1980;45:693–697.
21. Henry LW, Blasko JC, Griffin TW, Pancer, RG: Evaluation of fast neutron teletherapy for advanced carcinoma of the major salivary glands. Cancer 1979;44:814–818.
22. Errington RD, Catterall M: Re-irradiation of advanced tumors of the head and neck with fast neutrons. Int J Radiat Oncol Biol Phys 1986;12:191–195.
23. Leipzig B: Cisplatin Sensitization to radiotherapy of squamous cell carcinoma of the head and neck. Amer J Surgery 1983;145:462–465.
24. Coughlin CT, Grace M, O'Donnell JF: Combined modality approach in the management of locally advanced head and neck cancer. Cancer Treat Rep 1984;68:591–597.

# CHAPTER 21

# Clinical Results of Simultaneous Chemotherapy and Radiotherapy in Head and Neck Cancer

*Karen K. Fu, MD*

## INTRODUCTION

Chemotherapy has been combined with radiotherapy in the treatment of advanced head and neck cancer with the objectives of increasing local control, decreasing distant metastasis, and increasing survival. When chemotherapy is combined with radiotherapy, improved tumor control can result from the additive or direct interaction between the two modalities. Possible mechanisms of interaction between chemotherapy and radiotherapy that may result in an enhanced tumor cell kill include: (1) modification of the slope of the dose response curve, (2) decreased accumulation, or inhibition of repair of sublethal damage, (3) inhibition of recovery from potentially lethal damage, (4) perturbation in cell kinetics with an increase in the proportion of cells in the sensitive phases of the cell cycle and proliferative state, (5) decreased tumor bulk leading to improvement of blood supply, reoxygenation, recruitment, increased radiosensitivity, and chemosensitivity, and (6) increased drug delivery and uptake.[16] For a direct interaction to occur, it may require that the two modalities be administered simultaneously or in close temporal proximity.

Up to the late 1970s, in most studies combining radiotherapy and chemotherapy, only single agents were used and most often they were administered concurrently. More recently, multi-agent chemotherapy has been combined with radiotherapy either concurrently or sequentially. Most of the clinical trials combining radiotherapy and chemotherapy in head and

**321**

neck cancer have been nonrandomized.[17] Randomized studies are few and positive results are rare. This chapter will review the clinical advantages and toxic effects of simultaneous chemotherapy and radiotherapy in previously untreated head and neck cancer, with emphasis on randomized trials.

## CONCURRENT SINGLE AGENT CHEMOTHERAPY AND RADIOTHERAPY
### Bleomycin

Bleomycin has been the chemotherapeutic agent most frequently combined with radiotherapy in the treatment of head and neck cancer. There are at least 14 studies of simultaneous bleomycin and radiotherapy for head and neck cancer.[6,11,15,19,28,29,38,47,49,51,52,54,57,58] The complete response rates range from 38% to 79%, and the local control rates range from 31% at one year to 53% at 5 years. Six of these studies were randomized.[11,19,29,38,52,58] Results of randomized clinical trials of concurrent radiotherapy and bleomycin are summarized in Table 21.1. Although four of the studies showed an improved complete response rate and/or local-regional control rate,[19,29,38,52] only the trial on oral cavity cancer from India and the NCOG (Northern California Oncology Group) trial showed an advantage in survival with the combined treatment.[52,19]

With concurrent radiotherapy and bleomycin, increased acute toxicities such as radiation mucositis and skin reaction, dysphagia, weight loss, and weakness were observed in all these studies. A dose effect factor (DEF = isoeffect dose of radiation alone/isoeffect dose of radiation plus chemotherapy) of 1.5 for a 50% incidence of confluent mucositis has been reported.[38] The degree of acute toxicity varied with the bleomycin dose. With doses greater than five units twice weekly, severe mucositis often led to interruption of treatment and reduction of total radiation dose.[11,52] However none of the studies reported a significant increase of late normal tissue toxicity.

### 5-Fluorouracil (5-FU)

5-FU has been administered concurrently with radiotherapy in at least seven studies,[10,22,26,30,34,48,53] with complete response rates in the range of 40–69% and the 2-year local-regional control rates in the range of 38–49%. Two of these were randomized,[34,53] and the results are summarized in Table 21.2. In the randomized study from Japan,[53] 5-FU was infused intra-arterially during radiotherapy for maxillary sinus carcinomas. The non-recurrence rate of patients who received 5-FU was significantly better at one year but not at 2

**TABLE 21.1** Randomized Studies of Concurrent Radiotherapy and *Bleomycin* in Head and Neck Cancer

| Author/Date | Evaluable Patients | Complete Response Rate (1° ± N) | | % Local-Regional Control (yrs) | | % Survival (yrs) | | Significant |
|---|---|---|---|---|---|---|---|---|
| | | RT | RT + CT | RT | RT + CT | RT | RT + CT | |
| Cachin et al., 1977 (11) | 186 | 68% | 67% | N/A | N/A | 45% (2) | 42% (2) | No |
| Kapstad et al., 1978 (29) | 29 | 14% | 27% | N/A | N/A | N/A | N/A | No |
| Shanta and Krishnamurthis, 1980 (52) | 157 | 19% | 79% | N/A | N/A | 24% (5) | 66% (5) | Yes |
| Morita, 1980 (38) | 45 | N/A | N/A | 65% (2) | 73% (2) | N/A | N/A | No |
| Vermund et al., 1985 (58) | 222 | 58% | 63% | 58% (5) | 53% (5) | 42% (5) | 38% (5) | No |
| Fu et al., 1986 (19) | 96 | 45% | 67% | 26% (2) | 64.7% (2) | 25% (3) | 48% (3) | Yes |

1° = Primary; N = Node; yrs = Years; RT = Radiotherapy; CT = Chemotherapy

**TABLE 21.2** Randomized Studies of Concurrent Radiotherapy and 5-Fluorouracil in Head and Neck Cancer

| Author/Date | Evaluable Patients | Complete Response Rate (1° ± N) | | % Local-Regional Control (yrs) | | % Survival (yrs) | | Significant |
|---|---|---|---|---|---|---|---|---|
| | | RT | RT + CT | RT | RT + CT | RT | RT + CT | |
| Shigematsu et al., 1971 (53) | 63 | N/A | N/A | 29% (2) | 38% (2) | 59% (2) | 56% (2) | No |
| Lo et al., 1976 (34) | 138 | 32% | 44% | 18% (2) | 49% (2) | 13% (5) | 32% (5) | Yes |

1° = Primary; N = Node; yrs = Years; RT = Radiotherapy; CT = Chemotherapy

years, and the 2-year crude survival rate was similar for the study and control groups. The randomized study from the University of Wisconsin included patients with oropharygeal as well as oral cavity cancers.[34] Although the 2-year NED rate was significantly better in the combined treatment group (18% vs. 49%, p < 0.05), the 5-year survival was statistically significant only in patients with oral cavity cancer (13% vs. 40%, p < 0.05). However, the incidences of distant metastasis and second malignancies were similar for both the radiotherapy and combined treatment groups. 5-FU also increased the acute and late normal tissue effects of radiation. Major complications such as soft tissue or bone necrosis or fistula formation were seen only in the combined treatment group in this study.

In nonrandomized studies, acute and late injury to the eye, including keratoconjunctivitis, retinal and optic nerve damage, and blindness have been reported when 5-FU was infused intra-arterially during radiotherapy of carcinoma of the nasal cavity and paranasal sinuses.[22,48] However these effects might have occurred without the chemotherapy.

## Cisplatin

Recently, cisplatin has been used with increasing frequency in the treatment of advanced or recurrent head and neck cancer. Most often it has been used in combination with other chemotherapeutic agents and administered sequentially with radiotherapy. It has also been used as a single agent concurrent with radiotherapy in at least seven studies.[2,9,13,14,23,33,43] The only randomized trial was initiated by the ECOG (Eastern Cooperative Oncology Group), and now continued by both the ECOG and RTOG (Radiation Therapy Oncology Group). Although the ECOG pilot study showed a complete response rate of 83%,[23] and unpublished recent update of this trial showed a complete response rate of only 31% for the entire group of patients and no difference between radiotherapy and combined treatment groups.[43]

Cisplatin also increased radiation mucositis. The degree of enhancement varied with the drug dose. In the ECOG pilot study, marked increase of severe mucositis was observed with a cisplatin dose of 30 mg/m$^2$/week, but not with a dose of 10–20 mg/m$^2$/week. In their ongoing randomized trial, the dose of cisplatin is 20 mg/m$^2$/week.

## Methotrexate

There have been many studies combining methotrexate with radiotherapy for head and neck cancer. In most of these studies, methotrexate was administered primarily before radiotherapy. Concurrent radiotherapy and methotrexate were used in at least six studies,[4,12,31,35,37,42] however, only one of these was randomized.[12] Complete response rates were in the range of 20% to 68%, and local-regional control rates were in the range of 44% at 2 years to 32% at 3 years.

In the randomized study by Condit,[12] 40 patients with advanced head and neck cancer received split course radiotherapy alone or in combination with intravenous methotrexate every 2 weeks for four doses. Five patients in each treatment group failed to complete the planned treatment because of complications of advanced disease. The complete response rate was 60% with radiotherapy alone and 45% with the combined treatment. Survival rates were not reported.

Enhanced radiation mucositis was more often seen with concurrent than with sequential drug and radiation administration. Late normal tissue toxicity was also more common with concurrent drug and radiotherapy. Lustig et al. observed the following incidence rates with concurrent methotrexate and radiotherapy: 25% soft tissue complications, 25% severe edema, 4% bone necrosis and 6% severe fibrosis.[35] With sequential methotrexate and radiotherapy, the incidence of soft tissue complication decreased to 14%, severe edema decreased to 22% and there was no bone necrosis or severe fibrosis.

Thus, methotrexate appeared to increase the acute and late normal tissue toxicity of radiotherapy without improving the tumor response or patient survival when it was administered during the course of radiotherapy.

## Hydroxyurea

Hydroxyurea was used as a radiosensitizer in at least six studies.[25,32,44-46,56] The complete response rates were in the range of 42–73%. Three of the studies were randomized and the results are summarized in Table 21.3. Although one of these studies suggested an improved complete response rate,[44,45] subsequent trials failed to demonstrate any survival advantage for the combined treatment.[25,56] Hydroxyurea also enhanced radiation mucositis and to a lesser extent, skin reaction.

## Other Single Agents

A number of other single agents including 6-mercaptopurine, razoxane (ICRF 159) and BUdR have been used concurrently with XRT.[4,5] Most of these studies showed no significant improvement in local control or survival.

## MULTI-AGENT CHEMOTHERAPY AND RADIOTHERAPY

Various multi-agent chemotherapy regimens have been combined with radiotherapy and/or surgery for advanced head and neck cancer. In most

**TABLE 21.3** Randomized Studies of Concurrent Radiotherapy and Hydroxyurea in Head and Neck Cancer

| Author/Date | Evaluable Patients | Complete Response Rate (1° ± N) | | % Local-Regional Control (yrs) | | % Survival (yrs) | | Significant |
|---|---|---|---|---|---|---|---|---|
| | | RT | RT + CT | RT | RT + CT | RT | RT + CT | |
| Richards et al., 1969 (44) 1973 (45) | 40 | 20% | 65% | N/A | N/A | 35% (5) | 50% (5) | No |
| Stefani et al., 1971 (56) | 126 | 47% | 42% | N/A | N/A | 31% (2) | 22% (2) | No |
| Hussey et al., 1975 (25) | 40 | 56% | 67% | 28% (2) | 30% (2) | 27% (2) | 31% (2) | No |

1° = Primary; N = Node; yrs = Years; RT = Radiotherapy; CT = Chemotherapy

studies, chemotherapy was administered sequentially with radiotherapy. However, there were at least 12 studies in which chemotherapy was given during the course of radiotherapy.[1,7,8,20,21,24,27,36,39,40,41,50,55] Only one of the studies was randomized.[7] In this study, reported by Bezwoda et al., a seven-drug combination chemotherapy (vincristine, adriamycin, bleomycin, methotrexate, 5-FU, hydroxyurea and 6-MP) was administered before, during, and after a split course of radiotherapy. The complete response rate was 3.6% with radiotherapy alone and 3.3% with the combined treatment. Although the median survival was significantly better for the combined treatment group, it was only 56 weeks compared to 18 weeks for the radiotherapy group. Both the complete response rate and survival were lower than most reported series of advanced head and neck cancer treated with radiotherapy with or without chemotherapy.

In a nonrandomized study by O'Connor et al.,[40,41] 198 patients were treated with a combination chemotherapy regimen consisting of vincristine, bleomycin, and methotrexate with leucovorin rescue and synchronous radiotherapy. At 5 years, the probability of recurrence-free rate was 52%, the local control rate was 62%, and the crude actuarial survival was 41% (i.e., significantly better than that of the historical control group). However, there was also increased acute toxicity. Severe mucositis led to frequent treatment interruptions in many patients, and dysphagia and dehydration necessitated tube feeding in one third of the patients. There was also a 7.5% incidence of treatment related deaths.

In the other nonrandomized studies, either a three or two-drug combinations consisting of bleomycin, methotrexate, 5-FU, cisplatin, cyclophosphamide, vincristine, adriamycin, or mitomycin C were combined with concurrent radiotherapy. Although most of these studies suggested an enhanced tumor response, this was usually accompanied by an increased acute normal tissue toxicity. Treatment fatalities as high as 17% have also been reported.[55]

Thus, although multi-agent chemotherapy concurrent with radiotherapy may increase the local control rate, none of the studies to date has demonstrated a decreased incidence of distant metastasis or a significant increase of survival. Furthermore, treatment morbidity and mortality are also formidable.

## DISCUSSION

From the preceding review it is apparent that the results of most clinical studies of simultaneous chemotherapy and radiotherapy for head and neck cancer have been negative. Positive results have been demonstrated only with single agent chemotherapy (bleomycin, and 5-FU) and primarily for oral cavity cancer.[34,52] Although some combination chemotherapy regimens have produced encouraging complete response rates, randomized trials showing a significant improvement in long-term local-regional control or survival or decreased incidence of distant metastasis are not yet available.

One of the reasons for the failure of combined radiotherapy and chemotherapy to make a significant impact on the treatment of head and neck cancer may be the lack of effective chemotherapeutic agents and combination chemotherapy regimens. Continued search for new drugs with greater efficacy for this disease is needed.

Of the large number of chemotherapeutic agents being used clinically, only a few agents have been combined with radiotherapy. Further exploration of currently available but heretofore untested drugs for the combined treatment with radiotherapy in the laboratory and in the clinics may be worthwhile.

One of the aspects of combined modality treatment that has not been adequately clinically evaluated is the optimal time sequence of drug and radiation administration and the schedule of drug administration. Simultaneous chemotherapy and radiotherapy are usually associated with increased acute toxicity especially when multi-agent chemotherapy is used. On the other hand, sequential or alternating combination chemotherapy and radiotherapy may be better tolerated. For the optimal interaction with radiation, certain drugs may best be given by continuous infusion rather than by bolus injection.[10,18] The potential of combining chemotherapy with hyperfractionated radiotherapy also needs exploration. It is possible that certain schedules of drug and radiation administration exploiting the differences in repair and proliferative kinetics of tumor and normal tissues may yield the optimal therapeutic ratio. Further research into this aspect of combined modality studies in the laboratory, as well as in the clinic, may prove very fruitful.

In addition to searching for more effective chemotherapeutic drugs, other new treatment modifiers such as hyperthermia, radiosensitizers and radioprotectors, sublethal damage repair and potentially lethal damage repair inhibitors, and biological response modifiers may be incorporated into the combined treatment program to further enhance the efficacy of radiotherapy and/or chemotherapy and to minimize the treatment toxicity. Supportive care directed towards the improvement of the nutritional status of the patient may may also increase the patient responsiveness to the combined treatment.

One of the obstacles to progress in this area of clinical research may be the lack of good predictive assays of the response to chemotherapy. Experimental combined modality studies suggest that no enhanced tumor response can be expected when drugs are combined with radiotherapy unless the drugs are active against the tumor by themselves. Ideally, it would be more rational to determine which drugs are most effective for the individual patient before combining them with radiotherapy. Improvements in currently available stem cell assays and development of new assay techniques such as nuclear magnetic resonance spectroscopy may facilitate the selection of the best agents for the individual patient.

Predictive assays, preferably noninvasive, will also be useful in monitoring the response during the course of chemotherapy. Clinical assessment of complete response to treatment can be difficult and may not be possible until long after treatment has been completed. Reliable predictive assays may allow earlier evaluation of response so that changes in the treatment plan can be made promptly to avoid unnecessary side effects and alternative treatment regimens can be instituted.

It is interesting that positive results of combined chemotherapy and radiotherapy have only been demonstrated for carcinoma of the oral cavity,[34,52] and only for stage II disease in one trial.[3] It may be that the response to combined treatment is site- and stage-dependent. This can only be determined by randomized trials with stratification of patients by stage as well as by site. Because of the large number of patients required, such randomized trials should best be carried out through the intergroup cooperative trial mechanism.

## SUMMARY

The results of a majority of randomized trials of concurrent radiotherapy and chemotherapy have been negative. Enhancement of local-regional tumor response has been seen with bleomycin, 5-FU, and multi-agent chemotherapy concurrent with radiotherapy. Improved survival has been demonstrated only with single agent chemotherapy with bleomycin and 5-FU primarily for oral cavity cancer. There was no evidence of decreased distant metastasis.

Slight to moderate enhancement of normal tissue effects has been seen with most single agent chemotherapy concurrent with radiotherapy. Marked enhancement of treatment morbidity and mortality had been seen with multi-agent chemotherapy concurrent with radiotherapy. Further clinical trials using more effective drug combinations and chemotherapy and radiotherapy schedules with or without other new treatment modifiers are needed to improve the prognosis and quality of life of patients with advanced head and neck cancer.

# REFERENCES

1. Adelstein DJ, Sharan VM, Earle AS, et al: Combined modality therapy (CMT) with simultaneous 5-fluorouracil (5FU), cis-platinum (DDP) and radiation therapy (RT) in the treatment of squamous cell cancer of the head and neck. Proc ASCO 1985;4:131.
2. Al-Sarraf M, Kinzie J, Marcial V, et al: High local and regional complete remission with the combination of cis-platinum and radiotherapy in unresectable head and neck cancers. RTOG Study. Proc Internatl Conf Head Neck Cancer Vidockler HR (ed), Baltimore: Lancaster, 1984, p 50.
3. Arcangeli G, Nervi C, Righini R, et al: Combined radiation and drugs: The effect of intra-arterial chemotherapy followed by radiotherapy in head and neck cancer. Radiother Oncol 1983;1:101–107.
4. Bagshaw MA, Doggett RLS: A clinical study of chemical radiosensitization. Front Radiat Ther Oncol 1969;4:164–173.
5. Bakowski MT, Macdonald E, Mould RF, et al: Double blind controlled clinical trial of radiation plus razoxane (ICRF 159) versus radiation plus placebo in the treatment of head and neck cancer. Int J Radiat Oncol Biol Phys 1978;4:115–119.
6. Berdal P: Head and neck carcinoma: treatment with bleomycin and radiation. GANN Monograph on Cancer Research 1976;19:133–149.
7. Bezwoda WR, de Moor NG, Derman DP: Treatment of advanced head and neck cancer by means of radiation therapy plus chemotherapy—a randomized trial. Med Pediatr Oncol 1979;6:353–358.
8. Bitter K: Bleomycin-methotrexate-chemotherapy in combination with telecobalt-radiation for patients suffering from advanced oral carcinoma. J Maxillofac Surg 1977;5:75–81.
9. Bloom EJ, Green MD, Cooper JS, et al: Concomitant use of cis-platinum (CDDP) chemotherapy and radiation therapy (RT) in the treatment of advanced head and neck cancer. Proc ASCO 1985;4:137.
10. Byfield JE, Sharp TR, Frankel SS, et al: Phase I and II trial of five-day infused 5-fluorouracil and radiation in advanced cancer of the head and neck. J Clin Oncol 1984;2:406–413.
11. Cachin Y, Jortay A, Sancho H, et al: Preliminary results of a randomized EORTC study comparing radiotherapy and concomitant bleomycin to radiotherapy alone in epidermoid carcinomas of the oropharynx. Eur J Cancer 1977;13:1389–1395.
12. Condit PT: Treatment of carcinoma with radiation therapy and methotrexate. Mo Med 1968;65:832–835.
13. Coughlin CT, Grace M, O'Donnell JF, et al: Combined modality approach in the management of locally advanced head and neck cancer. Cancer Treat Rep 1984;68:591–597.
14. Coughlin CT, Richmond RC: Platinum based combined modality approach for locally advanced head and neck carcinoma. Int J Radiat Oncol Biol Phys 1985;11:915–919.
15. De-la-Garza JG, Garcia F, Armendariz C, et al: Simultaneous use of bleomycin and radiotherapy in malignant tumors of the head and neck. J Int Med Res 1976;4:158–164.
16. Fu KK: Biological Basis for the interaction of chemotherapeutic agents and radiation therapy. Cancer 1985;55:2123–2130.
17. Fu KK: Concurrent radiotherapy and chemotherapy, in Wittes RE (ed): Head and Neck Cancer, London: John Wiley & Sons, Ltd, 1985, pp 221–248.
18. Fu KK, Lam KN, Rainer PA: The influence of time sequence of cisplatin administration and continuous low dose rate irradiation (CLDRI) on their combined effects on a murine squamous cell carcinoma. Int J Radiol Oncol Biol Phys 1985;11:2119–2124.
19. Fu KK, Phillips TL, Silverberg IJ, et al: Combined radiotherapy and chemotherapy with bleomycin and methotrexate for advanced inoperable head and neck cancer: update of a Northern California Oncology Group (NCOG) randomized trial. J Clin Oncol (in press).

20. Fu KK, Silverberg IJ, Phillips TL, Friedman MA: Combined radiotherapy and multidrug chemotherapy for advanced head and neck cancer: results of a radiation therapy oncology group pilot study. Cancer Treat Rep 1979;63:351–357.
21. Glick JH, Fazekas JT, Davis LW, et al: Combination chemotherapy—radiotherapy for advanced, inoperable head and neck cancer. An RTOG pilot study. Cancer Clin Trials 1979;2:129–136.
22. Goepfert H, Jesse RH, Lindberg RD: Arterial infusion and radiation therapy in the treatment of advanced cancer of the nasal cavity and paranasal sinuses. Amer J Surg 1973;126:464–468.
23. Haselow RE, Adams GS, Oken MM, et al: Cis-platinum (DDP) and radiation therapy (RT) for locally advanced and unresectable head and neck cancer. Proc Amer Soc Clin Oncol 1983;2:160.
24. Hollmann K, Jesch W, Kuehboeck J, Dimopoulos J: Combined intra-arterial chemotherapy and radiation therapy of tumors in the maxillofacial region. J Maxillofac Surg 1979;7:191–197.
25. Hussey DH, Abrams JP: Combined therapy in advanced head and neck cancer: hydroxyurea and radiotherapy. Prog Clin Cancer 1975;6:79–86.
26. Jesse RH, Goepfert H, Lindberg RD, Johnson RH: Combined intra-arterial infusion and radiotherapy for the treatment of advanced cancer of the head and neck. Amer J Roentgenol 1969;105:20–25.
27. Kaplan MJ, Hahn SS, Johns ME, et al: Mitomycin and fluorouracil with concomitant radiotherapy in head and neck cancer. Arch Otolaryngol 1985;111:220–222
28. Kapstad B: Treatment of squamous cell carcinomas of the head and neck region with cobalt and bleomycin. Int J Radiat Oncol Biol Phys 1978;4:91–94.
29. Kapstad B, Bang G, Rennaes S, Dahler A: Combined preoperative treatment with colbalt and bleomycin in patients with head and neck carcinoma—A controlled clinical study. Int J Radiat Oncol Biol Phys 1978;4:85–89.
30. Komiyama S, Hiroto I Ryu S, Nakashima T, et al: Synergistic combination therapy of 5-fluorouracil, vitamin A and cobalt-60 radiation therapy upon head and neck tumors. Oncology 1978;35:253–257.
31. Kramer S: Use of methotrexate and radiation therapy for advanced cancer of the head and neck. Front Radiat Ther Oncol 1969;4:116–125.
32. Lerner HJ: Concomitant hydroxyurea and irradiation. Clinical experience with 100 patients with advanced head and neck cancer at Pennsylvania hospital. Amer J Surg 1977;134:505–509.
33. Leipzig B, Wetmore SJ, Klug D, Putzeys R: Cis-platinum sensitization to radiotherapy of squamous cell carcinomas in the head and neck, in Vidockler HR (ed): Proceedings of the International Conference on Head and Neck Cancer, Baltimore: Lancaster, 1984, p. 42.
34. Lo TCM, Wiley AL, Ansfield FJ, et al: Combined radiation therapy and 5-fluorouracil for advanced squamous cell carcinoma of the oral cavity and oropharynx: A randomized study. Amer J Roentgenol 1976;126:229–235.
35. Lustig RA, DeMare PA, Kramer S: Adjuvant methotrexate in the radiotherapeutic management of advanced tumors of the head and neck. Cancer 1976;37:2703–2708.
36. Malaker K, Robson F, Schipper H: Combined modalities in the management of advanced head and neck cancers. J Otolaryngol 1980;9:24–30.
37. Mason JH, Ediger AJ: Infusion chemotherapy. Proc Sixth Natl Cancer Conf 1970;6:621–625.
38. Morita K: Clinical significance of radiation therapy combined with chemotherapy. Strahlentherapie 1980;150:228–233.

39. Murthy AK, Taylor SG, Showel J, et al: Improved results with simultaneous chemotherapy and radiation in head and neck cancer. Proc ASCO 1985;4:138.
40. O'Connor AD, Clifford P, Dalley VM, et al: Advanced head and neck cancer treated by combined radiotherapy and VBM cytotoxic regimen — Four-year results. Clin Otolaryngol 1979;4:329–337.
41. O'Connor D, Clifford P, Edwards WG, et al: Long-term results of VBM and radiotherapy in advanced head and neck cancer. Int J Radiat Oncol Biol Phys 1982;8:1525–1531.
42. Pointon RCS, Askill C, Hunter RD, Wilkinson PM: Treatment of advanced head and neck cancer using synchronous therapy with methotrexate and irradiation. Clin Radiol 1983;34:459–462.
43. RTOG Meeting Book. (January 1987), p. 230.
44. Richards GJ, Chambers RG: Hydroxyurea: A radiosensitizer in the treatment of neoplasms of the head and neck. Amer J Roentgenol 1969;105:555–565.
45. Richards GJ, Chambers RG: Hydroxyurea in the treatment of neoplasms of the head and neck. A resurvey. Amer J Surg 1973;126:513–518.
46. Rominger CJ: Hydroxyurea and radiation therapy in advanced neoplasms of the head and neck. Amer J Roentgenol 1971;111:103–108.
47. Rygard J, Hansen HS: Bleomycin as adjuvant in radiation therapy of advanced squamous cell carcinoma in head and neck. Acta Otolaryngol (Suppl) 1979;360:161–166.
48. Sato Y, Morita M, Takashi HO, et al: Combined surgery, radiotherapy and regional chemotherapy in carcinoma of the paranasal sinuses. Cancer 1970;25:571–579.
49. Seagren SL, Byfield JE, Nahum AM, Bone RC: Treatment of locally advanced squamous cell carcinoma of the head and neck with concurrent bleomycin and external beam radiation therapy. Int J Radiat Oncol Biol Phys 1979;5:1531–1535.
50. Seagren SL, Byfield JE, Davidson TM, Sharp TR: Bleomycin, cyclophosphamide and radiotherapy in regionally advanced epidermoid carcinoma of the head and neck. Int J Radiat Oncol Biol Phys 1982;8:127–132.
51. Shah PM, Shukla SN, Patel KM, et al: Effect of bleomycin-radiotherapy combination in management of head and neck squamous cell carcinoma. Cancer 1981;48:1106–1109.
52. Shanta V, Krishnamurthi S: Combined bleomycin and radiotherapy in oral cancer. Clin Radiol 1980;31:617–620.
53. Shigematsu Y, Sakai S, Fuchihata H: Recent trials in the treatment of maxillary sinus carcinoma, with special reference to the chemical potentiation of radiation therapy. Acta Otolaryng 1971;71:63–70.
54. Silverberg IJ, Phillips TL, Fu KK, Chan PYM: Combined radiotherapy and bleomycin for advanced head and neck cancers: Results of a phase I pilot study. Cancer Treat Rep 1981;65:697–698.
55. Smith BL, Franz JL, Mira JG, et al: Simultaneous combination radiotherapy and multi-drug chemotherapy for stage III and stage IV squamous cell carcinoma of the head and neck. J Surg Oncol 1980;15:91–98.
56. Stefani S, Eells RW, Abbate J: Hydroxyurea and radiotherapy in head and neck cancer. Radiol 1971;101:391–396.
57. Tanaka Y, Wada T, Fuchihata H, et al: Combined treatment with radiation and bleomycin for intra-oral carcinoma. A preliminary report. Int J Radiat Oncol Biol Phys 1976;1:1189–1193.
58. Vermund H, Kaalhus O, Winther F, et al: Bleomycin and radiation therapy in squamous cell carcinoma of the upper aero-digestive tract: A phase III clinical trial. Int J Radiat Oncol Biol Phys 1985;11:1877–1886.

CHAPTER **22**

# Irradiation and Hyperthermia in Treatment of Locally Advanced and Recurrent Head and Neck Tumors

*Carlos A. Perez, MD, Bahman Emami, MD*
*Ronald S. Scott, MD, PhD,*
*Ned B. Hornback, MD,*
*Madeline Bauer, PhD,*
*Mary Ann Hederman, BS, and*
*Debbie VonGerichten, BS*

Biological data indicate that tumors may be more sensitive to heat because they are chronically oxygen deprived, nutritionally deficient, and have a low pH. Moreover, cells in the S-phase of the proliferative cycle, usually radioresistant, are known to be sensitive to hyperthermia. Tumors are less vascularized than normal tissues and will not dissipate heat as readily; these differences in microcirculation and blood flow accentuate the sensitivity of the tumors to heat. Temperature elevation within the tumor destroys existing blood vessels, further contributing to decreased vascularity and oxygen tension creating a low pH environment. Selective destruction of tumors occurs at about 42–45°C, whereas at higher temperatures, normal and tumor tissues may have the same response to heat. Further in vitro and in vivo experiments have demonstrated enhanced biological effects when heat is combined with irradiation and/or cytotoxic agents.[1] In this paper, we update a previous report describing the experience at the Mallinckrodt Institute of Radiology and data from multi-institutional trial on the use of irradiation and heat in the treatment of locally advanced or recurrent tumors of the head and neck.[2]

**334**

## TECHNIQUES

### Modalities of Heating

Physical agents currently used for power deposition in local and regional clinical hyperthermia include microwaves (MW), radiofrequencies (RF), and ultrasound (US). These modalities, which deposit thermal energy in tissues primarily by generating electromagnetic fields or mechanical ultrasonic motion, respectively, have different physical properties. Microwaves have limited penetration in soft tissues and greater propagation in fat; ultrasound will not propagate in media with a density different from that of water (such as bone or air). External contour and tissue composition of the anatomical area to be treated, as well as the size and depth of the tumor, determine the appropriate heating method to be used.

Depending on the anatomical area to be treated and the modality used, there are several methods for heat delivery. External hyperthermia can be administered with surface applicators for microwaves or external electrodes, coils, and plates for radiofrequency (RF), or piezo-crystal transducers for ultrasound.

Interstitial hyperthermia employs conducting electrodes or antennas implanted directly in the tissues for RF or microwaves, respectively. Intracavity antennas for microwaves or large electrodes for radiofrequency (encased in special applicators) can be introduced into natural cavities such as the oropharynx and larynx.

### Thermometry

At the present time all temperature measuring techniques are invasive, consisting of the introduction of sensors into the tumor and normal tissues.

Direct and continuous monitoring of temperatures in clinical applications of hyperthermia is mandatory for accurate thermal treatment verification at specific points. Subsurface thermometry is carried out with invasive probes in 20–29 gauge hypodermic needles or in 16 gauge plastic tubes. The most frequently used instruments are conducting probes—standard thermistors and thermocouples; minimally conducting probes—high resistivity thermistors (Bowman); and nonconducting optical probes—gallium arsenide (Christensen), or rare earth biophosphor sensors. Field-induced artifacts often occur when the conducting probes are used in electromagnetic fields, making high resistivity and optical probes preferable.

For satisfactory clinical thermometry, appropriate standard thermistors and probes must be used, and the temperature must be measured in at least two or three locations at the greatest possible depth of the tumor to permit adequate description of the thermal state of the tissue. One or more probes are placed on the skin to measure surface temperature.

Noninvasive thermometry techniques under development, not available for clinical applications today, include infrared and microwave thermography and ultrasound reconstruction.

Computer simulated thermal distribution can be obtained with methods based on the bio-heat equation.

## CLINICAL MATERIALS AND METHODS

Three different groups of patients with superficial metastatic or recurrent head and neck tumors were treated. A life expectancy of at least 3 months was anticipated for all patients. The investigational nature of the therapy was explained in detail and an informed consent form was signed by every patient.

### Group A — Local External Hyperthermia for Recurrent/Metastatic Tumors

A total of 117 tumors were treated with combinations of irradiation (Co60, 4 MV photons, 9 – 15 MeV electrons) and hyperthermia (915 MHz external microwaves) between March 1978 and December 1985 (minimum 3 month follow-up). Seventy percent of the patients had been previously treated with irradiation (from 5000 to 6500 cGy). Doses of irradiation ranging from 2000 to 4500 cGy in fractions of 400 cGy were delivered every 72 hours (twice weekly) followed by hyperthermia (41 – 43 °C, 60 minutes). The desired temperature was reached in the majority of patients in about 10 to 15 minutes. Fractionation every 72 hours was chosen to avoid the thermotolerance reported in some biological experiments.[5,6] Initially, microwave generators at 915 MHz (MCL 15222), specially modified for clinical use, were utilized, and later, commercially manufactured devices with dielectric filled waveguide applicators were employed. A plastic bag containing deionized water was used after one and one-half years to improve coupling of the applicators to irregular surfaces of the patient. Initially, a minimum of two thermistor probes (YSI, 524) encased in 24 gauge needles were used for continuous temperature monitoring during each hyperthermia session. The probes were inserted at the greatest possible depth of the tumor (one at the central axis, one peripheral, when possible) and one probe embedded in a 22 gauge plastic tube was placed at the skin surface during each treatment session. The temperature at these sites was recorded on a dual channel strip chart recorder. With the thermistors and thermocouples, temperatures were measured every 15 minutes with the power off. Variations of temperature of .5 to 2°C were noted with the RF generator power on or off and appropriate corrections were made to obtain the actual tissue temperature. Since 1981, high resistivity (Bowman) thermistors or gallium arsenide (Christensen) probes were used for measurements while the power remained on.

## Group B — Interstitial Thermoradiotherapy

From October 1981 to December 1985, 29 recurrent and/or persistent tumors were treated with interstitial thermoradiotherapy. The average dimensions of the tumors were calculated by the formula $A+B+C/3$. There were nine lesions less than 4 cm, and 20 lesions of 4 to 10 cm in average diameter. All patients had undergone previous definitive treatment by surgery and/or radiation therapy.

Interstitial irradiation was administered with $^{192}$I afterloading interstitial implant. The total dose was dependent upon initial radiotherapy dose, generally 4000–6000 cGy delivered in 4–7 days. The implantation was performed according to standard interstitial brachytherapy techniques following the Quimby system implantation technique.[7,8]

In the majority of the patients, interstitial hyperthermia was administered with coaxial microwave antennas (915 MHz) placed in teflon catheters (16 gauge angiocaths, Deseret Medical Inc, Sandy, Utah) that had been previously implanted in the tumor tissue under general anesthesia. The space between each teflon tube was 10 to 12 mm. The inner diameter of the teflon tubes was adequate for placement of both radioactive sources (ribbons) and microwave coaxial antennas. After the patient was transferred from the recovery room to the isolated floor room, $^{192}$I was loaded on the same day. The following day, the $^{192}$I wires were temporarily removed and the patient was transferred (with teflon catheters secured in place) to the radiotherapy department for a dosimetry procedure and then to the hyperthermia suite. The basic goal in the heating applications was the achievement of minimal tumor temperatures of 43°C for 60 minutes. This often required accepting temperatures, e.g., necrotic centers, above the protocol specified temperature of 43°C. In virtually all cases, the maximum measured tumor temperatue was less than 50°C. After completion of the hyperthermia, the patient was taken back to his room and the $^{192}$I wires were reinserted.[9] The second course of hyperthermia was administered at the completion of the $Ir^{192}$ implant when the radioactive sources were removed.

Heat was produced in a few patients through resistive heating inducted by radiofrequency electric currents (frequency range of 0.1–1.0 MHz) driven between pairs of electrically connected arrays of hollow stainless steel stylettes. The slabs of tissue between respective pairs of adjacent arrays were all heated simultaneously by connecting alternative arrays together to form a circuit with two "multi-electrode" planes. In all but one of the patients, the heating was performed in one session in the operating room, with the patient under general anesthesia. After completion of the hyperthermia session, the metallic guides were replaced with teflon tubes for routine afterloading $^{192}I$ implant. Hyperthermia was performed an average of 4 to 8 hours after loading the radioactive $^{192}I$ wires.

For most of the patients, steady state temperatures were mapped along at least one of the catheter tracks during each treatment. In carrying out thermometry with RF interstitial hyperthermia, standard thermistor probes were employed. For interstitial hyperthermia produced with microwave antennas, both high resistivity thermistors with carbon impregnated plastic leads and gallium arsenide "optical" thermometers were employed.

### Group C — Patients with Advanced Head and Neck Primary Malignant Tumors Treated with Definitive Doses of Radiotherapy and External Microwaves (RTOG Protocol No. 81–13)

A total of 48 patients with squamous cell carcinoma of the head and neck were treated with definitive radiotherapy, to a total dose of 6000 cGY delivered in 200 cGY TD daily fractions, five times weekly. A smaller group of patients, who could not be treated daily, received a total of 4800 cGY TD in fractions of 400 cGY TD per day, twice weekly. The two dose schedules are claimed to be equivalent.[10] Hyperthermia was delivered with 915 MHz external applicators twice weekly, within 30 minutes following radiotherapy. When the central tumor temperature was 42–43°C, 45 minute exposures were used. When the central tumor temperature reached 43–44°C, 30 minutes of exposure were used. All patients have been followed for at least 6 months after therapy and many for 1 year. Therefore, they are better suited for long term analysis of tumor control and late effects of radiotherapy and hyperthermia in normal tissues.

### RESULTS
### Group A — External Microwaves

Of 99 measurable epidermoid lesions in the head and neck (3 diffuse melanomas), 45 (45.5%) exhibited a complete response (CR) and 31 (31%) a partial response (PR), defined as more than 50% regression in all diameters (Table 22.1). Whereas only 39.5% of the squamous cell carcinomas had a CR, three sarcomas and 5/6 melanomas regressed completely after re-treatment. Approximately 84% of the epidermoid carcinomas, and all the sarcomas, melanomas, and adenocarcinomas that had a CR went on to exhibit

**TABLE 22.1** Head and neck Cancer—Group A: Irradiation and Hyperthermia Summary of Tumor Response—Control

| | No. of Lesions Treated | Tumor Regression | | Tumor Control in CR* |
|---|---|---|---|---|
| | | Complete | Partial (≥50%) | |
| Epidermoid ca (measurable) | 86 | 34 (39.5%) | 31 (36.0%) | 27/34 (79.4%) |
| Melanoma | 3 | 3 (100%) | — | 3/3 (100%) |
| Melanoma (extensive) | 3 | 2 (66.7%) | NA | 2/2 (100%) |
| Sarcoma | 3 | 3 (100%) | — | 3/3 (100%) |
| Adenocarcinoma | 3 | 2 (66.7%) | — | 2/2 (100%) |
| Basal cell ca | 1 | 1 | — | 1/1 (100%) |
| Total | 99 | 45 (45.5%) | 31 (31.3%) | 38/45 (84.4%) |

*No evidence of tumor recurrence.

**339**

control of the tumor (absence of recurrence) in the volume treated with irradiation and hyperthermia.

Seventy percent of the tumors less than 4 cm in thickness achieved satisfactory temperatures (over 42.5°C) in contrast to less than 10% of the tumors with depth greater than 4 cm. Of the 35 tumors less than 2 cm in depth reaching average tumor temperatures of 42.5°C, 25 (71.4%) had a complete regression, in contrast to 50% of 24 tumors 2–4 cm in thickness and 2/11 (18%) with greater depth. Each group showed better tumor regression rates with higher temperatures (Table 22.2). However, because of the small number of patients in the various groups, the differences are not statistically significant. This correlation must be analyzed in the light of the few temperature points taken and the variation in temperature throughout the tumor and during the daily hyperthermia sessions.

Greater proportions of complete regressions were noted in tumors measuring less than 2 cm in diameter (35/56 = 62.5%) or 2–4 cm in diameter (20/42 = 47.6%), whereas only 2/11 = 18%) of lesions larger than 4 cm diameter showed complete regression.

A correlation was made between tumor regression and irradiation doses. With doses over 3200 cGY, a higher incidence of complete tumor regression was noted in comparison with lower doses (Table 22.3). Further, greater tumor control was achieved with the higher irradiation doses in the tumors less than 3 cm in thickness (17/40 = 42.5%), or 3–5 cm in thickness (8/19 = 42.1%) in comparison with 1/11 (9%) of the tumors larger than 5 cm.

In 18 additional patients with non-measurable recurrent or metastatic epidermoid carcinoma diffusely infiltrating the neck, 13 (86.7%) showed tumor control (no evidence of recurrence) lasting several months after therapy or until the patient's death. One of these patients is alive, without tumor recurrence years after treatment, and three died of distant metastases with controlled tumor in the head and neck.

## SIDE EFFECTS OF THERAPY

Of the 114 sites treated, 25 (21.9%) developed tumor necrosis or ulcerations that did not heal spontaneously. Three patients (2.7%) showed a thermal burn that involved the skin and/or subcutaneous tissues. In most instances these burns healed with conservative management in 8 to 12 weeks. Other reactions of the skin and subcutaneous tissues, such as erythema, dry or moist desquamation, and fibrosis were observed in a proportion similar to those noted with irradiation alone, and indicated no significant enhanced normal tissue effects because of the hyperthermia (Table 22.4).

TABLE 22.2 Head and Neck Cancer—Group A: Irradiation and Hyperthermia Correlation of Average Temperature and Complete Tumor Response As a Function of Depth of Tumor

| Size of Tumor | <2 cm | | | 2.1–4 cm | | | >4 cm | | |
|---|---|---|---|---|---|---|---|---|---|
| Average Temperature °C | ≤41 | 41–42 | ≥42.5 | ≤41 | 42–42 | ≥42.5 | ≤41 | 41–42 | ≥42.5 |
| Measurable | 1/6 (16.7%) * | 5/10 (50%) * | 14/22 (63.6%) * | 2/5 (40%) | 6/13 (46.2%) | 12/24 (50%) | 0/3 | 0/1 | 2/11 (18.2%) |
| Non-measurable | 2/2 | 2/3 | 11/13 (84.6%) * | | | | | | |
| TOTAL | 3/8 (37.5%) | 7/13 (53.8%) | 25/35 (71.4%) | 2/5 (40%) | 6/13 (46.2%) | 12/24 (50%) | 0/3 | 0/1 | 2/11 (18.2%) |

*Denotes non-measurable patients with tumor control.

341

**TABLE 22.3** Head and Neck Recurrent Tumors: Tumor Control in Treated Field

| Depth of Recurrent Tumor | Dose | | | | |
|---|---|---|---|---|---|
| | 0–2000 | 2001–3000 | 3001–3999 | 4000–4500 | >4500 |
| ≤1 cm | 0/2 | 0/3 | 3/4 (75%) | 4/5 (80%) | |
| 1–3 cm | 0/4 | 2/7 (28.6%) | 5/17 (29.4%) | 11/22 (50%) | 1/1 |
| 3–5 cm | | | 1/5 (20%) | 7/13 (53.8%) | 0/1 |
| >5 cm | | | 0/2 | 1/8 (12.5%) | 0/1 |

## Group B — Interstitial Thermoradiotherapy

A total of 29 recurrent or metastatic lesions were treated. All but one were squamous cell carcinoma, the other being a mucoepidermoid carcinoma of the salivary gland. Nine of the tumors were less than 4 cm, whereas the remaining 20 lesions were 4 to 10 cm in average diameter (Table 22.5).

Twenty-one of the lesions were heated with microwave antennas while eight were treated with local RF interstitial electrodes. As in the patients treated with external hyperthermia, there was a significant correlation between the size of the tumor and the response to therapy. Six of nine lesions less than 4 cm in size showed a complete response and one partial response. Of 20 tumors with 4–10 cm average diameters, seven had a complete response and seven a partial response. There was no significant difference in the overall response depending on the type of heating.

Of the 21 patients receiving satisfactory heating (42.5°C for at least 30 minutes in both sessions), 13 exhibited a complete response and five a partial response. Only two showed no regression after therapy. In contrast, there were no complete responses in eight lesions with inadequate heating, and only one had a partial response.

In two of the patients, rapid tumor necrosis were observed. In such patients, after debridement of necrotic tissue, no gross tumor could be iden-

**TABLE 22.4** Irradiation and Hyperthermia Complications of Therapy: 114 Sites Treated

| Complications | No. | % |
|---|---|---|
| Ulceration | 20 | 17.5 |
| Dry desquamation | 20 | 17.5 |
| Subcutaneous fibrosis | 16 | 14.0 |
| Moist desquamation | 11 | 9.6 |
| Tumor necrosis | 5 | 4.4 |
| Thermal burn | 3 | 2.6 |

**TABLE 22.5** Hyperthermia and Interstitial Irradiation in Recurrent Head and Neck Tumors: Overall Response to Therapy (29 Lesions)

|  | Complete Response | Partial Response | No Response | Not Evaluable |
|---|---|---|---|---|
| <4 cm | 6 | 1 | 1 | 1 |
| ≥4 cm | 7 | 7 | 3 | 3 |

tified. Despite weekly debridement and conservative management, the ulceration took several months to heal.

Tumor necrosis resulted in a cutaneous sinus in one of the patients. In another patient with a massive floor of mouth tumor invading the skin of the submental region, the rapid tumor necrosis resulted in an oro-cutaneous fistula. The long delay in healing of the above process was most likely due to poor blood supply from extensive prior treatments such as surgery and/or radiation.

## Group C — Advanced Tumors Treated with Definitive Radiotherapy and External Microwaves

Of the 48 treated patients with squamous cell carcinoma of the head and neck (18 with a minimum of 6 months follow-up), 28 (58%) have shown a complete response and most of them have had partial tumor regression.

Of the 14 patients with lymph nodes less than 3 cm in size, seven were followed for 6 months and three (43%) are alive without recurrence in the neck (18 with a minimum of 6 months follow-up), 28 (58%) have shown a beyond 6 months; 2/11 (18%) are alive without neck recurrences. None of the patients with an initial complete nodal regression have progressed. Primary tumor control was not assessed.

Except for a few thermal burns, combined therapy has been well tolerated, and the late effects observed are similar to those from the surrounding radiotherapy fields. The sequelae of therapy in 46 evaluable patients is shown in Table 22.6.

## DISCUSSION

From preliminary data reported by us,[2,9-12] Arcangeli et al.,[13,14] and others,[15-23] it appears that a combination of irradiation and hyperthermia will produce more complete responses and better tumor control than comparable doses of irradiation alone.[8]

**TABLE 22.6** Definitive Irradiation and Hyperthermia in Locally Advanced Primary Head and Neck Tumor

| Most Severe Complications Reported Within 6 Months of RX Start | Cases Analyzed (%) (46 Evaluable Patients) |
| --- | --- |
| Skin pigmentation/fibrosis | 33 |
| Slight to severe erythema | 17 |
| Dry desquamation | 15 |
| Thermal blister | 14 |
| Moist desquamation | 7 |
| Persistent ulceration | 6 |
| Skin breakdown with ulceration | 4 |
| Skin/subcutaneous necrosis | 4 |

Arcangeli et al. noted greater tumor control with higher doses of irradiation and increasing numbers of hyperthermia treatments.[14] While these preliminary data are encouraging and certainly should support continued efforts in clinical evaluation of hyperthermia, it is imperative to develop stringent quality assurance programs to ensure the reliability of the treatments given and the data generated. Furthermore, preliminary results must be confirmed by clinical trials that randomly allocate patients with comparable lesions to be treated with irradiation alone or with irradiation and hyperthermia. The Radiation Therapy Oncology Group (RTOG) is conducting a large multi-institutional cooperative trial randomizing measurable recurrent superficial lesions (less than 4 cm in diameter) to be treated with irradiation alone (3200 cGY in eight fractions, twice weekly) or irradiation and hyperthermia (same dose of irradiation plus hyperthermia consisting of 42.5°–43°C for 60 minutes after each irradiation exposure).[24] Preliminary analysis showed greater complete tumor response in one of the arms, presumably the irradiation and heat (32%) compared to 16% in the other arm. The incidence of thermal burns has been 20%, the remaining morbidity being comparable in both arms.[24] In addition, a protocol to assess the effects of definitive doses of irradiation and hyperthermia (preliminary results of which were reported here), will be analyzed in the near future.[25] A prospective randomized study has been recently activated to compare the efficacy and morbidity of definitive irradiation and hyperthermia, in comparison with irradiation alone, in patients with palpable cervical lymph nodes from head and neck epithelial primary tumors.[26] Furthermore, a protocol to evaluate the efficacy of interstitial thermoradiotherapy compared with brachytherapy alone was activated.[27]

Patients with palpable neck nodes and large epidermoid carcinomas of the larynx, pyriform sinus, and pharynx have a high incidence of local and neck failures following combined therapy with surgery and irradiation. At Washington University, a protocol has been developed, based on preliminary results presented in this report, to deliver a combination of irradiation and hyperthermia to patients with advanced tumors of the larynx and pharynx following surgical resection of the primary tumor and radical neck dissection.[28]

The need to develop a reliable thermal dose expression and to accommodate variations in temperatures throughout the treatment sessions has been emphasized.[29] Dewhirst et al.,[30] in 130 tumors in pet animals, reported a significant correlation between the minimal temperature achieved during treatment and tumor response and control.

The results reported with interstitial irradiation and hyperthermia, using tumor control as an endpoint, are similar to those with irradiation alone. Emami and Marks observed a 52% CR in 25 patients with recurrent head and neck tumors treated with interstitial irradiation,[8] comparable to 63% CR in 29 patients reported by Syed et al.[31] Gelinas and Fletcher noted a 32% (32/106) surgical salvage for patients with similar recurrences.[32]

In our experience, the local tumor control (absence of relapse in the area treated) with irradiation and hyperthermia was 65%; this figure is superior to the 14% figure reported by Emami et al. in 95 patients treated with irradiation alone.[8]

A limited number of complete responses (ranging from 0% to 10% in most reports) have been described with combination chemotherapy (cisplatinum, Oncovin and bleomycin or high dose methotrexate with BCG).[33,34]

Donegan and Harris observed 3/15 (29%) CR's with intra-arterial combination of 5 FU, methotrexate, and bleomycin.[35]

Hyperthermia has the potential to significantly contribute to the management of primary or recurrent head and neck tumor patients who have high local or regional failure rate following treatment with existing modalities. Further improvements are needed in the selection of patients equipment, and techniques for heat delivery and temperature monitoring.[12]

Properly designed, prospective, randomized clinical trials in progress may objectively evaluate the efficacy of hyperthermia combined with irradiation as an adjuvant to surgery or as primary treatment of patients in high risk groups.

It will be imperative to develop well structured programs to adequately train physicians, physicists, technologists, and nurses who will be knowledgeable in the basic concepts and clinical administration of hyperthermia.

# REFERENCES

1. Dewey WC: Interaction of heat with radiation and chemotherapy. Cancer Res (suppl) 1984;44:4714S–4720S.
2. Perez CA, Emami B, Scott RS: Potential efficacy of hyperthermia in treatment of head and neck tumors, in Chretien PB, Johns ME, Shedd DP, Strong EW, Ward PH (eds): Head and Neck Cancer. Philadelphia: BC Decker Inc, 1985, pp 367–373.
3. Roemer RB, Cetas TC: Applications of bioheat transfer simulations in hyperthermia. Cancer Res (suppl) 1984;44:4788S–4798S.
4. Strohbehn JW: Calculation of absorbed power in tissue for various hyperthermia devices. Cancer Res (suppl) 1984;44:4781S–4887S.
5. Henle KJ, Bitner AF, Dethlefsen LA: Induction of thermotolerance by multiple heat fractions in Chinese hamster ovary cells. Cancer Res 1979;39:2486–2491.
6. Law MP, Ahier RG, Spomaia S. et al: The induction of thermotolerance in the ear of the mouse by fractionated hyperthermia. Int J Radiat Oncol Biol Phys 1984;10:865–873.
7. Hilaris BS, Henschke UK: General principles and techniques of interstitial brachytherapy, in Hilaris BS (ed): Handbook of Interstitial Brachytherapy. Publishing Sciences Group, Inc., 1975, pp 61–86.
8. Emami B, Marks JE: Retreatment of recurrent carcinoma of the head and neck by afterloading interstitial Iridium 192 implant. Laryngoscope 1983;93:1345–1347.
9. Emami B, Marks JE, Perez CA, et al: Interstitial thermoradiotherapy in the treatment of recurrent/residual malignant tumors. Amer J Clin Oncol 1984;7:699–704.
10. Scott RS, Johnson RJR, Story KV, Clay L: Local hyperthermia in combination with definitive radiotherapy: Increased tumor clearance, reduced recurrence rate in extended followup. Int J Radiat Oncol Biol Phys, 1984;10:2119–2123.
11. Emami B, Perez CA: Interstitial thermoradiotherapy: An overview. Endocurietherapy/Hyperthermia Oncology 1985;1:35–40.
12. Perez CA, Emami B, VonGerichten D: Clinical results with irradiation and local microwave hyperthermia in cancer therapy, In Overgaard J (ed): Proceedings of the 4th International Symposium of Hyperthermic Oncology, Vol I, London: Taylor & Francis, 1984, pp 398–402.
13. Arcangeli G, Cividalli A, Nervi C, et al: Tumor control and therapeutic gain with different schedules of combined radiotherapy and local external hyperthermia in human cancer. Int J Radiat Oncol Biol Phys 1983;9:1125–1134.
14. Arcangeli G, Nervi C, Cividalli A, Lovisolo GA: Problem of sequence and fractionation in the clinical application of combined heat and radiation. Cancer Res (suppl) 1984;44:4857S–4863S.
15. Cosset JM, Brule JM, Dutriex J, et al: Low frequency contact and interstitial hyperthermia association with brachytherapy. Int J Radiat Oncol Biol Phys 1984;10:307–312.
16. Kim SH, Hahn GM: Clinical and biological studies of localized hyperthermia. Cancer Res 1979;39:2258–2261.
17. Fazekas JT, Nerlinger RE: Localized hyperthermia adjuvant to irradiation in superficial recurrent carcinomas: A preliminary report on 46 patients. Int J Radiat Oncol Biol Phys 1981;7:1457–1463.
18. Hornback NB, Shype RE, Shidnia H, et al: Preliminary clinical results of combined 433 megahertz microwave therapy and radiation therapy on patients with advanced cancer. Cancer 1977;40:2854–2863.
19. Joseph C, Astrahan M, Lipsett J, et al: Interstitial hyperthermia and interstitial iridium 192 implantation. A technique and preliminary result. Int J Radiat Oncol Biol Phys 1981;7:827–833.

20. Oleson JR, Sim DA, Manning MR: Analysis of prognostic variables in hyperthermia treatment in 163 patients. Int J Radiat Oncol Biol Phys 1984;10:2231–2239.

21. Puthawala AA, Syed AMN, Sheikh KMA, et al: Interstitial hyperthermia for recurrent malignancies. Endocurietherapy/Hyperthermia Oncol 1985;1:125–134.

22. Vora N, Forell B, Joseph C, et al: Interstitial implant with interstitial hyperthermia. Cancer 1982;50:2518–2523.

23. Yabumoto E, Suyama S: Interstitial radio frequency hyperthermia combined with electron beam radiotherapy, in Overgaard J (ed): proceedings of the 4th International Symposium of Hyperthermic Oncology, Vol I, London: Taylor & Francis, 1984, pp 579–582.

24. Radiation Therapy Oncology Group Protocol 81–04: A randomized phase II study of efficacy of radiation and hyperthermia compared with irradiation alone in the treatment of some measurable human tumors. Carlos A. Perez, Study Chairman, Philadelphia, Pennsylvania 1981.

25. Radiation Therapy Oncology Group Protocol 81–13: Phase I/II study, combination of definitive radiotherapy and hyperthermia in patients with advanced malignant tumors. Carlos A. Perez and Ronald Scott, Study Co-Chairmen, Philadelphia, Pennsylvania, 1981.

26. Radiation Therapy Oncology Group Protocol No. 84–11: Phase III randomized study of definitive radiotherapy and hyperthermia versus radiotherapy alone in patients with advanced head and neck, breast, and suitable soft tissues for definitive radiotherapy. Ronald Scott, Study Chairman, Philadelphia, 1984.

27. Radiation Therapy Oncology Group Protocol No. 84–19: Randomized phase II study of interstitial thermoradiotherapy (43°C) compared with interstitial radiotherapy alone in the treatment of recurrent or persistent human tumors. Bahman Emami, Study Chairman, Philadelphia, 1984.

28. Washington University Intramural Protocol 85–05: Phase III randomized study of hyperthermia adjuvant to surgery and irradiation in cervical lymph node metastases from head and neck primaries. Bahman Emami, Study Chairman, 1985.

29. Sapareto SA, Dewey WC: Thermal dose determination in cancer therapy. Int J Radiat Oncol Biol Phys 1984;10:787–800.

30. Dewhirst MW, Sim DA, Sapareto S, Connor WG: The importance of minimum tumor temperature in determining early and long term responses of spontaneous pet animal tumors to heat and irradiation. Cancer Res 1984;44:43–50.

31. Syed AMN, Feder BH, George FW III: Persistent carcinoma of the oropharynx and oral cavity re-treated by afterloading interstitial $^{192}$Ir implant. Cancer 1977;39:2443–2450.

32. Gelinas M, Fletcher GH: Incidence and causes of local failure of irradiation in squamous cell carcinoma of the faucial arch, tonsillar fossa and base of the tongue. Diag Radiol 1973;380:383–387.

33. Amer MH, Izbicki RM, Vaitkevicius VK, et al: Combination chemotherapy with cis-diaminedichloroplatinum, Oncovin and bleomycin (COB) in advanced head and neck cancer. Phase II. Cancer 1980;45:217–223.

34. Buechler M, Mukherji B, Chasin W, et al: High dose methotrexate with and without BCG therapy in advanced head and neck malignancy. Cancer 1979;43:1095–1100.

35. Donegan WL, Harris P: Regional chemotherapy with combined drugs in cancer of the head and neck. Cancer 1976;38:1479–1483.

# Index

Page numbers followed by *f* indicate figures; page numbers followed by *t* indicate tables.

**349**